NOVEL APPROACHES TO SELECTIVE TREATMENTS OF HUMAN SOLID TUMORS

Laboratory and Clinical Correlation

ADVANCES IN EXPERIMENTAL MEDICINE AND BIOLOGY

NOVEL APPROACHES TO SELECTIVE TREATMENTS OF HUMAN SOLID TUMORS

Laboratory and Clinical Correlation

Edited by

Youcef M. Rustum

Grace Cancer Drug Center
Roswell Park Cancer Institute
Buffalo, New York

PLENUM PRESS • NEW YORK AND LONDON

Library of Congress Cataloging-in-Publication Data

Novel approaches to selective treatments of human solid tumors :
   laboratory and clinical correlation / edited by Youcef M. Rustum.
        p.   cm. -- (Advances in experimental medicine and biology ; v.
   339)
      Includes bibliographical references and index.
      ISBN 0-306-44592-1
      1. Fluorouracil--Congresses. 2. Folinic acid--Therapeutic use-
   -Congresses. 3. Cancer--Chemotherapy--Congresses.   I. Rustum,
   Youcef M. II. Series.
      [DNLM: 1. Neoplasms--drug therapy--congresses. 2. Fluorouracil-
   -therapeutic use--congresses. 3. Fluorouracil--metabolism-
   -congresses.   W1 AD559 v. 339 1993 / QZ 267 N9375 1993]
   RC271.F55N68 1993
   616.99'4061--dc20
   DNLM/DLC
   for Library of Congress   93-39406
                                                                  CIP

Proceedings of an international symposium on Novel Approaches to Selective Treatments of Human
Tumors: Laboratory and Clinical Correlation, held September 10–12, 1992, in Buffalo, New York

ISBN 0-306-44592-1

©1993 Plenum Press, New York
A Division of Plenum Publishing Corporation
233 Spring Street, New York, N.Y. 10013

Printed in the United States of America

PREFACE

The therapeutic efficacy of FUra has been attributed to its incorporation into cellular RNA and, to its inhibition of thymidylate synthase, leading to potent inhibition of DNA synthesis and DNA damage. Studies of cell lines *in vitro* and model systems *in vivo* have demonstrated that although mechanisms of sensitivity and resistance to FUra are multifactorial, in the presence of citrovorum factor (LV, CF, 5-formyltetrahydrofolate) the site of action of FUra becomes predominantly the pronounced and prolonged inhibition of thymidylate synthase. This action is the result of stabilization of the covalent ternary complex between FdUMP, an active metabolite of FUra, 5,10-methylenetetrahydrofolates, and thymidylate synthase. This effect of LV is thus an example of the concept of metabolic modulation.

CF is commercially available as a racemic mixture of diastereoisomers (6R and 6S). The 6R isomer is considered to be biologically inactive; the 6S isomer is the biologically active form that is metabolized intracellularly to form the various folate cofactor pools including 5,10-methylenetetrahydrofolates. Although the extent of metabolism of folates in normal and tumor tissues has not been clearly delineated, it has been determined that the formation of folypolyglutamates is primarily a function of schedule of CF administration, while the retention of significant concentrations of reduced folate is a function of the dose and also the schedule of LV. Thus, it appears that for optimal modulation of FUra activity several factors must be considered simultaneously. These include the dose and schedule of administration of CF, the initial intracellular concentrations of folylpolyglutamate forms, the level of thymidylate synthase, and the degree and duration of inhibition of thymidylate synthase. It has also become apparent that the schedule of administration of FUra could play an important factor in determining the therapeutic selectivity of the modulation. The latter is also influenced by the absolute and relative intracellular concentrations of FdUMP and the competing metabolite, dUMP.

In addition to CF, several other modulators of FUra were considered, including N-(phosphonacetyl)-L-aspartate (PALA), α-interferon (IFN) and combination of CF/PALA/ and/or INF. Although the precise mechanisms of IFN in the modulation of FUra are not clearly delineated, several possibilities were discussed, including effects on thymidine transport, alteration of the pharmacokinetic parameters of FUra, increase FUra incorporation into RNA and aberration of the observed *in vitro* increase in the level of thymidylate synthase following treatment with FUra. PALA, a potent inhibitor of pyrimidine biosynthesis via inhibition of aspartate transcarbomylase, potentiate the therapeutic selectivity of FUra by increasing its incorporation into cellular RNA, resulting in decreased level of thymidine kinase. As a consequence of these effects, utilization of salvage thymidine could be avoided, thus reducing the possibility of reversing the drug effect at the level of thymidylate synthase.

During this symposium, several drug combinations with FUra/modulator inhibitions, include cis-platinum, 5-fluoro-2'-deoxyuridine (FdUrd) were also discussed.

Furthermore, the role of continuous i.v. infusion of FUra and the role of chronobiology of FUra were also discussed.

Because of the results, FUra/CF modulation demonstrated that thymidylate synthase is an important target of antimetabolic action. As a result, several new, potent and specific thymidylate synthase inhibitors were also discussed. Some of these agents are at the preclinical development, while others have already entered Phase I and II clinical trials including ICI-D1694.

The major diseases of focus were advanced and adjuvant colorectal cancer, head and neck cancer and breast cancers.

This symposium addresses:

- What have we learned and where to go in further utilization of the concept of metabolic modulation?
- What is the therapeutic impact of altered modes of drug administration?
- Drug development: What are potential sites of intervention?

On the first day of this symposium, entitled "Novel Approaches to Selective Treatments of Human Tumors: Laboratory and Clinical Correlation" studies related to the mechanisms schedule association of FUra and FdUrd were discussed. It became apparent that the mechanisms of action of these agents is schedule dependent with FUra incorporation into RNA as the dominator of FUra action, when the drug was administered by i.v. push and thymidylate synthase and also when FUra was administered by continuous FU infusion. In contrast, thymidylate synthase inhibition appears to be the dominant site of action of FdUrd when administered by i.v. push and FUra incorporation into RNA appears to be the dominant site of action of FdUrd when administered by continuous i.v. infusion. Confirmation of the preclinical data could have significant inpact on the future development of clinical protocols with these agents when administered alone and/or in combination with modulators. In addition, during the first day of the symposium, clinical update of FUra modulation by various modulators in advanced and adjuvant colorectal cancer were discussed.

On the second day of the symposium, an update of the present status of FUra modulation in adult carcinoma, breast and head and neck carcinomas as well as the initial clinical experience with a new antifolate, ICI-D1694 were discussed. This new antifolate as well as others, including LY231514, AG331, appears to be very promising.

On the third day of this symposium, advances in the molecular biology of cancer and the discovery of new sites of intervention for drug development were discussed. This new and exciting area of research, although at its initial stages of clinical application, holds considerable promise for the future.

The encouraging clinical results based on strong rationales derived from *in vitro* and *in vivo* laboratory studies, reinforces the need for further laboratory investigations aimed at optimization of conditions and parameters responsible for selective modulation of FUra. It is clearly evident from the results of clinical trials conducted to date that by delineation of mechanisms associated with therapeutic selectivity of fluoropyrimidine and other thymidylate synthase inhibitors clinical protocols can be designed with the potential for therapeutic efficacy that can produce greater response rate of survivors of patients with advanced solid tumor malignancy.

On behalf of the organizing committee, I would like to take this opportunity to thank the speakers, discussants and attendees for their valuable contributions to this symposium. The success of this symposium should be credited to the tireless and unselfish efforts of Ms. Gayle Bersani and Ms. Geri Wagner to who I am greatly indebted. We would like also to thank Ms. Cheryl Melancon and Ms. Mae Brown for their help in typing manuscripts, transcribing the discussions, and preparing correspondence.

Major support of this symposium was generously provided by the Lederle Division of American Cyanamid, Taiho Pharmaceutical Co., of Japan, and US Bioscience. Without their generous financial support this 3-day symposium would not have been possible. Additional support was provided by Nippon-Roche, Burroughs Wellcome, Eli Lilly, and ICI Pharmaceuticals.

This symposium was held to honor David Machover, M.D. for his outstanding contributions to the clinical development of 5-fluorouracil/leucovorin modulation. Dr. Machover and his colleagues of Villijuif were the first to publish the positive results of 5-fluorouracil/leucovorin in patients with advanced colorectal cancer.

The manuscripts included in these proceedings do not represent contributions from all the symposium speakers.

Y.R. Rustum

Critical Questions for the Future Direction of FU/LV

Alternative Approaches to Modulation of Fluoropyrimidines

Update on Metabolic Modulation as a Therapeutic Approach for Adult Carcinomas

New Drugs

NEW SITES OF INTERVENTION IN THE DEVELOPMENT OF NEW DRUGS IN SOLID TUMORS

Concluding Remarks

5-FLUORO-2'-DEOXYURIDINE: ROLE OF SCHEDULE IN ITS

THERAPEUTIC EFFICACY

Shousong Cao, Zhanggeng Zhang, Patrick J. Creaven and
Youcef M. Rustum

Grace Cancer Drug Center
Roswell Park Cancer Institute
Buffalo, NY 14263

ABBREVIATIONS

5-Fluoro-2'-deoxyuridine (FdUrd); 5-fluorouracil (FUra); FdUrd monophosphate (FdUMP); FUra triphosphate (FUTP); thymidylate synthase (TS); 5-formyltetrahydrofolate (5-CHO-THF or LV); 5,10 methylenetetrahydrofolate $(5,10\text{-}CH_2THF)$; 5-methyltetrahydrofolate $(5\text{-}CH_3THF)$; tetrahydrofolate (THF); dihydrofolate (DHF); deoxythymidinemonophosphate (dTMP); deoxythymidine triphosphate (dTTP); fluorodeoxyuridine di and triphosphate (FdUDP and FdUTP, respectively); fluorouridine incorporation into DNA and RNA (F-DNA, F-RNA); fluorodihydrouracil (FUH_2); maximum tolerated dose (MTD); continuous infusion (C.I.); weekly (wk); area under the concentration time curve (AUC); complete tumor regression (CR); partial tumor response, greater than 50% tumor reduction (PR).

INTRODUCTION

The fluorinated pyrimidines 5-fluorouracil (FUra) and 5-fluoro-2'-deoxyuridine (FdUrd) are drugs that have been shown to have clinical activity against colorectal carcinoma and other malignancies. Attempts to enhance the effectiveness of FUra have been based on considerations of both the biochemical pathways of FUra activation and the site of FUra action, which in some cases involves inhibition of thymidylate synthase (TS) by 5-fluorodeoxyuridine monophosphate (FdUMP), the active metabolite of both FUra and FdUrd and in others involve the incorporation of 5-fluorouridine triphosphate (FUTP) into RNA.[1-4]

Thymidine rescue and protection studies have revealed that the inhibition of TS by FdUMP is the primary site of the growth inhibitory action of fluorinated pyrimidines in

Novel Approaches to Selective Treatments of Human Solid Tumors: Laboratory and Clinical Correlation Edited by Y. M. Rustum, Plenum Press, New York, 1993

many, although not in all cells[1-4]. In the presence of the cofactor N^5,N^{10}-methylenetetrahydrofolate (5,10-CH_2THF) FdUMP is a powerful inhibitor of TS, having a K_1 of 1.9 nM for the enzyme of human AML cells[5] and 0.05 nM for the L casei enzyme[6]. Waxman et al.[7] reported that incubation of Friend leukemia cells with high levels (10 μM) of leucovorin (LV) increased their sensitivity to FUra. According to Ullman et al.[8], the levels of folates which were sufficient for the normal growth of L-1210 cells did not provide for maximal binding of FdUMP to TS. These authors demonstrated a 3-fold increase in sensitivity of L-1210 cells to FdUrd when the LV concentration in the medium was raised from 0.01 to 1 μM.

The effect of excess LV on the sensitivity of human carcinoma cells (HEP-2) and mouse sarcoma cells (S-180) to FUra, with particular emphasis on the effect of TS inhibition was examined by Hakala and co-workers[9]. These two cell lines differ from each other not only in that S-180 cells are 50 times more sensitive to FUra than HEP-2 cells[10], but also in that TS inhibition is growth limiting in S-180 but not in HEP-2.[11]

In both cell lines, 10 μM LV (100 times more than that required for growth), potentiated 3-fold the growth inhibition by FUra. This excess did not affect the degree of TS inhibition by FUra when measured immediately after FUra. Instead, the potentiating effect of LV was due to the stabilization of the enzyme-FdUMP in the reduced folate complex.

Recent clinical phase I, II and III trials based on the initial laboratory data[7-12] demonstrated that indeed the response rate in patients with advanced colorectal cancer to FUra can be increased by LV[13,14]. Under these conditions, however, over 60% of these patients still remain unresponsive to FUra modulation by LV. Although mechanisms of resistance to FUra are multifactorial limited to FUra uptake and metabolism to the active metabolites FUTP and FdUMP have been implicated with resistance to FUra.

To maximize drug uptake into the cell and activation, specifically to increase the extracellular pools of FdUMP, FdUrd, the deoxyuridine nucleoside analog of FUra, has been evaluated as an alternative to FUra. The theoretical advantage of FdUrd over FUra is that it is only one metabolic step from the active metabolite FdUMP. Most on-going clinical studies utilize hepatic artery infusions of FdUrd with doses up to 0.3 mg/kg/day for 2 weeks[15,16]. The dose limiting toxicities are gastritis and chemical hepatitis. The two year survival rate for hepatic arterial infusion was 23% compared to 13% for systemic FUra in a study by Rougier et al.[15]

Several schedules of intravenous FdUrd have been evaluated. Curreri and Ansfield[17] used i.v. push of 30 mg/kg/day x 5 in the absence of toxicity. Sullivan et al.[18] reported decreased tolerance when FdUrd was given by continuous infusion. Severe toxicity was observed in three patients after three days of therapy with 30 mg/kg/day. (WBC nadir in 1 patient was 1000). At doses of 10 mg/kg/day severe toxicity was noted in two patients after five days of treatment. At doses of 1.5 and 3 mg/kg/day, moderate toxicity (2+ stomatitis, 1-2 + diarrhea, WBC nadir 3000 + 2600) was noted in two patients after seven days of therapy. It is possible that lower doses of FdUrd are tolerated when the drug is given by continuous infusion.

Ansfield et al.[19] reported their experience with twenty patients treated by continuous infusion of 3 mg/kg/day of FdUrd to the point of toxicity over an average of 5.5 days of therapy (range 4 - 6.5 days). Nineteen patients developed stomatitis, six had pharyngitis and esophagitis, twelve had diarrhea. WBC of 2000 - 3000/mm^3 occurred in four patients and <2000 in another four. Patients developed dermatitis and one nausea. "Many patients" required hospitalization for IV hydration.

Sullivan and Miller[20] subsequently reported results of continuous infusion in a larger series; doses as low as 0.5 - 1.0 mg/kg/day for 5 to 7 days resulted in moderate toxicity.

Lokich et al.[21] carried out phase I study to identify the maximally tolerated dose of FdUrd that could be administered for two weeks by constant intravenous infusion. Patients were monitored weekly and tolerance to treatment was determined by interview for the presence of gastrointestinal effects including nausea, vomiting or diarrhea and for stomatitis. Weekly CBC's were obtained. The drug infusion was discontinued at the first indication of toxicity.

At doses greater than 0.15 mg/kg/day the dose limiting toxicity was diarrhea with or without stomatitis. At doses of 0.125 mg/kg/24 hours or less, patients could be treated indefinitely without toxicity. On the basis of this study, a phase II dose of 0.125 - 0.15 mg/kg/day was recommended for a two week on treatment, two weeks off treatment schedule.

FdUrd by continuous IV infusion causes dose-limiting diarrhea. The other common toxicities of continuous infusion include nausea, anorexia, mucositis and possible skin alterations (hand-foot syndrome). Bone marrow toxicity is minimal. There appear to be no cumulative or long-term toxicities.[22]

In recent RPCI studies, we have examined modulation of FdUrd in in vitro and in vivo animal studies and in the clinic and have explored the role of dose and schedule in its toxicity, activity and interaction with leucovorin.

Growth Inhibition In Vitro

The growth inhibition of HCT-8 cells exposed for 3 and 72 h to FdUrd in vitro was evaluated with and without leucovorin using 3 h and 72 h continuous exposure schedules. The concentrations required for 50% inhibition of cell growth (IC_{50}) of FdUrd with and without 20 μM 6RS leucovorin (LV) are shown in Table 1. For the 3 h schedule, cells were exposed initially to LV alone for 21 h prior to exposure to the combination; for the 72 h schedule, both drugs were present for the duration of the experiment.

Table 1. IC_{50} (nm) of FdUrd î LV for HCT-8 cells.

LV (nm)	Exposure (h)	
	3	72
+	30 ±8	1.5 ± 0.6
-	115 ± 20	3.0 ± 1.0

Recent (RPCI) studies of FdUrd-LV in renal cell ca. using a 2 h infusion of LV and a 3 h infusion of FdUrd daily x 5 every 4 weeks found an MTD of FdUrd of 2000 mg/m²/d on this schedule.[23] This compared with an MTD of about 50 mg/m2/d when the drug is given by continuous infusion. In addition, a phase I clinical trial of weekly schedule of LV (500 mg/m2/2 h infusion) and i.v. push of FdUrd at 1 h indicate that the MTD's is approximately 1650 mg/m².[28]

The data in Table 1 confirm that FdUrd is markedly more active by prolonged exposure.

In Vivo Toxicity

1) Rats. The maximum tolerated dose (MTD) of FdUrd administered (i.v.) to normal rats was determined using 3 schedules: i.v. push x 1; continuous i.v. infusion for 4 d (C.I.); and weekly i.v. push for 3 weeks. The data are summarized in Table 2.

The data in Table 2 demonstrate the schedule dependency of FdUrd in this in vivo model system. With the i.v. weekly x 3 schedule, it was possible to deliver 3 times more drug than by the 4 day C.I. schedule. In rats, the dose limiting toxicity of FdUrd was mouth ulceration and diarrhea when given by C.I. and diarrhea when given by the weekly x 3 schedule, a profile of toxicity similar to what has been observed clinically.

2) Patients. FdUrd modulated by leucovorin has been explored in three phase I studies in different schedules. The results are given in Table 3.

Table 2. Maximum tolerated dose (MTD) of FdUrd in normal rats.

Schedule	MTD (mg/kg)	MTD (mg/m^2)	Dose/Course (mg/kg)
x 1 i.v. push	1300	7670	1300
C.I. x 4 d	100	590	400
Weekday x 3 (i.v. push)	400	2360	1200

Table 3. Clinical toxicity of FdUrd in combination with leucovorin (LV).

Schedule FdUrd	LV	LV dose (mg/m^2/d)	MTD of FdUrd (mg/m^2/8 weeks)
C.I.x5d[+]	C.I.x5.0d	500	1.33
3h inf.x5d[+]	2h inf. x5	200	20,000
i.v. pushx6[‡]	2h inf. wkx6	500	9,000

[+]Q 4 weeks; [‡]Q 8 weeks

The dose limiting toxicity was stomatitis for C.I. infusion x5d schedule was stomatitis[36], myelosuppression, stomatitis and diarrhea for the 3 h infusion x5d schedule[35] and diarrhea for the weekly x3 schedule.[28]

The data in Table 3 indicate that the amount of FdUrd in combination with leucovorin that is tolerated by patients is highly schedule dependent so that the dose limiting toxicity is also somewhat schedule dependent. Plasma FdUrd and FUra concentrations derived from FdUrd may be useful in warning of severe toxicity in patients receiving FdUrd i.v. push in combination with 2 h infusion of LV (500 mg/m^2/wk x 6). In patients with grade III and IV toxicity, the AUC for FdUrd was greater than 40 μM.h and for FUra was greater than 77 μM.h.[28]

Antitumor Activity of FdUrd in Rats Bearing Colon Carcinoma. The data in Table 4 is an outline of FdUrd, administered i.v. by different schedules, to rats bearing advanced colorectal cancer (about 3 gm tumor size). Response to FdUrd was calculated as: partial tumor regressing (PR) meaning >50% reduction in tumor size 3 weeks post therapy; and maintained complete regression (CR) for up to 3 months post therapy.

Table 4. Antitumor activity of FdUrd in rats bearing colon carcinoma: Role of drug scheduling.

Schedule	Dose[+] (mg/kg/d)	Response PR	CR
i.v. x 1	1300	0	6
i.v. x 4	100	25	8
c.i. x 4	100	58	17
wk x 3	400	87	13

[+]All treatment via the i.v. route

Table 5. In vitro metabolism of FdURd in HCT-8 cells.

Exposure time (h)	FdUMP (pmol/10^7 cells)	FUTP (pmol/10^7 cells)	F-RNA (pmol/mg/RNA)
3	340 ± 120	34 ± 12	3 ± 2
24	280 ± 108	103 ± 86	105 ± 30

In Vitro Metabolism of FdUrd. The in vitro metabolism of FdUrd to FdUMP, FUTP and the amount of drug incorporated into cellular RNA were investigated using HCT-8 cells in culture. Table 5 is an outline of the FdUMP and FUTP and F-RNA following 3 h and 24 h exposure to FdUrd.

The data in Table 5 indicate: 1) no significant change in FdUMP as function of time (3 vs 24 h), indicate rapid cellular metabolism to FdUMP; 2) the FUTP pools were increased with longer exposure, suggesting slow cellular conversion of FdUrd to FUra and subsequently to FUTP and 3) higher level of drug incorporation into cellular RNA with longer exposure. The increase in FUTP paralleled the observed increase in F-RNA. These data suggest, but do not prove that the primary site of action of FdUrd vary dependent on the mode of drug exposure, thymidylate synthase with short exposure and F-RNA with prolonged drug exposure.

CONCLUDING REMARKS

Based on laboratory and clinical results, several mechanisms of resistance to FUra alone and in combination with LV have been postulated. This includes overexpression of thymidylate synthase, the target enzyme for FdUMP; low level of FdUMP pools; increased levels of dUMP, the competing normal metabolite with FdUMP at the level of thymidylate synthase; limited drug incorporation into cellular RNA; and dissociation of the binary complex of FdUMP-thymidylate synthase due to significantly low level of 5,10-methylenetetrahydrofolate, resulting in rapid recovery of thymidylate synthase and consequently recovery of DNA synthesis.

Several approaches to overcome mechanisms associated with resistance to FUra have been investigated in preclinical and clinical settings with encouraging results. These include the use of N-phosphonoacetyl-L-aspartate (PALA)[29] to increase drug incorporation into cellular RNA; continuous i.v. infusion of FUra FdUrd[30,31] interferon found in vitro to reduce the incidence of overexpression of thymidylate synthase following FUra treatment.[32,33] Another possible approach to overcome resistance to FUra/LV modulation is the use of FdURd/LV. This agent is more rapidly transported into cells than FUra resulting in higher cellular pools of FdUMP.

The in vitro data with FdUrd in HCT-8 cells suggest that FdUrd offers several advantages over FUra. These include: 1) greater intracellular accumulation and retention of FdUMP as was demonstrated in our in vitro results; 2) FdUrd in a potent inhibitor of thymidylate synthase and DNA synthesis; 3) FdUrd produces significantly more single and double DNA strand breaks than FUra alone and in combination with LV[34]; and 4) thymidine rescue FdUrd cytotoxicity and DNA damage.[34]

Most of the recent clinical experience with FdUrd is via protracted continuous infusion demonstrating significant toxicity and limited response rate. The clinical data suggest that by altering the schedule of FdUrd administration the amount of drug that can be delivered was increased significantly. To test the therapeutic selectivity of this alternative mode of FdUrd administration, a phase I clinical trial of weekly i.v. push FdUrd in combination with 2 h infusion of LV (500 mg/m[2]) in patients with advanced colorectal cancer was designed and implemented at our Institute. Initial results indicate that indeed one can deliver significantly more drug with acceptable toxicity, diarrhea being the dose limiting toxicity. Response to this new mode of administration of FdUrd in combination with LV await further evaluation.

REFERENCES

1.   C. Heidelberger. Fluorinated pyrimidine. Prog. Nucl. Acid Res. Mol. Biol. 4:150 (1965).

2.   P. Reyes and C. Heidelberg. Fluorinated pyrimidines. XXXVI Mammalian thymidylate synthase. Its mechanism of action by fluorinated nucleotides. Mol. Pharmacol. 1:14 (1965).

3.   R.C. Sawyer, R.L. Stolfi, R. Nayak and D.S. Martin. Mechanism of cytotoxicity in 5-fluorouracil chemotherapy of two murine solid tumors, in: Nucleosides and Cancer Treatment, M.H.N. Tattersall and R.M. Fox, eds., Academic Press, Inc., New York (1981).

4.   S. Spiegelman, R. Nayak, R. Sawyer, R. Stolfi and D. Martin. Potentiation of the antitumor activity of 5-FU by thymidine and its correlation with the formation of (5-FU) RNA. Cancer 45:1129 (1980).

5. B.J. Dolnick and Y-C. Cheng. Human thymidylate synthetase derived from blast cells of patients with acute myelocytic leukemia. J. Biol. Chem. 252:7697 (1977).

6. D.V. santi, C.S. McHenry and H. Sommer. Mechanism of interaction of thymidylate synthetase with 5-fluorodoxyuridylate. Biochem. 13:471 (1974).

7. S. Waxman, H. Bruckner, A. Wagle and C. Schreiber. Potentiation of 5-fluorouracil (5-FU) antimetabolic effect by leucovorin (LV). Proc. AACR 19:149 (1978).

8. B. Ullman, M. Lee, D.W. Martin, Jr. and D.V. Santi. Cytotoxicity of 5-fluoro-2'-deoxyuridine: Requirement for reduced folate cofactors and antagonism by methotrexate. Proc. Natl. Acad. Sci. USA 75:980 (1978).

9. R.M. Evans, J.D. Laskin and M.T. Hakala. effect of excess folates and deoxyinosine on the activity and site of action of 5-fluorouracil. Cancer Res. 41:3288 (1981).

10. J.D. Laskin, R.M. Evans, H.K. Slocum, D. Burke, D. and M.T. Hakala. Basis for natural variation in sensitivity to 5-fluorouracil in mouse and human cells in culture. Cancer Res. 39:383 (1979).

11. R.M. Evans, J.D. Laskin and M.T. Hakala. Assessment of growth-limiting even thymidylate synthase caused by 5-fluorouracil in mouse cells and in human cells. Cancer Res. 40:4113 (1980).

12. J.A. Houghton, L.G. Williams, P.J. Cheshire, I.W. Weiner, P. Jadaud and P.J. Houghton. Influence of dose of [6RS] leucovorin on reduced folate pools and 5-fluorouracil mediated thymidylate synthase inhibition in human colon adenocarcinoma xenografts. Cancer Res. 50:3940 (1990).

13. N. Petrelli, L. Herrera, Y. Rustum, P. Burke, P.J. Creaven, J. Stulc, L.J. Emrich and A. Mittelman. A prospective randomized trial of 5-fluorouracil and methotrexate in previously untreated patients with advanced colorectal carcinoma. J. Clin. Oncol. 4:1559 (1987).

14. N. Petrelli, D. Stablein, H. Bruckner et al. A prospective randomized phase III trial of 5-fluorouracil (5FU) versus 5FU + high dose leucovorin (HDCF) versus 5FU + low dose leucovorin (LDCF) in patients (pts) with metastatic colorectal adenocarcinomas. A report of the Gastrointestinal Tumor Study Group. Proc. Am. Soc. Clin. Oncol. 7:94 (1988).

15. P. Rougier, A. Laplanche, M. Huguier and et al. Hepatic arterial infusion of floxuridine in patients with liver metastases from colorectal carcinoma: Long-term results of a prospective randomized trial. J. Clin. Oncol. 10:1112 (1992).

16. N. Kemeny, J. Daly, P. Oderman, and et al. Hepatic artery pump infusion: Toxicity and results in patients with metastatic colorectal carcinoma. J. Clin. Oncol. 2:595 (1984).

17. A.R.T. Curreri and F.J. Ansfield. Comparison of 5-fluorouracil and 5-fluoro-2'-deoxyuridine in the treatment of far advanced breast and colon lesions. Cancer Chemother. Rep. 16:287 (1962).

18. R.D. Sullivan, C.W. Young, E. Miller, N. Glathymidylate synthasetein, B. Clarkson and J.H. Burchenal. The clinical effects of the continuous administration of fluorinate pyrimidines (5-fluorouracil and 5-fluoro-2'-deoxyuridine). Cancer Chemother. Rep. 8:77 (1960).

19. F.J. Ansfield, J.M. Schroeder, J.M and A.R. Curreri. A preliminary comparison of 5-fluoro-2'-deoxyuridine administered by rapid daily intravenous injections and by slow continuous infusion. Cancer Chemother. Rep. 16:389 (1962).

20. R. Sullivan and E. Miller. The clinical effects of prolonged intravenous infusion of 5-fluoro-2'-deoxyuridine. Cancer Res. 25:1025 (1965).

21. J.L. Lokich, H. Sonneborn, S. Paul and Zipoli. Phase I study of continuous venous infusion of floxuridine (5-FUDR). Cancer Treat. Rep. 67:791 (1983).

22. D.C. Hohn, Royner, Cancer 57:465 (1986).

23. D. Raminski, P.J. Creaven, Y.M. Rustum and et al. Phase I clinical trial of floxuridine (FUdR) with leucovorin (LV) in patients (PTS) with advanced genitourinary cancer (AGC). Proc. ASCO 11:206 (19920.

24. M-B. Yin, M.A. Guimaraes, Z-Z. Zhang, M.A. Arredondo and Y.M. Rustum. Time-dependence of DNA lesions and growth inhibition by ICI D1694, a new quinazoline antifolate thymidylate synthase inhibitor. Cancer Res. 52:5900 (1992).

25. L.L. Danhauser and Y.M. Rustum. Chemotherapeutic efficacy of 5-fluorouracil with concurrent thymidine infusion against transplantable colon tumors in rodents. Can. Drug Del. 1:269 (1984).

26. L.L. Danhauser and Y.M. Rustum. A method for continuous drug infusion in unrestrained rats: Its application in evaluating the toxicity of 5-fluorouracil/thymidine combinations. J. Lab. Clin. Med. 93:1047 (1979).

27. D.W. Roberts. An isotopic assay for thymidylate synthase. Biochem.5:3546 (1966).

28. P.J. Creaven, Y.M. Rustum, N.J. Petrelli, N.J. Meropol. S.V. Udvari-Nagy and A. Proefrock. Floxuridine/leucovorin. A phase I and pharmacokinetic study. Proc. Am. Assoc. Cancer Res. 34 (1993).

29. P.J. O'Dwyer, A.R. Paul, J. Walczak, L.M. Weiner, S. Litwin and R.L.Comis. Phase II study of biochemical modulation of fluorouracil by low dose PALA in patients with colorectal cancer. J. Clin. Oncol. 8:1497 (1990).

30. N. Anderson, J. Lokich, M. Bern, S. Wallach, C. Moore and D. Williams. A phase I clinical trial of combined fluoropyrimidines with leucovorin in 14 days infusion. Cancer 15:233 (1989).

31. J.J. Lokich, A. Bothe, N. Fine and J. Perri. Phase I study of protracted venous infusion of floxuridine (5-FUdR) chemotherapy. Cancer Treat. Rep. 67:791 (1983).

32. E. Chu, S. Zinn, D. Boarman and jC.J. Allegra. The interaction of γ-interferon and 5-fluorouracil in H-630 human colon carcinoma cell line. Cancer Res. 50:5874 (1990).

33. S.M. Swain, M.E. Lipman, E.F. Egan, J.C. Drake, S.M. Steinberg and C.J. Allegra. Fluorouracil and high dose leucovorin in previously treated patients with metastatic breast cancer. J. Clin. Oncol. 7:890 (1989).

34. M-B. Yin and Y.M. Rustum. Comparative DNA strand breakage induced by FUra and FdUrd in human ileocecal adenocarcinoma (HCT-8) cells: Relevance to cell growth inhibition. Cancer Commun. 3:45 (1991).

35. D. Raminski, P.J. Creaven, Y.M. Rustum and et al. Phase I clinical trial of floxuridine with leucovorin in patients with advanced genitourinary cancer. Proc. ASCO 11:206, 1992.

36. P.J. Creaven, N. Petrelli and Y.M. Rustum. Modulation by 5-formyl-tetrahydrofolate of the activity of fluoropyrimidines in patients with colon carcinoma. 6th NCI EORTC Symposium, Amsterdam, 1989.

COMPARISON OF CONTINUOUS INFUSIONS AND BOLUS INJECTIONS

OF 5-FLUOROURACIL WITH OR WITHOUT LEUCOVORIN:

IMPLICATIONS FOR INHIBITION OF THYMIDYLATE SYNTHASE

Godefridus J. Peters, Giovanni Codacci-Pisanelli*,
Clasina L. van der Wilt, Jan A.M. van Laar, Kees Smid,
Paul Noordhuis, Herbert M. Pinedo**

Dept. Oncology, Free University Hospital, PO Box 7057, 1007 MB
Amsterdam, and **Netherlands Cancer Institute, the Netherlands;
*3rd Dept. Intern. Medicine, Univ. Roma "La Sapienza", Italy

INTRODUCTION

Although 5-fluorouracil (5FU) is in clinical use for more than three decades, it is not clear what is the most efficacious schedule of 5FU administration [1, 2]. For systemic treatment with 5FU a number of different schedules are in clinical use (Table 1). The two major schedules for bolus injections do not show significant differences in either toxicity or antitumor activity. For the prolonged administration schedules, however, the pattern of toxicity changes. For weekly bolus injections, myelotoxicity (mainly leukopenia) is usually dose-limiting; however, at the prolonged administration schedules the pattern of toxicity changes with mucositis and diarrhea as serious site-effects for continuous infusions. In addition, the hand-foot syndrome is frequently observed at protracted infusions of several weeks, as well as other skin lesions (see ref. in Table 1). Interestingly the addition of LV to both the bolus injections and the continuous infusions, caused a marked increase in gastrointestinal toxicity. In several schedules this increase of toxicity was the only result of the modulatory agent, with no apparent effect on the antitumor activity.

Most studies on protracted infusion have been performed as Phase II trials. In a large randomized trial Lokich et al [24] compared bolus injections (daily times 5) of 5FU with protracted infusion for 10 weeks. A significantly higher response rate (30%) was observed in the infusional arm compared with the bolus arm (7%), with no significant differences in the survival. A similar pattern has been observed for the comparison of bolus 5FU with LV-5FU; increased response for LV-5FU but no significant effect on survival [2, 4]. The addition of LV to the protracted infusion did however in most studies only result in an increased toxicity [18,19,25,27], as well as that of interferon-α [26]. An additional administration of interferon-α to the

*Novel Approaches to Selective Treatments of Human Solid Tumors: Laboratory
and Clinical Correlation* Edited by Y. M. Rustum, Plenum Press, New York, 1993

Table 1.   Doses and schedules used for systemic administration of single agent 5FU in various malignancies

Injections:	1.	Weekly i.v. push at 500-800 mg/m^2 [1-3]
	2.	Daily times 5 repeated every 3-4 weeks at 300-500 mg/m^2/day [1, 2, 4]
Infusions:	3.	24 hr infusion at high dose (2400; tested from 750-3400 mg/m^2) [5,6,21,22]
	4.	3-5 day infusion at 1000 (varying from 185-3600) mg/m^2 [7-11, 20, 23]
	5.	Protracted infusions varying from 1 week to 10 weeks at 200-750 mg/m^2/day, depending on length of infusion period [12-19, 24- 27]

Many of these schedules are being used in combination with single modulators, such as LV [2, 18, 19], dypiridamol [10, 20], interferon-α [26], PALA [5, 6], 6-methylmercaptopurine riboside [7, 22], uridine [3], cisplatinum [11, 23], irradiation [8] or multiple modulators. A large number of different schedules was used for the modulators. For combinations with *e.g.* LV and/or interferon the dose of 5FU in the continuous infusions had to be reduced.

continuous infusion schedule with LV did not indicate a substantial improvement in treatment results [28].

A scientific rationale for an improved effect of 5FU administered as continuous infusion was already formulated several years ago. Several investigators have pointed out that continuous *in vitro* exposure of cells to 5FU is much more effective than short 1-hr exposure periods followed by culture in drug-free medium [29, 30]. For some of our human colon cancer cell lines we have observed a similar pattern; a 50% growth inhibition (IC50) for the 1-hr exposure was observed at about 300 μM [32], while for a continuous exposure of 24-72 hr an IC50 of 2-10 μM was observed [31-33]. During continuous exposure to 5FU a constant high level of the active metabolite of 5FU, FdUMP, would be present in order to facilitate maximum inhibition of thymidylate synthase (TS), the target for FdUMP. TS was inhibited almost completely during exposure to 5FU, but recovered after removal of the drug [34].

The study of prolonged infusion of cytostatics in animal model systems has been hampered by the lack of reliable infusion systems. Short term infusions (24 hr) can be carried out by catherisation of the tail vein, while for longer periods (3-7 days) osmotic pumps can be applied. For very long infusion periods one has to rely on slow-release forms of 5FU. We compared weekly i.p. bolus injections of 5FU with s.c. continuous infusions for three weeks in mice bearing subcutaneously implanted colon tumors. Both schedules were given at their maximum tolerated doses (MTD), at which the toxicity profile, 5FU plasma pharmacokinetics, and thymidylate synthase (TS) inhibition in the tumors were evaluated.

MATERIALS AND METHODS

Materials

5FU for bolus treatment of animals was obtained from Hoffmann-La Roche, Mijdrecht, the Netherlands, and was formulated as a 10 mg/ml solution. Slow-release pellets containing 5FU and intended for continuous infusions were obtained from Innovative Research of America, Toledo, OH, USA. [6-^{3}H]-dUMP was from Radiochemical Center Amersham, England and [6-^{3}H]-FdUMP from Moravek, Brea, CA, USA. All other chemicals were of analytical grade.

Treatment of mice and blood sampling

All mice were kept in an area with standardized light-dark cycle for at least 10-14 days prior to the beginning of an experiment. Mice had access to food and water *ad libitum*. For each treatment dose limiting toxicity was determined in healthy mice (female Balb/c and C57Bl/6 mice) before applying the schedule to tumor-bearing animals. As parameters for the MTD we used a weight loss not exceeding 15% and/or a lethality of less than 10%. Investigations on toxicity have been performed essentially as previously described [35-38]. For determination of the antitumor activity female Balb/c and C57Bl/6 mice were transplanted with two murine colon adenocarcinomas, Colon 26 and Colon 38, respectively.

For weekly bolus treatment, mice received intra-peritoneal bolus injections of 5FU. For continuous infusions slow release pellets containing 5FU (5, 10, 15, 20 mg) were implanted subcutaneously in ether anesthetized mice. After three weeks the pellets were detoriated. Blood sampling in these mice was done at the same time point of the day and was performed by retro-orbital bleeding under slight ether anesthesia with heparinized hematocrit capillaries; plasma samples were frozen and 5FU was measured with gas-chromatography coupled to mass spectrometry, as described [39, 40]. Plasma pharmacokinetics of 5FU after bolus injections and continuous infusions have been studied in normal C57Bl/6 mice, essentially as has been described previously [40]. Because of the sensitive analytical procedure only small blood samples were required for a reliable analysis.

Enzyme assays

The activity of thymidylate synthase was measured after treatment with 5FU using two assays, the FdUMP ligand binding assay and the catalytic assay (conversion of dUMP to dTMP), as previously described [37]. Mice were killed by cervical dislocation, tumors were excised immediately and directly frozen in liquid nitrogen. The frozen tumors were pulverized using a micro-dismembrator and supernatants were prepared as described [37]. For measurement of the total TS activity in tumors from treated mice, the ternary complex consisting of FdUMP, TS and 5,10-methylene-tetrahydrofolate (CH_2-THF), was dissociated followed by a neutral charcoal wash.

RESULTS

Pharmacokinetics

The MTD for 5FU administered as weekly bolus injections was comparable to that reported previously [35-37], 100 mg/kg. The MTD for continuous infusions (administered as subcutaneously implanted pellets) was 10 mg/21 days per mouse, equivalent to 23.8 mg/kg/day assuming an initial mouse weight of 20 g. In order to determine whether the pellets indeed have a constant release of 5FU during the period indicated by the manufacturer, we measured the plasma 5FU concentrations during the infusion period. Plasma 5FU concentrations have been measured in the same mice sampled repeatedly during 21 days at the same time point of the day. The plasma 5FU concentrations varied between 0.1 and 1.0 µM, much lower than the peak plasma 5FU concentrations in mice after bolus injections (Fig. 1). Plasma concentrations dropped below detectable levels at 22 days after implantation of the pellets, indicating that release of 5FU was completed. The total area under the

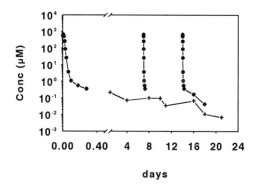

Figure 1.   Plasma 5FU concentrations in mice after administration of bolus injections of 5FU at 100 mg/kg (-●-) to C57Bl/6 and Balb/c mice, or implantation of slow-release pellets containing 10 mg 5FU (-+-) in C57Bl/6 mice [40,47]. For the bolus injections no difference was observed between the two mouse strains. Values are means of at least 6 mice. SD was less than 30%. For the bolus injections it was assumed that repeated administration did not affect the plasma pharmacokinetics [39] and the same curve was plotted three times.

plasma concentration *vs* time (AUC) curve was 37 μmol.hr/l for the continuous infusions, that for one bolus injection was 285 μmol.hr/l [40]. For three weekly bolus injections this would have been about 855 μmol.hr/l, assuming no effect of repeated administration on plasma pharmacokinetics [39].

Toxicity

Continuous infusions caused a delayed, but considerable weight loss leading to death at the higher doses; at the 10 mg dose a maximum of 15% was observed after 11 days. After bolus injections the maximal weight loss was observed at the first days after administration of 5FU and did not exceed 10% [35-37]. In addition to the weight loss we also determined the myeloid toxicity of continuous infusions of 5FU (Fig. 2). For mice treated with saline or implanted with the carrier material of the pellets, no significant effect on blood cell count was observed. Bolus injections of 5FU caused a severe leukopenia in contrast to the decrease in leucocyte count observed in mice treated with continuous infusions. In both treatment modalities these decreases were followed by a rebound in leucocytes which was more pronounced in mice treated with a continuous infusion. The other parameters measured, thrombocytes and hematocrit, decreased to 43 and 31% of the pretreatment values.

Antitumor activity

The antitumor activity of continuous infusions was determined both in mice bearing Colon 26 (Fig. 3) and compared in the same experiment with the antitumor effect of bolus injections. In the 5FU-insensitive Colon 26 continuous infusion with 5FU resulted in a significant growth arrest in the first week after implantation of the pellet, bolus injections of 5FU only resulted in a small growth delay. After 8 days, however, the tumors resumed growth in the animals treated with a continuous

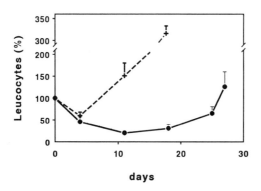

Figure 2. Comparison of the myelotoxicity of weekly bolus injections of 5FU (-•-) at 100 mg/kg and continuous infusion of 5FU (-+-) at a total dose of 10 mg per mouse. Leucocyte counts relative to the value before treatment are given. Values are means ± SD of at least 6 mice and are from [35,36,38,47].

infusion; the ultimate life-span of mice treated with a continuous infusion was comparable to that in mice treated with a bolus injection. Against Colon 38, a 5FU-sensitive tumor, continuous infusions resulted in unmeasurable tumor load in several mice. However, in these mice tumors also resumed growth after 8 days and there was no difference in the overall antitumor effect of continuous infusions compared to bolus injections (data not shown).

Since LV was able to potentiate the antitumor activity of 5FU both in Colon 26 and Colon 38, we combined LV with the continuous infusion of 5FU in Colon 26. Since no clear advantage for any of the LV schedules has become apparent, we compared various schedules and doses of LV administration, weekly (d 1, 7 and 14) bolus injections at 100 mg/kg, daily (d 1-5, 8-12, 15-19) bolus injections of 5 mg/kg and three times weekly (days 1,3,5 and 8,10 ,12 and 15,17, 19) of 10 mg/kg. However, neither of these schedules was able to enhance the antitumor activity. In contrast these schedules appeared to be more toxic than the continuous infusion of 5FU alone, as was manifested by an increased weight loss and lethality.

Activity of thymidylate synthase

For bolus injections of 5FU we obtained evidence that the antitumor activity of 5FU was related to the extent and long-term duration of TS inhibition. A resumed tumor growth was associated with an increase in the total activity of TS in these tumors [37]. This effect was more pronounced for the catalytic activity of TS than for the FdUMP binding of TS. In mice treated with a continuous infusion of 5FU we determined the activity of TS in Colon 26 tumors (Fig. 4). The extent of TS inhibition was comparable with that observed after a bolus injection. After 11 days, however, the activity of TS in the tumors recovered and exceeded that of tumors from untreated mice. The total increase in enzyme activity was comparable to that observed after treatment of mice with weekly bolus injections of 5FU, whereas this increase was not present in tumors of mice treated with LV and bolus 5FU [37].

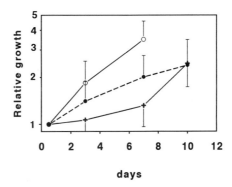

Figure 3. Comparison of the antitumor effect of bolus injections of 5FU at weekly doses of 100 mg/kg (-●-) and continuous infusion (-+-) of 5FU administered as slow-release pellets containing 10 mg 5FU. Growth of control tumors is depicted as -o-. Values are means ± SE of 6 mice and were calculated relative to the tumor volume at the first day of treatment. Implantation of the carrier material did not affect tumor growth. The maximal T/C value (ratio between tumor size from treated and control mice) for continuous infusions was 0.35 compared to 0.7 for bolus treatments (means of at least 4 separate experiments). The overall survival for both groups was comparable.

DISCUSSION

Continuous infusions in mice; effect of leucovorin

Continuous exposure of tumor cells to 5FU has shown to be more effective than short-term treatment, based on IC50 values. In this study we demonstrate that continuous infusion of 5FU to mice can indeed enhance the antitumor activity of 5FU when evaluation is based on tumor size, criteria comparable to that used clinically for complete and partial response. However, when the long term effects, such as survival, are being considered this difference is not present anymore.

Continuous administration of 5FU to mice using slow-release pellets appeared to be a feasible treatment modality. The pellets released 5FU at a constant rate since the plasma 5FU concentrations were in the same range during the whole treatment period of 21 days. These plasma levels of 5FU were comparable with levels observed in patients during protracted infusion measured in this laboratory [25] and in other studies [41-43] and with that in rats [44]. 5FU plasma concentrations measured during relatively short-term infusions (3-7 days) [10, 41, 43] tended to be higher than that measured during longer infusion periods. However, this may well be related to the higher dose which can be applied at the shorter infusion periods and the fact that a number of investigators used 5FU in combination with a modulator [10, 43]. In these studies a clear relationship between dose and steady-state 5FU concentrations was observed. However, at a dose (370 mg/m²/day) comparable with our studies [10, 25], similar 5FU concentrations were observed. Considering the plasma pharmacokinetics, our murine model seems to have a number of similarities compared to continuous infusion schedules applied in the clinic.

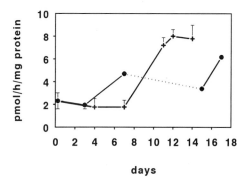

Figure 4. Comparison of the inhibition of TS after administration of 5FU as a weekly bolus injection (-●-) at 100 mg/kg [37] and as a continuous infusion of 5FU (-+-) at a total dose of 10 mg per mouse. The absolute residual TS activity is depicted. For the bolus injections the line between days 7 and 15 is discontinued because no measurements were performed, while treatment of mice was continued at days 7 and 14. Values are means ± SD of 4-6 separate tumors.

The overall dose of 5FU administered to mice during the continuous administration was 10 mg. When compared with the weekly bolus treatment this is about twice the amount of 5FU administered as bolus injection; for a weekly bolus injection of 5FU at 100 mg/kg this would have been 6 mg of 5FU for a mouse of 20 g. This higher amount of 5FU which can be administered as a continuous infusion is consistent with the clinical protocol in which enormous amounts of the drug can be delivered using protracted infusion (about 7000 mg in 4 weeks when a dose of 300 mg/m^2/day is given compared to 2 x 1000 mg for two weekly bolus injections). It has been suggested from clinical studies that dose-intensity is related with the response of 5FU [45, 46]. However, the higher dose intensity of the continuous infusion did not result in a higher exposure based on the AUC; at repeated administration of 5FU the AUC was higher than for the continuous infusion (Fig. 1). Values for the AUC based on plasma levels measured during a two week continuous infusion of 300 mg/m^2/day [25] were compared with the AUC of bolus injections [39], and no advantage for the continuous infusion in view of the AUC could be demonstrated. However, measurement of plasma levels has limited value considering the relation with antitumor activity, although a relation with hematological side effects has been demonstrated [39].

Administration of 5FU as a continuous infusion was able to inhibit the TS activity in tumor to a similar extent as a bolus injection. These data support the observation of others [48] that for a maximal inhibition of TS a relatively low dose is sufficient, which would provide FdUMP levels above a threshold required to inhibit the enzyme. Recently Chen & Erlichman [49] demonstrated that in a biochemical modulation schedule higher concentrations of FdUMP did not enhance the inhibition of TS. Continued exposure of the tumor to 5FU did, however, not support a prolonged inhibition of TS, despite the presence of 5FU in the tumor at concentrations (about 1 µmol/kg) sufficient to support TS inhibition *in vitro*. The most likely explanation for the decreased enzyme inhibition is an enhanced enzyme synthesis. Addition of LV to the weekly bolus treatment with 5FU seemed to abrogate such an enzyme synthesis *in vivo* [37] explaining the increase in therapeutic efficacy of the LV-5FU schedule.

Administration of LV did not enhance the antitumor effect of continuous infusion of 5FU. Several schedules mimicking either a continuous exposure to LV or peak exposure were used. The only modulating effect, however, was an increase in toxicity manifested as increased weight loss due to diarrhea. This phenomenon is comparable to clinical studies in which only minimal amounts of LV (as low as 5 mg daily given orally for two weeks) increased toxicity [25], as well as other schedules of LV [18,19]. This increased toxicity is possibly due to damage to normal mucosal tissues affecting the physiological function of gut mucosa such as reabsorption of nutrients and fluids. Co-administration of LV is very likely to enhance the inhibition of TS in normal mucosa, affecting normal functioning of this tissue. Folate pools in these tissues are very low and only minimal amounts of additional folate might be responsible for such an enhanced inhibition.

Continuous infusions or bolus injections of 5FU?

The *in vitro* evidence of a enhanced efficacy of continuous exposure has led to a number of clinical studies in which patients have been treated with protracted infusions of 5FU varying from one week to several months (see Table 1). Despite a number of Phase I and II trials in which 5FU was given as a continuous infusion convincing evidence for a better antitumor activity was not present [1]. Only recently Lokich et al [24] reported an increased response rate of 30% for the protracted infusion compared to 7% for the daily administration (*x* 5) of bolus 5FU treatment. However, this treatment was not more efficacious considering survival, which was similar in both treatment arms. These results are comparable with the present data in mice, in which the initial better anti-tumor effect was not associated with an increase in life span. These overall clinical results are comparable to that observed for the combination of 5FU with LV (Table 2), in which a higher response rate was observed consistently for a number of randomized trials irrespective of the 5FU schedule [2, 4, 28]. However, the effect of the combination regimen of LV-5FU on survival is negligible. This has led to the question which schedule would be preferable from a therapeutic point of view; protracted continuous infusions with 5FU or biochemical modulation of 5FU with LV?

There seems to be no preference for any of these two schedules, when the available data are being considered of large randomized trials in which one of these treatment regimens was included (Table 2). It should, however, be noted that not only criteria such as response and survival, but also quality of life, costs and feasibility of the treatment should be taken in consideration [13]. Generally, continuous infusion will require hospitalization for implantation of the pump; subsequent treatment can be performed on a out-patient basis. However, both the LV-5FU combinations (5FU given as a bolus) and the protracted infusions have a limited value with regard to the overall survival of the patients and most patients do not respond. The use of multiple modulators [2] such as the combination of 5FU with PALA, LV, interferon and/or uridine may be another step forward. It is, however, remarkable that these modulators have shown their efficacy mainly when 5FU was given as a bolus injection or a short-term infusion at a high dose. A flat rate continuous infusion of 5FU may not prove to be the first choice of systemic treatment for colorectal cancer but have certainly shown their value in the treatment of other malignancies [13] especially in combination with cisplatinum in

Table 2. Comparison of the therapeutic efficacy of bolus schedules and protracted infusions against advanced colorectal cancer

Treatment modality	Response rate		Dose-limiting toxicity	Ref.
Bolus 5FU*	12%	(44/366)	leukopenia	2,4,28
Bolus 5FU with LV*	34%	(155/457)	gastro-intestinal	2,4,28
PALA with high dose 5FU**	36%	(40/110)	myelosuppression, diarrhea	5,6,50
Interferon-α with 5FU@	39%	(44/112)	myelosuppression, mucositis neurological	51,52,53
Protracted infusion#	40%	(160/399)	mucositis, HFS, diarrhea	54
Protracted infusion with LV##	30%	(16/48)	mucositis, HFS, diarrhea	18,19

*Summary of controlled randomized trials comparing 5FU with LV-5FU using various schedules.
**, 5FU given as a bolus or a high dose at 24 hr infusion.
@, 5FU was given as a loading dose of 5 days continuous infusion (750 mg/m^2) followed by weekly bolus at 750 mg/m^2, with IFNα.
#, compilation of Phase II trials and one randomized trial [24] as summarized by Ahlgren [54]. Various lengths and intensities of the 5FU schedules were used. HFS, hand-foot syndrome.
##, compilation of Phase I and II trials, using different length and dosages of 5FU infusion as well as that of LV. Generally the dose of 5FU was decreased in the presence of LV, since the grade of toxicity was enhanced in the presence of LV.

head and neck cancer. However, other treatment modalities might find their application in the treatment of colorectal cancer. It has for instance been shown that a continuous exposure to 5FU is essential in combination with radiation [55]. Also chronomodulation of 5FU administration might enable to reduce the toxicity and enhance the antitumor effect [56]. However, only a randomized comparison of the possibly active schedules can give the answer.

ACKNOWLEDGEMENTS

This research was supported by a grant from the Dutch Cancer Society IKA-VU 88-20 and by Cyanamide Lederle BV, Etten-Leur, the Netherlands. GJP is the recipient of a senior fellowship of the Royal Netherlands Academy of Sciences.

REFERENCES

1. H.M. Pinedo and G.J. Peters. 5-Fluorouracil: biochemistry and pharmacology, *J. Clin. Oncol.* 6:1653-1664 (1988).
2. G.J. Peters and C.J. van Groeningen, Clinical relevance of biochemical modulation of 5-fluorouracil, *Ann. Oncology* 2:469-480 (1991).
3. C.J. van Groeningen, G.J. Peters, and H.M. Pinedo, Modulation of 5-fluorouracil toxicity with uridine. *Sem. Oncology* 19 (Sup 3):148-154 (1992).
4. P. Piedbois, M. Buyse, Y. Rustum, D. Machover, C. Erlichman, R.W. Carlson, F. Valone, R. Labianca, J.H. Doroshow, and N. Petrelli, Modulation of Fluorouracil by Leucovorin in Patients With Advanced Colorectal Cancer: Evidence in Terms of Response Rate, *J. Clin. Oncol.* 10:896-903 (1992).
5. P.J. O'Dwyer, A.R. Paul, J. Walczak, L.M. Weiner, S. Litwin, and R.L. Comis, Phase II study of biochemical modulation of fluorouracil by low-dose PALA in patients with colorectal cancer, *J. Clin. Oncol.* 8:1497-1503 (1990).
6. B. Ardalan, S. Gurckarn, and H. Silberman, A randomized phase I and II study of short-term infusion of high-dose fluorouracil with or without N-(Phosphonacetyl)-L-aspartic acid in patients with advanced pancreatic and colorectal cancer, *J. Clin. Oncol.*, 6:1053-1058 (1988).

7. W.P. Peters, G. Weiss, and D.W. Kufe, Phase-I trial of combination therapy with continuous-infusion MMPR and continuous-infusion 5FU, *Cancer Chemother. Pharmacol.* 13:136-138 (1984).

8. P.I. Raju, Y. Maruyama, J. MacDonald, and P. DeSimone, Treatment of Unresectable Pancreatic Carcinoma Using Irradiation with Concurrent Intravenous 5-FU Infusion Therapy, *Cancer Invest.* 6:263-266 (1988).

9. A. Shah, W. MacDonald, J. Goldie, G. Gudauskas, and B. Brisebois, 5-FU Infusion in Advanced Colorectal Cancer: A Comparison of Three Dose Schedules, *Cancer Treatment Rep.* 69:739-742 (1985).

10. D.L. Trump, M.J. Egorin, A. Forrest, J.K.V. Willson, S. Remick, and K.D. Tutsch, Pharmacokinetics and Pharmacodynamic Analysis of Fluorouracil During 72-Hour Continuous Infusion With and Without Dipyridamole, *J. Clin. Oncol.* 9:2027-2035 (1991).

11. A. Thyss, G. Milano, N. Renée, J. Vallicioni, M. Schneider, and F. Demard, Clinical pharmacokinetic study of 5-FU in continuous 5-day infusions for head and neck cancer, *Cancer Chemother. Pharmacol.* 16:64-66 (1986).

12. Ph. Rougier, H. Ammarguellat, M. Ghosn, G. Piot, M. Benhamed, J.M. Tigaud, Ph. Laplaige, C. Theodore, J. Kac, J. Goldberg, P. Carde, and J.P. Droz, Phase II Trial of 7-Day Continuous 5-Fluorouracil Infusion in the Treatment of Advanced Colorectal Carcinoma, *Oncology* 49:35-39 (1992).

13. J.S. Macdonald, Continuous Low-Dose Infusion of Fluorouracil: Is the Benefit Worth the Cost? *J. Clin. Oncol.* 7(4):412-414 (1989).

14. S.M. Grunberg, C. Clay, and D.V. Spicer, Tolerance of Extended (28 Day) Continuous Infusion of 5-Fluorouracil in Advanced Head and Neck Cancer, *Sel. Cancer Ther.* 7:17-21 (1991).

15. V.P. Barbounis, H.P. Kalofonos, A.J. Munro, C.G. McKenzie, J.M. Sackier, and A.A. Epenetos, Treatment of Colorectal Cancer and Other Malignancies with Continuous Infusion of 5-Fluorouracil, *Anticancer Res.* 9:33-40 (1989).

16. S. Huan, R. Pazdur, A. Singhakowinta, B. Samal, and V.K. Vaitkevicius, Low-Dose Continuous Infusion 5-Fluorouracil: Evaluation in Advanced Breast Carcinoma, *Cancer* 63:419-422 (1989).

17. R. Hansen, E. Quebbeman, P. Ritch, C. Chitambar, and T. Anderson, Continuous 5-Fluorouracil (5FU) Infusion in Carcinoma of the Pancreas: A Phase II Study, *Am. J. Med. Sci.* 295:91-93 (1988).

18. C.G. Leichman, L. Leichman, C.P. Spears, P.J. Rosen, F. Muggia, S. Jeffers, and W. Waugh, Biological Modification of protracted infusion of 5-fluorouracil with weekly leucovorin: A dose seeking clinical trial for patients with disseminated gastrointestinal cancers, *Cancer Chemother. Pharmacol.* 26:57-61 (1990).

19. H.A.M. Sinnige, A.G. Nanninga, R.C.J. Verschueren, D.Th. Sleijfer, E.G.E. de Vries, P.H.B. Willemse, and N.H. Mulder, A Phase I-II Study of 14-days Continuous Infusion of 5-Fluorouracil with Weekly Bolus Leucovorin in Metastatic Colorectal Carcinoma, *Eur. J. Cancer* 28A:885-888 (1992).

20. S.C. Remick, J.L. Grem, P.H. Fischer, K.D. Tutsch, D.B. Alberti, L.M. Nieting, M.B. Tombes, J. Bruggink, J.K.V. Willson, and D.L. Trump, Phase I Trial of 5-Fluorouracil and Dipyridamole Administered by Seventy-two-Hour Concurrent Continuous Infusion, *Cancer Res.* 50:2667-2672 (1990).

21. B. Ardalan, K. Stridhar, R. Reddy, P. Benedetto, S. Richman, S. Waldman, L. Morrell, L. Feun, N. Savaraj, and A. Livingstone, Phase I Study of High Dose 5-Fluorouracil and High Dose Leucovorin with Low Dose Phosphonacetyl-L-Aspartic Acid in Patients with Advanced Malignancies, *Int. J. Radiation Oncology Biol. Phys.* 22:511-514 (1992).

22. P.J. O'Dwyer, G.R. Hudes, J. Colofiore, J. Walczak, J. Hoffman, F.P. LaCreta, R.L. Comis, D.S. Martin, and R.F. Ozols, Phase I Trial of Fluorouracil Modulation by N-Phosphonacetyl-L-aspartate and 6-Methylmercaptopurine Riboside: Optimization of 6-Methylmercaptopurine Riboside Dose and Schedule Through Biochemical Analysis of Sequential Tumor Biopsy Specimens, *J. Natl. Cancer Inst.* 83:1235-1240 (1991).

23. J.A. Kish, J.F. Ensley, J. Jacobs, A. Weaver, G. Cummings, and M. Al-Sarraf, A randomized trial of cisplatin (CACP) + 5-fluorouracil (5-FU) infusion and CACP + 5-FU bolus for recurrent and advanced squamous cell carcinoma of the head and neck, *Cancer* 56:2740-2744 (1985).

24. J.J. Lokich, J.D. Ahlgren, J.J. Gullo, J.A. Philips, and J.G. Fryer, A Prospective Randomized Comparison of Continuous Infusion Fluorouracil With a Conventional Bolus Schedule in Metastatic Colorectal Carcinoma: A Mid-Atlantic Oncology Program Study, *J. Clin. Oncol.* 7:425-432 (1989).

25. C.H.N. Veenhof, R.L. Poorter, P.J.M. Bakker, D.M.J. Biermans-Van Leeuwe, P. Noordhuis, G. Codacci-Pisanelli, and G.J. Peters, Fourteen days continuous 5-Fluorouracil (5-FU) infusion and low dose oral calcium leucovorin (LV) in patients with gastrointestinal cancer. *Proc. Amer. Soc. Clin. Oncol.* 11:181 (Abstract 539) (1992).

26. R.M. Hansen, P.S. Ritch, J.A. Libnoch, and T. Anderson, Continuous 5-Fluorouracil Infusion and Alpha Interferon in Advanced Cancers: A Report of Initial Treatment Results, *Am. J. Med. Sci.* 301:246-249 (1991).

27. N. Anderson, J. Lokich, M. Bern, S. Wallach, C. Moore, and D. Williams, A Phase I Clinical Trial of Combined Fluoropyrimidines With Leucovorin in a 14-Day Infusion: Demonstration of Biochemical Modulation, *Cancer* 63:233-237 (1989).

28. C-H. Köhne-Wömpner, H-J. Schmoll, A. Harstrick, and Y.M. Rustum, Chemotherapeutic Strategies in Metastatic Colorectal Cancer: An Overview of Current Clinical Trials, *Sem. Oncol.* 19 (Suppl 3):105-125 (1992).

29. B. Drewinko and L.-Y. Yang, Cellular Basis for the Inefficacy of 5-FU in Human Colon Carcinoma, *Cancer Treatment Rep.* 69:1391 1398 (1985).

30. P.M. Calabro-Jones, J.E. Byfield, and J.F. Ward, Time-dose relationships for 5-fluorouracil cytotoxicity against human epithelial cancer cells in vitro, *Cancer Res.* 42:4413-4420 (1982).

31. G.J. Peters, E. Laurensse, A. Leyva, J. Lankelma, and H.M. Pinedo, Sensitivity of human, murine and rat cells to 5-fluorouracil and 5'deoxy-5-fluorouridine in relation to drug metabolizing enzymes, *Cancer Res.* 46:20-28 (1986).

32. Y.P.A.M. Keepers, P.E. Pizao, G.J. Peters, J. van Ark-Otte, B. Winograd, and H.M. Pinedo, Growth-inhibition kinetics - schedule and concentration dependency - of anticancer agents in colon cancer cells, *Proc. Amer. Assoc. Cancer Res.* 32:386 (Abstract 2292) (1991).

33. C.L. van der Wilt, H.M. Pinedo, J. Cloos, P. Noordhuis, K. Smid, and G.J. Peters, Effect of folinic acid on 5-fluorouracil activity and expression of thymidylate synthase. *Sem. Oncology* 19 (Sup 3):16-25 (1992).

34. G.J. Peters, E. Laurensse, A. Leyva, and H.M. Pinedo, Purine nucleosides as cell-specific modulators of 5-fluorouracil metabolism and cytotoxicity, *Eur. J. Cancer Clin. Oncol.* 23:1869-1881 (1987).

35. J.C. Nadal, C.J. van Groeningen, H.M. Pinedo, and G.J. Peters, Schedule-dependency of in vivo modulation of 5-fluorouracil by leucovorin and uridine in murine colon carcinoma, *Invest. New Drugs* 7:163-172 (1989).

36. G.J. Peters, J. van Dijk, E. Laurensse, C.J. van Groeningen, J. Lankelma, A. Leyva, J.C. Nadal, and H.M. Pinedo. In vitro biochemical and in vivo biological studies of the uridine "rescue" of 5-fluorouracil, *Brit. J. Cancer* 57:259-265 (1988).

37. C.L. van der Wilt, K. Smid, H.M. Pinedo, and G.J. Peters, Elevation of thymidylate synthase following 5-fluorouracil treatment is prevented by addition of leucovorin in murine colon tumors, *Cancer Res.* 52:4922-4928 (1992).

38. C.L. van der Wilt, J. van Laar, F. Gyergyay, K. Smid, and G.J. Peters, Biochemical modification of the toxicity and antitumor effect of 5-fluorouracil and cis-platinum by WR-2721 (ethiofos) in mice, *Eur. J. Cancer*, in press.

39. C.J. van Groeningen, H.M. Pinedo, J. Heddes, R.M. Kok, A.P.J.M. de Jong, E. Wattel, G.J. Peters and J. Lankelma, Pharmacokinetics of 5-fluorouracil assessed with a sensitive mass spectrometric method in patients during a dose escalation schedule, *Cancer Res.* 48:6956-6961 (1988).

40. G.J. Peters, J. Lankelma, R.M. Kok, P. Noordhuis, C.J. van Groeningen, S. Meijer, and H.M. Pinedo, Long retention of high concentrations of 5-fluorouracil in human and murine tumors compared to plasma, *Cancer Chemother. Pharmacol.*, in press.

41. T. Yoshida, E. Araki, M. Iigo, T. Fujii, M. Yoshino, Y. Shimada, D. Saito, H. Tajiri, H. Yamaguchi, S. Yoshida, M. Yoshino, H. Ohkura, M. Yoshimori, and N. Okazaki, Clinical significance of monitoring serum levels of 5-fluorouracil by continuous infusion in patients with advanced colonic cancer, *Cancer Chemother. Pharmacol.* 26:352-354 (1990).

42. M. Slavik, J. Wu, D. Einspahr, and C. Riley, Clinical pharmacokinetics of 5-fluorouracil low dose continuous intravenous infusion, *Proc. Amer. Assoc. Cancer Res.* 32:173 (Abstract 1030) (1991).

43. C. Erlichman, S. Fine, and T. Elhakim, Plasma Pharmacokinetics of 5-FU Given by Continuous Infusion With Allopurinol, *Cancer Treatment Rep.* 70:903-904 (1986).

44. S. Fujii, Y. Shimamoto, H. Ohshimo, T. Imaoka, M. Motoyama, M. Fukushima, and T. Shirasaka, Effects of the Plasma Concentration of 5-Fluorouracil and the Duration of Continuous Venous Infusion of 5-Fluorouracil with an Inhibitor of 5-Fluorouracil Degradation on Yoshida Sarcomas in Rats, *Jpn. J. Cancer Res.* 80:167-172 (1989).

45. W.M. Hryniuk, A. Figueredo, and M. Goodyear, Applications of Dose Intensity to Problems in Chemotherapy of Breast and Colorectal Cancer, *Semin. Oncol.* 14 (Suppl 4):3-11 (1987).

46. S.G. Arbuck, Overview of Clinical Trials Using 5-Fluorouracil and Leucovorin for the Treatment of Colorectal Cancer, *Cancer* 63:1036-1044 (1989).

47. G. Codacci-Pisanelli, C.L. van der Wilt, P. Noordhuis, R. Kok, F. Franchi, H.M. Pinedo, and G.J. Peters, Pharmacodynamics and antitumour activity of continuous infusion (c.i.) of 5-Fluorouracil in mice, *Proc. Amer. Assoc. Cancer Res.* 33:533 (Abstract 3184) (1992).

48. L.D. Nord and D.S. Martin, Loss of Murine Tumor Thymidine Kinase Activity *in vivo* Following 5-Fluorouracil (FUra) Treatment by Incorporation of FUra into RNA, *Biochem. Pharmacol.* 42:2369-2375 (1991).

49. T.-L. Chen and C. Erlichman, Biochemical modulation of 5-fluorouracil with or without leucovorin by a low dose of brequinar in MGH-U1 cells, *Cancer Chemother. Pharmacol.* 30:370-376 (1992).

50. N. Kemeny, J.A. Conti, K. Seiter, D. Niedzwiecki, J. Botet, D. Martin, P. Costa, J. Wiseberg, and W. McCulloch, Biochemical Modulation of Bolus Fluorouracil by PALA in Patients With Advanced Colorectal Cancer, *J. Clin. Oncol.* 10:747-752 (1992).

51. S. Wadler, B. Lembersky, M. Atkins, J. Kirkwood, and N. Petrelli, Phase II trial of fluorouracil and recombinant interferon alfa-2a in patients with advanced colorectal carcinoma: an Eastern cooperative oncology group study, *J. Clin. Oncol.* 9:1806-1810 (1991).

52. R. Pazdur, J.A. Ajani, Y.Z. Patt, R. Winn, D. Jackson, B. Shepard, R. DuBrow, L. Campos, M. Quaraishi, J. Faintuch, J.L. Abruzzese, J. Gutterman, and B. Levin, Phase II study of fluorouracil and recombinant alfa-2a in previously untreated advanced colorectal carcinoma. *J. Clin. Oncol.* 8:2027-2031 (1990).

53. N. Kemeny, A. Younes, K. Seiter, D. Kelsen, P. Sammarco, L. Adams, S. Derby, P. Murray, and C. Houston, Interferon alfa-2a and 5-fluorouracil for advanced colorectal carcinoma. Assessment of activity and toxicity. *Cancer* 66:2470-2475 (1990).

54. J.D. Ahlgren, O. Trocki, J.J. Gullo, R. Goldberg, W.A. Muir, R. Sisk, and L. Schacter, Protracted Infusion of 5-FU with Weekly Low-Dose Cisplatin as Second-Line Therapy in Patients with Metastatic Colorectal Cancer Who Have Failed 5-FU Monotherapy, *Cancer Invest.* 9:27-33 (1991).

55. J.E. Byfield, 5-Fluorouracil radiation sensitization: A brief review, *Invest. New Drugs* 7:111-116 (1989).

56. W.J.M. Hrushesky, More Evidence for Circadian Rhythm Effects in Cancer Chemotherapy: The Fluoropyrimidine Story, *Cancer Cells* 2:65-68 (1990).

DISCUSSION OF DR. RUSTUM'S/DR. PETER'S PRESENTATION

Dr. Charles Young: Could you comment further on the interface between leucovorin and the weekly i.v. push of FdUrd?

Dr. Rustum: The trial we are doing now Charley is the 2 hr continuous infusion of leucovorin 500 mg/M^2 with i.v. push FdUrd at 1 hr. So that's the schedule we are evaluating. We have evaluated continuous infusion of FdUrd with continuous infusion of leucovorin and the toxicity was enormous. The toxicity of i.v. push FdUrd with 2 h infusion of leucovorin is quite manageable according to the weekly schedule of RPCI.

Dr. Allegra: Joe, recently Dr. Bertino's lab published some data suggesting that cells become resistant in vitro to continuous infusion via a DNA directed mechanism whereas cells exposed to pulse exposures to fluorouracil become resistant via decrease in RNA incorporation. Those data are very different in fact they're exactly opposed to the data you have presented. Do you have any comment?`

Dr. Rustum: The data obtained by Drs. Sobrero and Bertino were with FUra. Our data with FUra are consistent with their findings. With respect to FdUrd, however, our in vitro data indicate that the mechanism of action of FdUrd administered by short-term exposure (2h) is primarily via DNA directed mechanisms. In contrast, long-term exposure of cells to FdUrd, RNA directed mechanisms appear to dominate.

CELLULAR INTERACTIONS BETWEEN THE NATURAL AND UNNATURAL ISOMERS OF 5-FORMYLTETRAHYDROFOLATE

Jacques Jolivet and Richard Bertrand

Montreal Cancer Institute
1560 Sherbrooke St. East
Montréal (Québec)
Canada H2L 4M1

INTRODUCTION

Leucovorin is a pharmaceutical preparation containing a mixture of the natural and unnatural diastereomers of 5-formyltetrahydrofolate (N^5-HCO-H_4PteGlu). All reduced folates have an S chirality at the 6 carbon of the tetrahydropterine ring and the natural and unnatural isomers of 5-formyltetrahydrofolate are designated respectively as (6S)- and (6R)-N^5-HCO-H_4PteGlu[1-4]. After being used for many years as a rescue agent following high doses of the antifolate methotrexate (MTX)[5], leucovorin is now also administered clinically in combination with 5-fluorouracil (5-FU) to enhance its antitumor activity, an effect dependent on the replenishment of intracellular folate pools by the reduced folate[6,7]. Following intravenous leucovorin administration, the 6S isomer disappears rapidly from plasma with a mean elimination half-life of 20 to 30 minutes while the 6R compound has a much slower clearance (half-lives of 7.5 to 11 hours) and persists at high concentrations for prolonged periods[6,8]. Consequently, the possible interactions between the natural and unnatural N^5-HCO-H_4PteGlu isomers have been studied both experimentally and in the clinic. This paper will summarize available data on the isomers' cellular interactions.

IS THE UNNATURAL ISOMER TRANSPORTED INTO CELLS?

Sirotnak et al. first examined stereospecific N^5-HCO-H_4PteGlu transport in L1210, S180 and Ehrlich murine tumor cells and found that the unnatural isomer was 20-fold less effective than the natural isomer as a competitive inhibitor for MTX influx with K_i values of 35.2 to 53.8 μM[9] in anionic buffers. Furthermore, K_i values derived from a mixture containing equal amounts of the natural and unnatural isomer were twofold greater than the values derived using the pure natural reduced folate suggesting no significant interactions between

Novel Approaches to Selective Treatments of Human Solid Tumors: Laboratory and Clinical Correlation Edited by Y. M. Rustum, Plenum Press, New York, 1993

23

the isomers. We reexamined (6R)-N5-HCO-H4PteGlu transport characteristics in the human leukemia CCRF-CEM cell line[10]. Time-dependent uptake experiments illustrated in figure 1 revealed that total intracellular folates were significantly lower in CCRF-CEM cells after exposure to the 6R than the 6S isomer with greater levels obtained in anion-free (Panel A) compared to anionic buffers (Panel B).

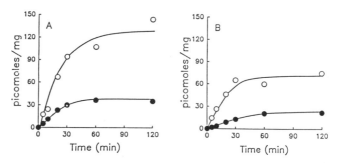

Fig.1 **Time-dependent uptake of (6R) and (6S)-N5-HCO-H4PteGlu by CCRF-CEM cells.** CCRF-CEM cells were exposed to 5μM [^{3}H]-(6R)-N5-HCO-H4PteGlu (closed circles) or 5μM [^{3}H]-(6S)-N5-HCO-H4PteGlu (open circles) for up to 120 minutes in the anion-free (panel A) or anionic buffer (panel B) as described[10]. Uptake is expressed in pmoles/mg and represents the mean results of duplicate experiments.

To determine if the lower intracellular folate levels observed after exposure of the CCRF-CEM cells to the 6R isomer was secondary to poor membrane transport or deficient intracellular metabolism, uptake of both isomers at various concentrations was determined during 5 minute exposures, a period too short for significant intracellular metabolism to occur. As illustrated in figure 2, intracellular N5-HCO-H4PteGlu uptake was consistently higher after exposures to the natural compared to the unnatural isomer with greater uptake again seen under anion-free conditions. Separate 5 minute uptake inhibition studies indicated that the 6R isomer was a competitive inhibitor of the 6S compound, (6S)-N5-CH3-H4PteGlu, folic acid and methotrexate influx. Results are summarized in Table I.

V_{max} values for all folates and methotrexate influx in the presence of the unnatural isomer were very similar to those reported previously[11] in the same buffers, indicating specific binding of the unnatural isomer to the reduced folate transport protein. The uptake inhibition of folates by (6R)-N5-HCO-H4PteGlu was decreased greater than tenfold by adding anions to the extracellular buffer demonstrating, as already described for other folates and antifolates[11], the great dependence on the composition of extracellular anions to the unnatural isomer's binding efficiency to the transport protein. These results were comparable to those obtained in the murine tumor cells[9] and in HT-29 human colon

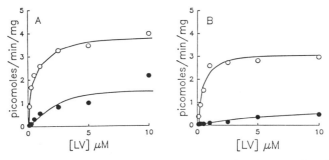

Fig.2 **Concentration-dependent uptake of (6R) and (6S)-N⁵-HCO-H₄PteGlu by CCRF-CEM cells.** Cells were exposed for 5 minutes at various [³H] (6R)-N⁵-HCO-H₄-PteGlu (closed circles) or [³H]-(6S)-N⁵-HCO-H₄PteGlu (open circles) concentrations in the anion-free (panel A) or anionic buffer (panel B) as described[10]. Results are expressed in pmoles/min/mg and represent the mean of duplicate experiments.

carcinoma cells[12] and confirmed that $(6R)-N^5-HCO-H_4PteGlu$ was a much poorer substrate than the natural isomer for the transmembrane transport protein, did not seem to be extensively metabolised intracellularly but could possibly hinder the cellular uptake of $(6S)-N^5-HCO-H_4PteGlu$ at high concentrations. It was thus important to further examine the unnatural isomer's intracellular fate and effects on the natural isomer's cellular effects.

IS THE UNNATURAL ISOMER METABOLISED INTRACELLULARLY AND DOES IT AFFECT INTRACELLULAR FOLATE POOLS?

$(6R)-N^5-HCO-H_4PteGlu$ could theoretically be metabolised on the pteridine ring and/or polyglutamylated and consequently perturb intracellular folate metabolism. The unnatural isomer is not a substrate however for methenyltetrahydrofolate synthetase, the enzyme responsible for the stereospecific transformation of $(6S)-N^5-HCO-H_4PteGlu$ to $N^{5-10}-CH^+-H_4PteGlu$[13]. Indeed, we have used this characteristic to purify the unnatural isomer by incubating leucovorin with methenyltetrahydrofolate synthetase until all the $(6S)-N^5-HCO-H_4PteGlu$ present in the leucovorin preparation was consumed[10]. Although there is no other known enzyme for which the unnatural isomer is or could be a substrate, Lee and Schilsky have shown that the unnatural isomer could at high concentrations competitively inhibit *Lactobacillus casei* thymidylate synthase in a cell free system with a K_i of 1.59 mM[14]. An early preliminary report also suggested that the unnatural isomer could be a substrate for mouse liver folylpolyglutamate synthetase although with 15-fold poorer affinity than the natural isomer[15]. Since the inhibition of thymidylate synthase by the unnatural isomer or possible inhibition of other folate-dependent enzymes by $(6R)-N^5-HCO-H_4PteGlu$ polyglutamates could perturb intracellular folate metabolism, the potential effects of $(6R)-N^5-HCO-H_4PteGlu$ on intracellular folate pools was directly examined in tumor cells. Boarman and Allegra determined in HCT 116 colon cells that up to a

Table 1. (6R)-N[5]-HCO-H$_4$PteGlu as an inhibitor of the uptake of various folates and methotrexate.

Substrate	Anion-free buffer			Anionic buffer		
	K_t	V_{max}	K_i	K_t	V_{max}	K_i
(6S)-N[5]-HCO-H$_4$-PteGlu[a]	0.3	4.0	1.9	1.0	4.3	30
(6S)-N[5]-CH$_3$-H$_4$PteGlu[b]	0.2	3.9	1.6	1.2	4.6	25
Folic acid[c]	16	4.3	3.0	56	4.7	45
Methotrexate[d]	0.7	4.0	2.2	4.4	4.5	28

K_i values (μM) for (6R)-N[5]-HCO-H$_4$PteGlu were derived from Dixon plots constructed from experiments in which the uptake of tritiated folates in CCRF-CEM cells was inhibited by fixed concentrations of unlabelled (6R)-N[5]-HCO-H$_4$PteGlu. K_t and V_{max} values for each labelled competing compound are expressed in μM and pmoles/mg/min and were determined from Lineweaver-Burke plots. All values represent the mean result of duplicate experiments. Experiments were performed in both anion-free and anionic buffers as described[10].

[a] [^{3}H]-(6S)-N[5]-HCO-H$_4$PteGlu was varied from 0.25 to 1.0 μM in the anion-free and 0.5 to 1.5 μM in the anionic buffer.
[b] [^{3}H]-(6S)-N[5]-CH$_3$-H$_4$PteGlu was varied from 0.2 to 0.8 μM in the anion-free and 0.4 to 2.0 μM in the anionic buffer.
[c] [^{3}H]-Folic acid was varied from 5 to 20 μM in the anion-free and 10 to 50 μM in the anionic buffer.
[d] [^{3}H]-MTX was varied from 0.4 to 1.5 μM in the anion-free and 2.0 to 5.0 μM in the anionic buffer.

20:1 ratio of the unnatural to natural isomer resulted in no significant effects both on the metabolism of the natural isomer into the one-carbon substituted folate pools and on their metabolism to polyglutamate forms[16]. Furthermore, McGuire et al. have recently reported that the unnatural isomer was essentially inactive both as a substrate and as an inhibitor of rat and human folylpolyglutamate synthetase[17]. One possible explanation to explain the discrepancy between this and the earlier report[15] is a possible species difference in the substrate specificity of folylpolyglutamate synthetase. Another possibility is contamination of the unnatural isomer preparation by (6R)-N[10]-HCO-H$_4$PteGlu, a good substrate for polyglutamylation which can be formed at low levels during the carbodiimide reaction used to formylate the unnatural isomer in the earlier report. One can thus conclude that at the present time, there is no firm evidence that the unnatural isomer can be metabolised intracellularly or interfere with intracellular folate metabolism in human cells.

DOES THE UNNATURAL ISOMER HAVE ANY EFFECT ON CELL GROWTH OR MTX AND 5-FU CYTOTOXICITY ?

The possibility that (6R)-N5-HCO-H4PteGlu could support cell growth or influence cell growth support by the natural isomer has been investigated by a number of authors. We examined this possibility using human leukemia CCRF-CEM cells[10]. (6R)-N5-HCO-H4-PteGlu failed to promote the cell growth of folate-depleted cells at 10 μM while the same concentration of either the 6S isomer or leucovorin supported cell growth. Furthermore, the unnatural isomer failed to interfere with cell growth supported by the natural compound as folate-depleted cells maintained normal cell growth when refed with at least 0.1 μM of the 6S isomer despite co-exposure with up to 100 μM 6R isomer. Similar negative results were also obtained in the HCT-8 human colon cancer cell line[18]. Early reports that the unnatural isomer could support cell growth at high concentrations[12] again probably reflected contamination by (6S)-N5-HCO-H4PteGlu.

The effects of (6R)-N5-HCO-H4PteGlu on MTX rescue by the natural isomer have been studied by a number of investigators. Sirotnak et al originally reported that the unnatural isomer was 200-fold less effective than the natural isomer in preventing MTX cytotoxicity in L1210 cells[9]. In mice, a natural isomer preparation was at least twice as effective as leucovorin in reversing MTX toxicity[19] while in vitro the mixture of isomers was again as effective but no less so than as an equimolar preparation of the pure natural isomer in reversing MTX cytotoxicity in a number of human cell lines[20]. Using a deoxyuridine (dU) suppression test in human leukemia CCRF-CEM cells, Zittoun et al determined that (6R)-N5-HCO-H4PteGlu could revert MTX-induced dU suppression when cells were co-incubated with 10^{-3} M of the unnatural isomer and 10^{-7} M MTX. No rescue could be seen when using either higher MTX or lower (6R)-N5-HCO-H4PteGlu. Furthermore, two other groups reported that the unnatural isomer could not impair the natural isomer's capacity to protect CCRF-CEM cells from the growth inhibitory effects of MTX in tissue culture[17,22]. Again, contamination with the natural isomer was probably responsible for the weak rescue potential observed with the unnatural isomer preparations used in the L1210 cell experiments[9] while contamination or more likely uptake competition with MTX can explain the prevention of dU suppression by MTX observed with co-exposure to 10,000-fold higher (6R)-N5-HCO-H4PteGlu concentrations. One can thus conclude that experimentally the unnatural isomer has no significant impact on MTX rescue by the natural isomer. Early evidence suggests that this conclusion will also be valid in the clinic. Eighteen children with acute lymphocytic leukemia were rescued from MTX in a crossover clinical trial with either oral preparations of (6S)- or (6R,S)-N5-HCO-H4PteGlu[23]. Both reduced folate preparations resulted in comparable blood folate profiles and equivalent treatment tolerance.

The effects of (6R)-N5-HCO-H4PteGlu on the potentiation of 5-FU cytotoxicity by the natural isomer have also been extensively examined. We examined this possible interaction in human leukemia CCRF-CEM cells[10]. As illustrated in Fig. 3, simultaneous cell exposure to 1mM 6R isomer had no effect on the enhancement of the growth inhibitory effects of

5-fluorouracil observed with 1μM leucovorin, the lowest folate concentration at which enhanced 5-FU activity could be detected. Equally negative results were obtained in CCRF-CEM cells[17,21] and in human colon cancer cells HCT-8[18] by other investigators. It thus seems unlikely that the 6R isomer detected in plasma following intravenous leucovorin administration[6] will impair the potentiation of 5-fluorouracil cytotoxicity by the natural 6S isomer.

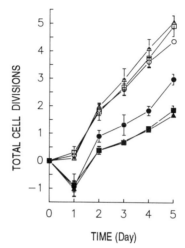

TIME (Day)

Fig.3 **Effects of (6R)-N⁵-HCO-H₄-PteGlu on 5-fluorouracil (5-FU) cytotoxicity.** CCRF-CEM cells at a density of 2.10^5/ml were grown in RPMI-1640 medium for 4 hrs without (open circles) or with 100 μM 5-FU (closed circles) for the last two hours; added 1 μM leucovorin without (open triangles) or with 5-FU (closed triangles) and 1 μM leucovorin and 1 mM (6R)-N⁵-HCO-H₄-PteGlu without (open squares) or with 5-FU (closed squares). After drug exposure, cells were washed twice, resuspended in drug-free medium at a density of 2.10^4/ml and their growth followed daily for 5 days. Cell counts were determined visually using an hemocytometer. Growth curves were generated by plotting Total Cell Divisions (TCD) vs time. TCD was calculated from the formula[24]:

$$TCD= \log_{10} (N^t/N^0)/\log_{10}2$$

where N^0 is the initial cell number following resuspension and N^t is the cell number at time t. Points represent the mean and standard deviation of six experiments.

CONCLUSIONS

Although (6R)-N⁵-HCO-H₄-PteGlu can be transported intracellularly and is a weak inhibitor of (6S)-N⁵-HCO-H₄PteGlu uptake, the unnatural isomer has no measurable impact on the natural isomer's replenishment of intracellular folate pools, support of cell growth, rescue from MTX or potentiation of 5-FU cytotoxicity. The available experimental evidence strongly support the conclusion that (6R)-N⁵-HCO-H₄-PteGlu is a biologically inert compound.

REFERENCES

1. H.E. Sauberlich and C.A. Baumann. A factor required for the growth of Leuconostoc citrovorum. J Biol Chem 176: 165-173 (1948).
2. T.J. Bond, T.J. Bardos, M. Sibley, W. Shive. The folinic acid group, a series of new vitamins related to folic acid. J Amer Chem Soc 74: 3852-3853 (1949).
3. D.B. Cosulish, J.M. Smith, H.P. Broquist. Diastereomer of leucovorin. J Amer Chem Soc 74: 4215-16 (1952).
4. J.C. Fontecilla-Camps, C.E. Bugg, C. Temple, J.C. Rose, J.A. Montgomery, R.L. Kisliuk. Absolute configuration of biological tetrahydrofolate. A crystallo-graphic determination. J Amer Chem Soc 101: 6114-6115 (1979).
5. J. Jolivet, K.H. Cowan, G.A. Curt, N.J. Clendoninn, B.A. Chabner. The pharmacology and clinical use of methotrexate. N Engl J Med 309: 1094-1104 (1983).
6. D. Machover, E. Goldschmidt, P. Chollet, G. Metzger, J. Zittoun, J. Marquet, J.M. Vandenbulcke, J.L. Misset, L. Scharzenberg, J.B. Fourtillan, H. Gaget, G. Mathe. Treatment of advanced colorectal and gastric adenocarcinomas with 5-fluorouracil and high-dose folinic acid. J Clin Oncol 4: 685-696 (1986).
7. B. Ullman, M. Lee, D.W. Martin Jr, D.V. Santi. Cytotoxicity of 5-fluoro-2'-deoxyuridine: Requirement for reduced folate cofactors and antagonism by methotrexate. Proc Natl Acad Sci USA 75: 980-983 (1978).
8. J.A. Straw, D. Szapary, W.T. Wynn. Pharmacokinetics of the diastereomers of leucovorin after intravenous and oral administration to normal subjects. Cancer Res 44: 3114-3119 (1984).
9. F.M. Sirotnak, P.L. Chello, D.M. Moccio, R.L. Kisliuk, G. Combepine, Y. Gaumont, J.A. Montgomery. Stereospecificity at carbon 6 of formyltetrahydrofolate as a competitive inhibitor of transport and cytotoxicity of methotrexate in vitro. Biochem Pharmacol 28: 2993-2997 (1979).
10. R. Bertrand and J. Jolivet. Lack of interference by the unnatural isomer of 5-formyltetrahydrofolate in leucovorin preparations. J Natl Cancer Inst. 81: 1175-1178 (1989).
11. G.B. Henderson, J.M. Tsuji, H.P. Kumar. Characterization of the individual transport routes that mediate the influx and efflux of methotrexate in CCRF-CEM human lymphoblastic cells. Cancer Res 46: 1633-1638 (1986).
12. R.L. Shilsky, G.B. Kay and K.E. Choi. Uptake and biological activity of the stereoisomers of leucovorin in human colon cancer cells. Proc Annu Meet Am Assoc Cancer Res 29: A1989 (1988).
13. R. Bertrand, R.E. MacKenzie and J. Jolivet. Human liver methenyltetrahydrofolate synthetase: improved purification and increased affinity for folate polyglutamate substrates. Biochim Biophys Acta 911: 154-161 (1987).
14. P.P. Lee and R.L. Schilsky. Inhibition of thymidylate synthase by the diastereoisomers of leucovorin. Cancer Chemoth Pharmacol 26: 273-277 (1990).
15. J.K. Sato and R.G. Moran. Interaction of methotrexate and citrovorum factor at folylpolyglutamate synthetase. Proc Annu Meet Am Assoc Cancer Res 25: A1234 (1984).

16. D.M. Boarman and C.J. Allegra. Intracellular metabolism of 5-formyltetrahydrofolate in human breast and colon cell lines. Cancer Res 52: 36-44 (1992).

17. J.J. McGuire and C.A. Russell. Biological and biochemical properties of the natural (6S) and unnatural (6R) isomers of leucovorin and their racemic (6R,S) mixture. J Cell Pharmacol 2: 317-323 (1991).

18. Z.-G. Zhang and Y.M. Rustum. Effects of diastereoisomers of 5-formyltetrahydrofolate on cellular growth, sensitivity to 5-fluoro-2'-deoxyuridine, and methenyltetrahydrofolate polyglutamate levels in HCT-8 cells. Cancer Res 51: 3476-3481 (1991).

19. C. Temple Jr, J.D. Rose, W.R. Laster and J.A. Montgomery. Reversal of methotrexate toxicity in mice by a calcium salt of citrovorum facor and related compounds. Cancer Treat Rep 65: 1117-1119 (1981).

20. S. Bernard, M.C. Etienne, J.L. Fischel. P. Formento and G. Milano. Critical factors for the reversal of methotrexate cytotoxicity by folinic acid. Br J Cancer 63: 303-307 (1991).

21. J. Zittoun, J. Marquet, J.J. Pilorquet, C. Tonetti, E. De Gialluly. Comparative effect of 6S, 6R and 6RS leucovorin on methotrexate rescue and on modulation of 5-fluorouracil. Br J Cancer 63: 885-888 (1991).

22. K.E. Choi, R.L. Schilsky, S.C. McGrath, C.A. VanKast. Purification and biological activity of the steroisomers of leucovorin. Proc Annu Meet Am Assoc Cancer Res 28: A1089 (1987).

23. M.-C. Etienne, A. Thyss, Y. Bertrand, R. Touraine, H. Rubie, A. Robert, G. Milano. l-folinic acid versus d,l-folinic acid in rescue of high-dose methotrexate therapy in children. J Natl Cancer Inst 84: 1190-1195 (1992).

24. E. Mini, B.A. Moroson, J.R. Bertino. Cytotoxicity of floxuridine and 5-fluorouracil in human T-lymphoblast leukemia cells: enhancement by leucovorin. Cancer Treat Rep 71: 381-9 (1987).

LEUCOVORIN AS A PRODRUG[1]

D.G. Priest[2], J.C. Schmitz[2], and T. Walle[3]

[2]Department of Biochemistry and Molecular Biology
[3]Department of Pharmacology
Medical University of South Carolina
Charleston, SC 29425

INTRODUCTION

To exert its antitumor effects, leucovorin must ultimately become activated by conversion to CH_2FH_4.[*] Elevation of this reduced folate cofactor stabilizes the inhibitory ternary complex formed between the FU active metabolite, FdUMP and thymidylate synthase, resulting in suppression of DNA synthesis or repair.[1-4] It has been demonstrated both in animal models[5] and in humans[6] that administration of leucovorin results in intratumor elevation of CH_2FH_4 and the closely related reduced folate, FH_4. However, precisely when and where the metabolic activity causing this elevation occurs remains in question. Further, while enzyme activities have been reported[7-9] that could sustain the interconversions shown below, the precise metabolic pathways used have not been defined.

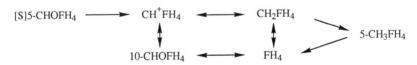

Leucovorin, as well as its major circulating metabolite, $5-CH_3FH_4$, have been shown to modulate FU activity in culture systems,[10-12] but it remains unclear the extent to which tumor tissue itself participates in metabolic activation in humans or animal models. Following IP administration of leucovorin to mice with implanted adenocarcinoma 38 solid tumors, leucovorin itself became elevated in the tumor

---

[1]This work was supported by Grant No. CH461 from the American Cancer Society, Grant No. CA22754 from the National Cancer Institute, and Grant No. RR-01070 from the National Institutes of Health, Division of Research Services.
[*]The abbreviations used are: CH_2FH_4, 5,10-methylenetetrahydrofolate; FH_4, tetrahydrofolate; [S]5-$CHOFH_4$, 5-formyltetrahydrofolate, leucovorin; CH^+FH_4, 5,10-methenyltetrahydrofolate; 10-$CHOFH_4$, 10-formyltetrahydrofolate; $5-CH_3FH_4$, 5-methyltetrahydrofolate; FU, fluorouracil; FdUMP, fluorodeoxyuridine monophosphate.

Novel Approaches to Selective Treatments of Human Solid Tumors: Laboratory and Clinical Correlation Edited by Y. M. Rustum, Plenum Press, New York, 1993

more profoundly than other metabolites, suggesting limited metabolic activity of this folate form within the tumor.[13] There are several sites of leucovorin metabolism which are alternatives to the tumor. Liver, with a high level of the enzyme that acts on leucovorin, methenyltetrahydrofolate synthase,[14] as well as other folate metabolizing enzymes,[15,16] has been presumed to make an important contribution to the metabolism of IV administered leucovorin. Red blood cells, on the other hand, have also been shown to be active *in vitro* but the quantitative contribution of this tissue remains unclear.[17] Intestinal tissue was shown by analysis of portal vein metabolites to be a rich source of activity for orally administered leucovorin.[18] Overall, it appears likely that sites other than the tumor could contribute substantially to leucovorin metabolism making metabolic products available to the tumor through prior activation.

To address questions of systemic disposition and metabolic activity, several pharmacokinetic studies have undertaken examination of the behavior of both the parent compound and metabolites thereof in plasma following oral and IV administration of leucovorin.[19-23] Studies based on HPLC separation followed by microbiological identification[19] have shown that the active [S]-isomer of leucovorin is cleared rapidly ($t_{1/2} \sim 1/2$ hr) and $5\text{-}CH_3FH_4$ accumulates extensively ($t_{1/2} \sim 6$ hrs) following IV administration of [R,S]leucovorin. However, while modulation of FU activity by $5\text{-}CH_3FH_4$ has been shown in culture systems,[12] this folate was relatively ineffective in elevating human tumor xenograph CH_2FH_4 and FH_4 in immune compromised mice.[24] The presence of metabolites other than $5\text{-}CH_3FH_4$ have been detected in human plasma following leucovorin administration, but their identification was not fully addressed using the HPLC/microbiological methodology. Using an analytical approach based on cycling of folates to CH_2FH_4 followed by entrapment into a stable ternary complex with *L casei* thymidylate synthase and $[^3H]FdUMP$,[25,26] we have observed significant, dose dependent elevation of relatively labile metabolites, including the active metabolite for FU modulation, CH_2FH_4, and the closely related folate FH_4, following both oral and IV administration of leucovorin[26] and folic acid.[27]

MATERIALS AND METHODS

Thymidylate synthase was purified from an *E. coli* strain that over produces *L. casei* thymidylate synthase as previously described.[28] 5,10-methylenetetrahydrofolate reductase,[15] 10-formyltetrahydrofolate deacylase,[16] dihydrofolate reductase,[29] and methenyltetrahydrofolate synthase[7] were purified from pig liver, beef liver, *L. casei* and rabbit liver, respectively, as described previously. Folic acid was obtained from Lyphomed (Deerfield, IL). [R,S]5-CHOFH$_4$ (Leucovorin Calcium) was a gift from Burroughs Wellcome Company (Research Triangle Park, NC). $[^3H]FdUMP$ (20 Ci/mmol) was purchased from Moravek Biochemicals (Brea, CA). Other reagents were purchased from Sigma Chemical Company (St. Louis, MO).

Drug Administration

Twenty five volunteers, after signing informed consent agreements, were randomly separated into groups of five each for administration of leucovorin at doses of 10, 25, 125, 250, and 500 mg/m². Each group was administered leucovorin both orally and IV with a 30 day wash-out period between. Oral doses were given as 5 and 25 mg tablets and IV doses were given by syringe in a 10 mg/ml aqueous solution at a rate of approximately 100 mg/min. Following administration, blood samples were collected over a period of 24 hr but most intensively for the first 9 hr. Folic acid was administered, at a dose of 25 mg/m² in saline solution both orally and IV, to an additional group of 5 volunteers who had signed informed consent agreements. Blood samples were again collected over a 24 hr period with the most intensive collection over the first 12 hours.

Plasma Preparation

Immediately following blood withdrawal by continuous IV access, samples (7ml) were centrifuged at 400g for 5 min at 4°C and resultant plasma diluted into an equal volume of cold 50 mM Tris HCl buffer (pH 7.4) which contained 100 mM sodium ascorbate and 1 mM EDTA for storage at -20°C until analysis. After being thawed, diluted plasma samples were placed in a boiling water bath for 3 min and centrifuged to remove precipitated protein. Supernatant (0.1-100 μl) was used to estimate reduced folates. Analysis of reference folates, added to plasma samples, resulted in recovery of 70-97%. Because the boiling step caused dissociation of reference CH_2FH_4 to quantitatively yield FH_4, these two pools have been summed. However, studies with unboiled plasma indicate that at least 1/3 of this combined pool is CH_2FH_4.

Reduced folate estimation

The ternary complex assay is based upon enzymatic cycling of reduced folates to CH_2FH_4 followed by entrapment into a stable ternary complex with excess thymidylate synthase and [3H]FdUMP.[25] Methods have been described previously for the estimation of tissue levels of CH_2FH_4, FH_4, $5-CH_3FH_4$, $10-CHOFH_4$, FH_2, and $[S]5-CHOFH_4$.[26] Reaction mixtures for analysis of CH_2FH_4 typically contained 20 mU thymidylate synthase and 125 nM [3H]FdUMP (20 Ci mM) in 200 μl of a buffer which contained 50 mM Tris HCl, 50 mM sodium ascorbate, and 1mM EDTA (pH 7.4). Other folates were estimated in the same system but with the addition of reagents and enzymes necessary for their conversion to CH_2FH_4. Following incubation at 25° for 30 min reactions were stopped by the addition of 1% SDS and the mixture boiled for 5 min. Aliquots (25 μl) were eluted over 400 μl minicolumns of Sephadex G25 by centrifugation and the excluded complex (25 μl) was diluted into scintillation cocktail and counted to determine bound [3H]FdUMP and hence, CH_2FH_4.

The linear trapezoidal method was used to estimate area under the curve (AUC) for each folate from concentration vs time plots.

RESULTS

The ternary complex-based assay has been used to evaluate the plasma pharmacokinetics of leucovorin and its metabolites. Following IV administration of 25 mg/m² leucovorin to healthy volunteers, the parent drug is rapidly cleared from plasma and metabolites appear (Fig. 1). The predominant metabolite is $5\text{-}CH_3FH_4$. This folate reaches the highest peak levels and has the longest half-life resulting in the greatest AUC of any metabolite. However, CH_2FH_4 and FH_4, which were treated together because of dissociation of CH_2FH_4 during analysis, are also present. This pool reaches a peak level which is approximately 30% that of the $5\text{-}CH_3FH_4$ peak level. However, the half-life is much shorter than for $5\text{-}CH_3FH_4$ resulting in an AUC which is only approximately 7% that of the more stable metabolite (Table 1). $10\text{-}CHOFH_4$ is also present at readily detectable levels but only achieves a peak concentration that is approximately 10% that of the $CH_2FH_4 + FH_4$ pool.

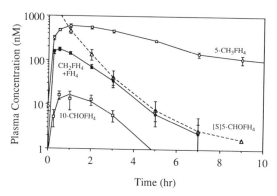

Figure 1. Plasma levels of $[S]5\text{-}CHOFH_4$ (Δ), $5\text{-}CH_3FH_4$ (O), $CH_2FH_4 + FH_4$ (●) and $10\text{-}CHOFH_4$ (□) following IV administration of 25 mg/m^2 [R,S]leucovorin. The ternary complex based methodology was used for estimation of plasma folates. Points represent the mean from duplicate analyses of samples from five volunteers. Error bars represent SEM.

Leucovorin dose dependence studies over the range 10-500 mg/m^2 show that there is a linear relationship between IV dose and AUC for the sum of all metabolites (Fig. 2). However, examination of individual folates within the total metabolite pool, showed that the relative amount of $5\text{-}CH_3FH_4$ diminished with increasing dose (Fig. 3) while $CH_2FH_4 + FH_4$ and $10\text{-}CHOFH_4$ increased. This result suggests that some degree of saturation is reached with regard to the transformation of $10\text{-}CHOFH_4$ and $CH_2FH_4 + FH_4$ to $5\text{-}CH_3FH_4$ even though conversion of the parent compound to its metabolites is directly dependent on dose.

Oral administration of the same 25 mg/m^2 leucovorin dose results in slightly less elevation of $5\text{-}CH_3FH_4$ than observed after IV administration (Fig. 4). The parent compound $[S]5\text{-}CHOFH_4$ was present at readily detectable, but relatively low levels. $CH_2FH_4 + FH_4$ and $10\text{-}CHOFH_4$ were also present although at lower levels than following IV administration. For example, $CH_2FH_4 + FH_4$ AUC was only 4% as large as the $5\text{-}CH_3FH_4$ AUC (Table 1).

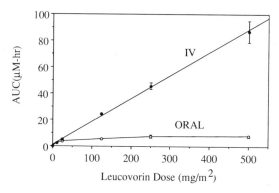

Figure 2. Dependence on dose of AUC for the sum of all leucovorin metabolites following IV (●)and oral (○) administration of [R,S]leucovorin. Each point represents the mean ± SEM of estimates from five volunteers.

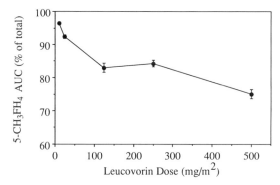

Figure 3. Dose dependence of 5-CH$_3$FH$_4$ as a percentage of total leucovorin metabolites after IV leucovorin administration. Each point represents the mean ± SEM of estimates from five volunteers.

The dose dependence of AUC for the sum of all metabolites following oral administration shows clear saturation behavior (Fig. 2). When the AUC for total folate, including parent compound and metabolites, is compared to the AUC for total folate following IV administration, an estimate of the percentage of each oral dose absorbed can be calculated. It can be seen in Table 2 that absorption decreases significantly as the dose is raised. Comparison of the AUC for the parent compound alone between oral and IV administration, provides a means to estimate the oral bioavailability of the parent species. It can be seen in Table 2 that [S]5-CHOFH$_4$ bioavailability is only 2.8% at the lowest dose and decreases even further as the dose is elevated. Absorption of total folate and parent compound bioavailability taken together were used to estimate "first pass" metabolism of leucovorin (Table 2). An extremely high value of 96% was seen at the lowest dose that showed clear evidence of decline as the dose was

Table 1. Comparison of Metabolite AUC after Administration of Leucovorin and Folic Acid

Folate Administered	Dose (mg/m^2)	CH$_2$FH$_4$+FH$_4$ AUC (nM-hr)[1]		5-CH$_3$FH$_4$	
		IV	Oral	IV	Oral
Leucovorin	25	351 ± 24	160 ± 11	4820 ± 447	3675 ± 237
Folic Acid	25	584 ± 55	350 ± 41	2115 ± 316	1893 ± 315

[1] AUC values represent the mean ± SEM of estimates from five volunteers.

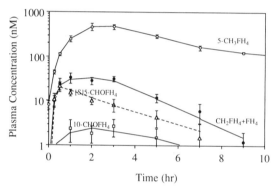

Figure 4. Plasma levels of [S]5-CHOFH$_4$ (Δ), 5-ĊH$_3$FH$_4$ (O), CH$_2$FH$_4$ + FH$_4$ (●) and 10-CHOFH$_4$ (□) following oral administration of 25 mg/m^2 [R,S]leucovorin. Conditions are the same as in Figure 1 except leucovorin was administered orally.

increased. Thus, the parent drug bioavailability is a composite of low and saturable absorption as well as high and saturable "first pass" metabolism.

For the purpose of comparison, a pharmacokinetic study of folic acid, administered both orally and IV, has also been undertaken. At an oral dose of 25 mg/m^2, total absorption, as determined from comparison with the same dose administered IV, was about the same as for leucovorin (Table 2). On the other hand, bioavailability of the fully oxidized parent compound was much greater, and "first pass" metabolism was much less, than for leucovorin. The total accumulation of 5-CH$_3$FH$_4$ following folic acid administration both orally and IV was less than following leucovorin while the CH$_2$FH$_4$ + FH$_4$ pool AUC was approximately twice as great (Table 1).

Table 2. Absorption and Metabolism of Orally Administered Leucovorin and Folic Acid

	Dose (mg/m^2)	Total Absorption[1] (%)	Parent Compound Bioavailability[2] (%)	"First Pass" Metabolism[3] (%)
Leucovorin	10	72	2.8	96
	25	55	2.6	95
	125	14	0.7	95
	250	10	0.8	92
	500	5	0.4	91
Folic Acid	25	65	60.3	7.7

[1] Absorption = [(oral total folate AUC/IV total folate AUC)x100%]
[2] Bioavailability = [(oral LV AUC/IV LV AUC)x100%]
[3] First Pass Metabolism = [100% - {(Bioavailability/Absorption)x100%}]

DISCUSSION

Several studies of the human plasma pharmacokinetics of leucovorin, using microbiological detection techniques, have centered on evaluation of the parent compound and the major metabolite, 5-CH$_3$FH$_4$.[19,22,23] Although other folate species were detected, their identification and quantitation was generally not fully addressed with this analytical approach. Studies presented here using the ternary complex-based assay were entirely consistent with earlier studies with regard to [S]5-CHOFH$_4$ and 5-CH$_3$FH$_4$ levels, but also could be used to show substantial elevation of CH$_2$FH$_4$ + FH$_4$, and 10-CHOFH$_4$. The presence of CH$_2$FH$_4$ and FH$_4$ in the circulatory system could provide a means to elevate intratumor levels of the active metabolite for FU modulation without requiring extensive leucovorin metabolism within the tumor itself. Orally administered leucovorin, while it is almost completely metabolized presystemically, results in clinical responses. This supports the concept that metabolites, as opposed to the parent compound, play an important role in FU modulation and this would be particularly true for the active species itself.[30,31]

Dose dependence studies of IV administered leucovorin show that the AUC for the sum of all metabolites is directly proportional to dose. However, the proportion of total metabolites attributable to 5-CH$_3$FH$_4$ diminishes at higher doses, while other metabolites become relatively elevated, suggesting metabolic saturation at the point where 5-CH$_3$FH$_4$ is formed. This result is consistent with those of Newman and coworkers who observed disproportionately low 5-CH$_3$FH$_4$ at higher doses during infusion of leucovorin.[32] Presumedly, 5-CH$_3$FH$_4$ is a terminal metabolite of leucovorin, while 10-CHOFH$_4$, CH$_2$FH$_4$, and FH$_4$ are intermediates. These intermediates could become elevated in plasma as a result of escape from the compartment where metabolism occurs prior to complete transformation to 5-CH$_3$FH$_4$. Further metabolism to 5-CH$_3$FH$_4$ would presumably require that they be taken up again. The observation that less extensive accumulation of 5-CH$_3$FH$_4$, relative to the other metabolites, occurs as the leucovorin dose is raised suggests that the final step in formation of this metabolite is most sensitive to dose elevation and is probably the overall rate limiting process. The specific nature of the rate limiting effect could be at either the metabolic or transport level. The metabolic limitation could reside in methy-lenetetrahydrofolate reductase, the enzyme most likely to play a dominant role in $5\text{-}CH_3FH_4$ formation. Transport limitation could be the result of saturation of carrier sites or competition by other folates, as precursor folates are reacquired by the cell system responsible for metabolism.

Oral administration of [R,S]leucovorin has been considered as an alternative to IV administration.[19] In this study the same metabolites were identified following oral leucovorin administration as after IV administration. Low oral doses yielded only slightly less total plasma folate levels as when the same dose was administered IV, indicating relatively efficient absorption. However, clear saturation of absorption occurs as the dose is increased such that at 500 mg/m^2 only 5% of an oral dose can be found in the circulatory system either as the parent compound or metabolites. The relatively low oral bioavialibility of the parent compound is a function of both incomplete absorption and high presystemic metabolism. The intestine is the primary site of presystemic metabolism, as reported by Whitehead et al.,[18] and it is likely that this is the site of metabolic saturation as well.

Folic acid, at least at low dose, behaves similarly to leucovorin with regard to total absorption, but parent compound bioavailability is much higher and "first pass" metabolism is much lower. Both of these observations are consistent with generally lower metabolic reactivity of the fully oxidized folate which is due presumably to its relative poor substrate properties for the enzyme, dihydrofolate reductase. Accumulation of $CH_2FH_4 + FH_4$, both in absolute terms and relative to $5\text{-}CH_3FH_4$ is significantly higher following folic acid administration vs leucovorin. This suggests that, providing plasma $CH_2FH_4 + FH_4$ plays a role in FU modulation, this may be a superior folate source for some therapies.

REFERENCES

1. P.V. Danenberg and K.D. Danenberg, Effect of 5,10-methylene-tetrahydrofolate on the dissociation of 5-fluoro-2'-deoxy-uridylate from thymidylate synthetase: evidence for an ordered mechanism, *Biochemistry*, 17:4018 (1978).

2. B. Ullman, M. Lee, and D.W. Martin, Jr, et al., Cytotoxicity of 5-fluoro-2'-deoxyuridine: requirement for reduced folate cofactors and antagonism by methotrexate, *Proc. Natl. Acad. Sci.*, 75:980 (1978).

3. J.A. Houghton, C. Schmit, and P.J. Houghton, The effects of derivatives of folic acid on the fluorodeoxyuridylate thymidylate synthetase covalent complex in human colon xenografts, *Eur. J. Can. Clin. Oncol.*, 18:347 (1982).

4. R.M. Evans, J.D. Laskin, and M.T. Hakala, Effect of excess folates and deoxyinosine on the activity and site of action of 5-fluorouracil, *Cancer Res.* 41:3288(1981).

5. J.A. Houghton, L.G. William, and S.S. DeGraaf, et al., Relationship between dose rate of 6[RS]leucovorin administration, plasma concentrations of reduced folates, and pools of 5,10-methy-lenetetrahydrofolates and tetrahydrofolates in human colon adenocarcinoma xenografts, *Cancer Res.*, 50:3493 (1990).

6. F. Trave, Y.M. Rustum, and N.J. Peterelli, Plasma and tumor tissue pharmacology of high-dose intravenous leucovorin calcium in combination with fluorourouracil in patients with advanced colorectal carcinoma, *J. Clin. Oncol.*, 6:1184 (1988).

7. S. Hopkins and L.V., 5,10-methenyltetrahydrofolate synthetase. Purification and properties of the enzyme from rabbit liver, *J. Biol. Chem.*, 259:5618 (1984).

8. R.E. MacKenzie, Biogenesis and interconversion of substituted tetrahydrofolates, *in*: "Folates and Pterins", R.L. Blakley and S.J. Benkovic, eds., Wiley-Interscience, New York (1984).

9. L.V. Schirch, Folates in serine and glycine metabolism, *in*: "Folates and Pterins", R.L. Blakley and S.J. Benkovic, eds., Wiley-Interscience, New York (1984).

10. B. Ullman, M. Lee, D.W. Martin, Jr., and D.V. Santi, Cytotoxicity of 5-fluoro-2'-deoxyuridine: requirement for reduced folate cofactors and antagonism by methotrexate, *Proc. Natl. Acad. Sci.,U.S.A.* 75:980 (1978).

11. R.M. Evans, J.D. Laskin, and M.T. Hakala, Effects of excess folates and deoxyinosine on the activity and site of action of 5-fluorouracil, *Cancer Res.* 41:3288 (1981).

12. E. Mini, T. Mazzei, M. Coronnello, L. Criscuoli, M. Gualtieri, P. Periti, and J.R.. Bertino, Effects of 5-methyltetrahydrofolate on the activity of fluoropyrimidines against human leukemia (CCRF-CEM) cells, *Biochem. Pharmac.*, 36:2905 (1987).

13. R.J. Mullin, B.R. Keith, and D.S. Duch, Distribution and metabolism of calcium leucovorin in normal and tumor tissue, *in*: "The expanding role of folate and fluoropyrimidines in cancer chemotherapy", Y. Rustum and J.J. McGuire, eds., Plenum Press, New York (1988).

14. R. Bertrand, R.E. Mackenzie, and J. Jolivet, Human liver methenyltetrahydrofolate synthetase: improved purification and increased affinity for folate polyglutmate substrates, *Biochim. Biophys. Acta*, 911:154 (1987).

15. R.G. Matthews, Methylenetetrahydrofolate reductase from pig liver, *Methods Enzymol.*, 122:372 (1986).

16. F.M. Huennekens and K.G. Scrimgeor, N-10-formyltetrahydrofolic deacylase, *Methods Enzymol.*, 6:373 (1963).

17. M.S. Bunni and D.G. Priest, Human red blood cell-mediated metabolism of leucovorin [(R,S)5-formyltetrahydrofolate], *Arch. Biochem. Biophys.*, 286:633 (1991).

18. V.M. Whitehead, R. Pratt, A. Viallet, and B.A. Cooper, Intestinal conversion of folinic acid to 5-methyltetrahydrofolate in man, *Br. J. Haematol.*, 22:63 (1972).

19. J.A. Straw, D. Szapary, and W.T. Wynn, Pharmacokinetics of the diastereomers of leucovorin after intravenous and oral administration to normal subjects, *Cancer Res.*, 44:3114 (1984).

20. R.L. Schilsky and M.J. Ratain, Clinical pharmacokinetics of high-dose leucovorin calcium after intravenous and oral administrations, *J. Natl. Cancer Inst.*, 82:1411 (1990).

21. A. Schalhorn, M. Kühl, and G. Stupp-Poutot, et al., Pharmacokinetics of reduced folates after short-term infusion of d,1-folinic acid, *Cancer Chemother. Pharmacol.*, 25:440 (1990).

22. B.W. McGuire, L.L. Sia, and J.D. Haynes, et al., Absorption kinetics of orally administered leucovorin calcium, *NCI Monogr.* 5:47 (1987).

23. P.O. Greiner, J. Zittoun, and J. Marquet, et al., Pharmacokinetics of (-)-folinic acid after oral and intravenous administration of the racemate, *Br. J. Clin. Pharmac.*, 28:289 (1989).

24. J.A. Houghton and L.G. William, et al., Comparison of the conversion of 5-formyltetrahydrofolate and 5-methyltetrahydrofolate to 5,10-methylenetetrahydrofolates and tetrahydrofolates in human colon tumors, *Can. Comm.*, 1:167 (1989).

25. D.G. Priest and M.T. Doig, Tissue folate polyglutamate chainlength determination by electrophoresis as thymidylate synthase-fluorodeoxyuridylate ternary complexes, *Methods Enzymol.*, 122:313 (1986).

26. D.G. Priest, J.C. Schmitz, M.A. Bunni, and R.K. Stuart, Pharmacokinetics of leucovorin metabolites in human plasma as a function of dose administered orally and intravenously, *J. Natl. Can. Inst.*, 83:1806 (1991).

27. J.C. Schmitz, R.K. Stuart, J.C. Barredo, and D.G. Priest, Interconversion of folates in human plasma and red blood cells, *Pro. Am. Asso. Can. Res.*, 33:410 (1992).

28. K. Pinter, V.J. Davisson, and D.V. Santi, Cloning, sequencing, and expression of the *Lactobacillus casei* thymidylate synthase gene, *DNA*, 7:235 (1988).

29. R.B. Dunlap, N.G.L. Harding, and F.M. Huennekens, Thymidylate synthetase from aminopterin-resistant *Lactobacillus casei, Biochemistry* 10:88 (1971).

30. J.D. Hines, D.J. Adelstein, J.L. Spiess, P. Giroski, and S.G. Carter, Efficacy of high-dose oral leucovorin and 5-fluorouracil in advanced colorectal carcinoma, *Cancer*, 63:1022 (1989).

31. L.R. Laufman, W.D. Brenckman, Jr., and K.A. Stydnicki, et al., Clinical experience with leucovorin and 5-fluorouracil, *Cancer*, 63:103 (1989).

32. E.M. Newman, S.A. Akman, and J.S. Harrison, et al., Pharmacokinetics and toxicity of continuous infusion (6S)-folinic acid and bolus 5-fluorouracil in patients with advanced cancer, *Cancer Res.*, 52:2408 (1992).

DISCUSSION OF DR. JOLIVET'S/DR. PRIEST'S PRESENTATION

Dr. Allegra: I have a question for Dave. The formation of the 5,10 pools in plasma is really spectacular, it's enormous amounts of the compound that seem to get formed very quickly, 40% of the concentrations of leucovorin that you're pushing. Given the 5,10-methylene is a relatively minor component, intracellularly probably around 5%, and given this, Dr. Houghton and others have shown that even with high concentrations of leucovorin, the ability to expand that pool was 3 or 4-fold at most. How to explain that apparent discrepancy in such an enormous conversion preferably, relatively small conversions in the cells? Secondly, could you speculate as to where this conversion is occurring?

Dr. Priest: I'll speculate on the second one, it's the easier one. We have seen some metabolism also in red blood cell system which is substantial, quantitatively a substantial organ in the body probably even larger than the liver but we're still unsure about the relative contribution of the red blood cell system. White has also shown that a lot of the metabolism of oral dose occurs prior to the liver and portal vein. I suspect that metabolism goes on in the intestine and probably at different places systemically. With regard to the high accumulation, that was a bolus dose and we did get very high accumulation. The specific role of the circulating pool of methylenetetrahydrofolate, tetrahydrofolate, in the elevating tumor pool of methylenetetrahydrofolate of course remains speculative and that's a much more difficult question. I do know that there is apparently stabilizing factors in the plasma for the dissociation of methylenetetrahydrofolate into tetrahydrofolate. It's about 6 or 7 times slower in plasma. This could account at least in part for the persistance of these agents in plasma.

Audience: To Dr. Jolivet. To say that the 6R leucovorin is not cytotoxic doesn't necessarily mean that it's biologically inactive in the whole organism. For example, Barry Shane reported that there is a metabolism to some as yet unidentified compound which is not a folate. I wonder if you could comment on that when you say it's biologically inert.

Dr. Jolivet: Well, let me qualify this. In all the biological experimental in vitro data in which it is tested it doesn't seem at least reproducibly to influence cell growth, it cannot support cell growth in most systems, it cannot influence cell growth in or modify or impair cell growth by the naturalized isomer, cannot prevent methotrexate rescue and it cannot prevent or change 5-FU potentiation. Similar results were obtained by a number of investigators in a number of in vitro systems. Obviously the proof of the pudding is in clinical trial and we'll hear about those later. There might be some aspects with unknown metabolism and some known aspects in man that might make a difference but clearly my point was that this was a review of the cellular pharmacology. From what's been published, in the cells it doesn't seem to have any influence in cellular systems.

Dr. Machover: The enzyme methylenetetrahydrofolate sythetase seems to have a very high activity throughout the body because of the rapid metabolism of formylmethylenetetrahydrofolate. Do you have an idea about the differences in different organs or among tumors? This could be a key for explaining some resistance.

Dr. Jolivet: Well, David eluded to a study by Dr. Duch who showed in a murine tumor system that activity of that specific enzyme, was low and that in one murine model system the lack of potentiation of FU by leucovorin seems to be related to the comparative activity of this initial enzymatic step. We have been working for years to get probes to answer that question and now we have the probes and we are going to start looking at tissue level of the enzyme. This might be one factor at least explaining sometimes the lack of potentiation of FUra action by leucovorin.

CLINICAL USE OF LEUCOVORIN: INTRACELLULAR METABOLISM

Carmen J. Allegra and Donna Voeller

NCI-Navy Medical Oncology Branch
National Cancer Institute
Bethesda, MD 20889-5105

INTRODUCTION

5-fluorouracil is a frequently used and central agent in the treatment of certain malignancies including those of the breast, gastrointestinal tract, and upper aerodigestive system. While many analogs of 5-fluorouracil have been synthesized since the early 1960's none has supplanted 5-fluorouracil for general clinical use. One of the major focal points of recent investigative work has been efforts to enhance the activity of 5-fluorouracil through biochemical modulation. The mechanisms by which malignant cells become resistant to the cytotoxic effects of 5-fluorouracil are manifold[1]. Resistance mechanisms in in vitro model systems have included alternations in the anabolism and catabolism of 5-fluorouracil, decreased incorporation of 5-fluorouracil into nucleic acids, a relative deficiency in intracellular folates, and qualitative or quantitative alterations in the target enzyme thymidylate synthase. While each of these mechanisms has been documented to occur in preclinical model systems, few have been shown to be responsible for clinical insensitivity to 5-fluorouracil. Since the underlying molecular mechanism of the catalytic function of thymidylate synthase has been disclosed, several investigators have recognized the need for adequate intracellular levels of the folate substrate 5,10-methylenetetrahydrofolate, to optimize the cytotoxic effects of 5-fluorouracil via ternary complex formation with thymidylate synthase and the fluorinated nucleotide FdUMP[2,3]. Early investigations demonstrated that malignant cells were capable of growth with intracellular levels of folates that were suboptimal for ternary complex formation with fluoropyrimidines[2]. In these cells the addition of endogenous folates could be used to markedly enhance ternary complex formation and thus the cytotoxicity of fluoropyrimidines. These observations have since been extended to clinical trials which have demonstrated the clinical benefit of leucovorin given concurrently with the fluoropyrimidine agents[4-7]. The relative success of these clinical investigations strongly suggest that relative intracellular folate depletion is an important mechanism by which malignant cells become resistant to fluoropyrimidines in patients and that thymidylate synthase is a critical chemotherapeutic target. Given the merits of leucovorin, recent preclinical and clinical investigations have focused on optimizing the dose and scheduling of leucovorin. Our laboratory has used a human colon (HCT-116) and a human breast (MCF-7) carcinoma cell lines as in vitro model systems to investigate the cellular metabolism of leucovorin[8]. A series of investigations by Houghton and colleagues using a human colon xenograft model in immune-deprived mice suggests that the critical tetrahydrofolate and 5,10-methylene-tetrahydrofolate intracellular pools may be increased by up to 4-fold using prolonged (24 hrs.) infusions of leucovorin[9,10]. When compared to short, high dose leucovorin exposure, these authors concluded that prolonged infusional exposure to leucovorin was optimal for increasing the intracellular pools of tetrahydrofolate and 5,10-methylenetetrahydrofolate and represented the most efficient means of generating

Novel Approaches to Selective Treatments of Human Solid Tumors: Laboratory and Clinical Correlation Edited by Y. M. Rustum, Plenum Press, New York, 1993

the higher polyglutamate forms of these folates. Several investigations have demonstrated that the higher polyglutamates of 5,10-methylenetetrahydrofolate are 50 to 100-fold more potent in potentiating ternary complex formation with thymidylate synthase and FdUMP when compared with the mono- and diglutamate forms of this folate [11,12]. It has also been demonstrated that the higher polyglutamate forms of both folates and antifolates have a prolonged intracellular retention[8,13]. These findings suggest that schedules which optimize the formation of higher polyglutamates of tetrahydrofolate and 5,10-methylenetetrahydrofolate would be optimal for the modulation of 5-fluorouracil. This concept is further supported by an investigation by Romanini and colleagues which demonstrated that leucovorin was ineffective in increasing the cytotoxicity of 5-fluorouracil in cells incapable of metabolizing folates to the higher polyglutamate forms.

The goal of the present investigations were to identify the critical factors that determine metabolism of leucovorin to the higher polyglutamates of 5,10-methylenetetrahydrofolate in human malignant cells.

MATERIALS AND METHODS

Cell Lines

Human breast cancer (MCF-7) and human colon cancer (HCT-116) cell lines were used for these experiments. The cells were grown in minimal essential media without folic acid and supplemented with 10% fetal calf serum, 2 mM glutamine, and 50 nM leucovorin.

Intracellular Folate Pool Measurements

The breast and colon cells were exposed to various concentrations of radiolabeled leucovorin or 5-methyltetrahydrofolate for various time intervals up to 24 hrs. Following drug exposure, the cells were washed and harvested. The intracellular folates were then extracted, separated by high-performance liquid chromatography, and quantitated using previously published techniques[8,15]. In addition to folate metabolism during the leucovorin exposures, we also examined the retention of intracellular folates following leucovorin exposure.

Intracellular Folate Polyglutamate Measurements

Following exposure of the breast and colon cells to radiolabeled leucovorin or 5-methyltetrahydrofolate, the cells were washed, harvested, and the intracellular folate polyglutamates were then extracted by boiling for 90 seconds in 2 ml of a 2% ascorbate, 2% mercaptoethanol solution, pH 6.0. The extracted folate polyglutamates were concentrated by a solid phase extraction, then separated and quantitated by high-performance liquid chromatography. We found that the various intracellular folate polyglutamates could be separated by high-performance liquid chromatography without the need for prior degradation to paraaminobenzoic acid polyglutamates[8]. Using this technique, we were able to quantitate the formation of the various folate polyglutamate forms as well as their intracellular retention following leucovorin exposure. We found that the polyglutamated forms of the various one-carbon substituted intracellular folates could be separated based on the length of the polyglutamate tail as this was the major factor responsible for their retention time.

RESULTS

We first examined the metabolism of leucovorin in the MCF-7 breast carcinoma cell line exposed to a 500-fold concentration range of leucovorin from 0.1 to 50 μM. We found that 5-methyltetrahydrofolate, 10-formyltetrahydrofolate and tetrahydrofolate each constituted approximately one-third of the total intracellular folate pool in these cells and that the intracellular level of these folates increased in proportion with the concentration of leucovorin in the media. We noted a 6-fold increase in total intracellular folate pools over the 500-fold leucovorin concentration. Of note was the absence of intracellular leucovorin (5-formyltetrahydrofolate) at all exposure concentrations suggesting that cellular transport

Table 1. Intracellular Folate Pools in Human MCF-7 Breast Cancer Cells Exposed to Various Concentrations of Leucovorin.

	Tetrahydrofolate folate	10-Formyl-tetrahydrofolate	5-Methyl-tetrahydrofolate	5,10-methylene-tetrahydrofolate
Leucovorin (μM)		pmol/mg		
0.1	8	13	12	2
1	36	33	31	3
10	82	70	29	6
50	109	107	24	18

rather than intracellular metabolism of leucovorin was rate-limiting (Table 1). Of particular note, was the 10-fold increase in 5,10-methylenetetrahydrofolate which occurred in cells exposed to 50 μM leucovorin as shown in Table 1.

The polyglutamates of 5,10-methylenetetrahydrofolate have been shown by several investigators to be more potent in ternary complex formation when compared with the monoglutamated form of this folate. The increased potency of the polyglutamates combined with their prolonged intracellular retention, makes metabolism to this form of folate of primary importance in defining the optimal dose and scheduling of leucovorin. We investigated the degree of polyglutamation in both the breast and colon cancer cell lines exposed to 10 μM leucovorin for up to 24 hrs. of exposure. We also investigated the intracellular retention of the polyglutamate forms once formed in the colon cell line. We found that formation of the higher polyglutamate forms was principally time-dependent as shown in Table 2.

While both short and long exposures to a high concentration of leucovorin (10 μM) resulted in a greater intracellular concentration of the lower polyglutamate forms when compared with exposures to 1 μM, the intracellular amounts of the higher polyglutamates in cells exposed to 1 μM leucovorin were not significantly different than in cells treated with a higher leucovorin exposure. Conversely, a prolonged exposure (24 hrs.) to a low concentration of leucovorin (1 μM) results in a substantially higher polyglutamate formation when compared to brief exposures (2 hrs.) to even the higher 10 μM concentration of leucovorin. As illustrated in Table 2, a 24 hr. exposure to 1 μM leucovorin in the colon carcinoma cells results in approximately 109 pmol/mg of higher polyglutamate forms while a 2 hr. exposure to 10 μM leucovorin results in approximately 6-fold lower amounts of higher polyglutamates despite a similar concentration x time exposure, these data suggest that duration of exposure to leucovorin appears to be the principal factor in the formation of the higher folate polyglutamates.

As illustrated in Table 3, we found that the intracellular retention of the various polyglutamate forms of intracellular folates was directly proportional to the polyglutamate chain length. The pentaglutamates were retained with a half-life of 19.5 hrs. compared with 1.2 hr. for the monoglutamate forms.

Given that the common commercially available form of leucovorin is provided as a racemic mixture of biologically active and inactive forms, we also investigated the impact of the inactive stereoisomer on the intracellular metabolism of the active form of leucovorin. We studied ratios of up to 20:1 inactive to active stereoisomers of leucovorin and found that the inactive stereoisomer did not alter the intracellular metabolism of the active isomer to either the various one-carbon substituted folate forms or to the various polyglutamate states during 24 hour leucovorin exposures.

Since 5-methyltetrahydrofolate is the predominant folate in mammalian plasma and undergoes cellular metabolism through pathways that are distinct from those utilized by

Table 2. Polyglutamation of Intracellular Folates in Colon and Breast Cancer Cells Exposed to Leucovorin.

	Intracellular Polyglutamates (pmol/mg)	
	Glu-1 + Glu-2	Glu-3 - Glu-5
Human Colon Cancer Cells (HCT-116)		
Leucovorin 10 µM		
2 hrs.	77	18
24 hrs.	110	147
Leucovorin 1 µM		
2 hrs.	21	22
24 hrs.	15	109
Human Breast Cancer Cells (MCF-7)		
Leucovorin 10 µM		
2 hrs.	82	22
24 hrs.	124	172

Table 3. Intracellular Half-Life of Folate Polyglutamates.

Folate Polyglutamate Chain Length	Intracellular Half-Life (hrs.)
Glu-1	1.2
Glu-2	2.2
Glu-3	2.4
Glu-4	5.5
Glu-5	19.5

leucovorin, we felt it would be important to investigate the relative merits of this form of reduced folate versus leucovorin in its ability to expand the 5,10-methylenetetrahydrofolate pools. We found that the predominant intracellular folate in MCF-7 breast cancer cells exposed to 5-methyltetrahydrofolate was 5-methyltetrahydrofolate as opposed to the extensive metabolism of leucovorin by these cells. Approximately 15% of the intracellular 5-methyltetrahydrofolate was metabolized to either tetrahydrofolate or 10-formyltetrahydrofolate. In contrast to the expansion of 5,10-methylenetetrahydrofolate which we noted with leucovorin exposure, we found that 5-methyltetrahydrofolate exposures resulted in no detectable intracellular 5,10-methylenetetrahydrofolate even in cells exposed to 10 µM 5-methyltetrahydrofolate.

DISCUSSION

Our investigations concerning the metabolism of leucovorin in the human breast (MCF-7) and colon (HCT-116) cell lines suggest that metabolism to the various one-carbon substituted forms of folate is both time- and dose- dependent. Since no intracellular leucovorin was detected in cells exposed to even the highest concentrations of leucovorin, it would appear that the rate-limiting step in the intracellular metabolism of leucovorin is the transmembrane transport rather than its interconversion through the various biosynthetic pathways. Of interest was the finding that in the breast cancer cell line, the 5,10-methylenetetrahydrofolate pools could be markedly expanded (10-fold) by exposure of cells to high concentrations of leucovorin. It is not possible to assess the degree of expansion in 5,10-methylenetetrahydrofolate pool in the colon carcinoma cell line since the level of this folate fell below the detection limits of the assay at all concentrations of leucovorin.

The polyglutamated form of 5,10-methylenetetrahydrofolate has been described as having an enhanced ability to participate in ternary complex formation when compared with the monoglutamated form of this folate[11,12]. The ability of pentaglutamated 5,10-methylenetetrahydrofolate to participate in ternary complex formation is approximately 50 to 100-fold greater than that of the monoglutamate. The present report demonstrates that the higher polyglutamates particularly the pentaglutamate, has a prolonged intracellular half-life of approximately 19.5 hrs. compared to 1.2 hr. for the monoglutamated folates. These two facts, taken together, support the concept that formation of 5,10-methylenetetrahydrofolate polyglutamates would be the desired metabolite for optimizing the interaction between leucovorin and the fluoropyrimidines. Formation of the higher folate polyglutamates in both the breast and colon cell lines appear to be time- and dose-dependent; however, the duration of exposure to leucovorin appeared to be of greater importance than the absolute concentration of leucovorin to which the cells are exposed. This conclusion is supported by data shown in Table 2 for the colon cells treated with either 10 or 1 µM leucovorin. Prolonged exposure to either of these leucovorin concentrations resulted in a similar intracellular level of the higher polyglutamates while exposure for 24 hrs. to the lower concentration of leucovorin resulted in approximately 6-fold greater amounts of higher polyglutamates compared to cells treated with the higher concentration of leucovorin for only 2 hrs. Both of these exposure conditions result in similar concentration x time exposures (24 µM - hrs. and 20 µM - hrs., respectively). These data would support the use of continuous infusion or multiple repetitive dosing schedules as the optimal means of expanding the 5,10-methylenetetrahydrofolate polyglutamate pools with the use of exogenous leucovorin. It is of interest that clinical trials utilizing the daily for five day regimens of 5-fluorouracil plus leucovorin given at either 20 or 200 mg/m^2 result in a similar increase in response rate and an increase in survival of patients with advanced colorectal carcinoma[4]. Conversely, while trials utilizing the weekly schedule of 5-fluorouracil and leucovorin have resulted in an enhanced response rate, they have not resulted in prolongation of survival[5]. It may be speculated that the activity of the daily for 5 day regimens utilizing either high or low doses of leucovorin may be related to frequent daily dosing with leucovorin which would allow adequate time for cellular metabolism to the optimal 5,10-methylenetetrahydrofolate polyglutamates prior to the next daily dose of 5-fluorouracil. Biochemical data from the tumor of patients with advanced breast cancer treated with the daily for 5 day regimen of 5-fluorouracil plus leucovorin clearly demonstrate that the addition of leucovorin was capable of stabilizing ternary complex formation for up to 24 hrs. following the fluorouracil dose[7]. The importance of folate polyglutamation is echoed in a study by Romanini and colleagues which demonstrates that cells incapable of polyglutamating exogenously administered folates did not share the enhanced cytotoxicity of simultaneously administered 5-fluorouracil with cells that were capable of polyglutamation[14]. Studies from Houghton and colleagues clearly support the role of prolonged exposure of malignant cells to leucovorin as being the preferred mode for expansion of the critical 5,10-methylenetetrahydrofolate polyglutamate pools[9,10].

Leucovorin for clinical use is available as a racemic mixture of active and inactive diastereomers. Since the inactive stereoisomer has a prolonged serum half-life when compared with the biologically active form of leucovorin and is capable of achieving concentrations in the plasma that exceed those of the active isomer[16], it has been speculated that the inactive stereoisomer isomer of leucovorin may diminish the activity of the biologically active form of leucovorin. It has been hypothesized that these two isomers of leucovorin could compete at the level of cellular transport or at various steps along the biosynthetic pathways. Our data demonstrates that ratios of inactive to active stereoisomers of leucovorin of up to 20:1 have no impact on the uptake or metabolism of the active form of leucovorin to either the one-carbon metabolites or polyglutamates. A recent report by Machover and colleagues suggest that the use of the pure biologically active form of leucovorin is associated with a high response rate (52%) when used with 5-fluorouracil for the treatment of patients with advanced colorectal carcinoma[16]. Our preclinical data suggests that the use of the pure active stereoisomer of leucovorin would have activity similar to that of racemic leucovorin. The response rate of 52% reported by Machover and colleagues using biologically pure leucovorin is similar to that previously reported by these investigators using racemic leucovorin 39% for the treatment of patients with advanced colorectal carcinoma[17]. The clinical utility of the pure biologically active stereoisomer of leucovorin will await future randomized investigations. While 5-methyltetrahydrofolate would not appear to be as useful an agent as leucovorin for the expansion of 5,10-methylenetetrahydrofolate, it is conceivable that other forms of reduced folate such as 5,10-methylenetetrahydrofolate may prove to be of clinical value provided these forms of folate can be handled in a manner which would allow preservation of their reduced and therefore active state.

Since 5-methyltetrahydrofolate is the predominant folate in mammalian plasma, we hypothesized that this folate may be more efficient in its conversion to the 5,10-methylenetetrahydrofolate polyglutamates given that mammalian cells have developed specific mechanisms for handling this folate in contrast with leucovorin. Our data suggests that 5-methyltetrahydrofolate is less efficient when compared with equivalent doses of leucovorin in its ability to expand the 5,10-methylenetetrahydrofolate pool and that the metabolism of 5-methyltetrahydrofolate to the polyglutamate forms is qualitatively and quantitatively distinct from that of leucovorin.

In summary, our preclinical investigations suggest that the intracellular metabolism of leucovorin to the active 5,10-methylenetetrahydrofolate polyglutamates is most efficiently accomplished through prolonged exposure to even relatively low doses of leucovorin. These findings support the use of either continuous infusion or multiple frequent dosing schedules as the optimal means of combining leucovorin with the fluoropyrimidines. Our data does not support the use of 5-methyltetrahydrofolate as a potential alternative to leucovorin. Furthermore, racemic leucovorin appears to be biologically equal to the pure active leucovorin with regard to its cellular metabolism.

REFERENCES

1. J.L. Grem, Fluorinated Pyrimidines, in: "Cancer Chemotherapy," B.A. Chabner, and J.M. Collins, eds., J.B. Lippincott Co., Philadelphia, (1990).

2. M.-B. Yin, S.F. Zakrzewski, M.T. Hakala, Relationship of cellular folate cofactor pools to the activity of 5-fluorouracil, Mol. Pharmacol. 23:190 (1983).

3. B. Ullman, M. Lee, D.W. Martin Jr., D.V. Santi, Cytotoxicity of 5-fluoro-2'-deoxyuridine: requirement for reduced folate cofactors and antagonism by methotrexate, Proc. Natl. Acad. Sci. USA 75:980 (1978).

4. M.A. Poon, M.J. O'Connell, C.G. Moertel, et. al., Biochemical modulation of fluorouracil: Evidence of significant improvement of survival and quality of life in patients with advanced colorectal carcinoma. J. Clin. Oncol. 7:1407 (1989).

5. N. Petrelli, H.O. Douglass, Jr., L. Herrera, et. al., The modulation of fluorouracil with leucovorin in metastatic colorectal carcinoma: A prospective randomized phase III trial. J. Clin. Oncol. 7:1419 (1989).

6. C. Erlichman, S. Fine, A. Wong, et. al., A randomized trial of fluorouracil and folinic acid in patients with metastatic colorectal carcinoma. J. Clin. Oncol. 6:469 (1988).

7. S.M. Swain, M.E. Lippman, E.F. Egan, J.C. Drake, S.M. Steinberg, and C.J. Allegra, 5-Fluorouracil and high-dose leucovorin in previously treated patients with metastatic breast cancer, J. Clin. Oncol. 7:890 (1989).

8. D.M. Boarman, and C.J. Allegra, Intracellular metabolism of 5-formy-tetrahydrofolate in human breast and colon cell lines, Cancer Res. 52:36 (1992).

9. J.A. Houghton, L.G. Williams, P.J. Chesire, I.W. Wainer, P. Jadaud, P.J. Houghton, Influence of dose of [6RS] leucovorin on reduced folate pools and 5-fluorouracil-mediated thymidylate synthase inhibition in human colon adenocarcinoma xenografts. Cancer Res. 50:3940 (1990).

10. J.A. Houghton, L.G. Williams, S.S.N. de Graaf, P.J. Chesire, J.H. Rodman, D.C. Maneval, I.W. Wainer, P. Jadaud, P.J. Houghton, Relationship between dose rate of [6RS] leucovorin administration, plasma concentrations of reduced folates, and pools of 5,10-methylenetetrahydrofolates and tetrahydrofolates in human colon adenocarcinoma xenografts. Cancer Res. 50:3493 (1990).

11. C.J. Allegra, B.A. Chabner, J.C. Drake, R. Lutz, D. Rodbard, J. Jolivet, Enhanced inhibition of thymidylate synthase by methotrexate polyglutamates, J. Biol. Chem. 260:9720 (1985).

12. S. Radparvar, P.J. Houghton, J.A. Houghton, Effect of polyglutamation of 5,10-methylenetetrahydrofolate on the binding of 5-fluoro-2'-deoxyuridylate to thymidylate synthase purified from a human colon adenocarcinoma xenograft, Biochem. Pharmacol. 38:335 (1989).

13. D.G. Kennedy, R. Clarke, H.W. Van denBerg, R.F. Murphy, The kinetics of methotrexate polyglutamate formation and efflux in a human breast cancer cell line (MD.MB.436): the effect of insulin, Biochem. Pharmacol. 32:41 (1983).

14. A. Romanini, J.T. Lin, D. Niedzwiecki, M. Bunni, D.G. Priest, J.R. Bertino, Role of folypolyglutamates in biochemical modulation of fluoropyrimidines by leucovorin,Cancer Res. 51:789 (1991).

15. C.J. Allegra, R.L. Fine, J.C. Drake, and B.A. Chabner, The effect of methotrexate on intracellular folate pools in human MCF-7 breast cancer cells: evidence for direct inhibition of purine synthesis. J. Biol. Chem. 261:6478 (1986).

16. D. Machover, X. Grison, E. Goldschmidt, J. Zittoun, J.-P. Lotz, G. Metzger, J. Richaud, L. Hannoun, J. Marquet, T. Guillot, R. Salmon, A. Sezeur, S. Mauban, R. Parc, V. Izrael, Fluorouracil combined with the pure (6S)-stereoisomer of folinic acid in high doses for treatment of patients with advanced colorectal carcinoma: A phase I-II study, J. Natl. Cancer Inst. 84:321 (1992).

17. D. Machover, E. Goldschmidt, P. Chollet, et. al., Treatment of advanced colorectal and gastric adenocarcinomas with 5-fluorouracil and high-dose folinic acid. J. Clin. Oncol. 4:685 (1986).

SOME CONSIDERATIONS CONCERNING THE DOSE AND SCHEDULE OF 5FU AND LEUCOVORIN: TOXICITIES OF TWO DOSE SCHEDULES FROM THE INTERGROUP COLON ADJUVANT TRIAL (INT-0089)

Daniel G. Haller, Myrto Lefkopoulou,
John S. Macdonald, Robert S. Mayer

University of Pennsylvania Cancer Center, Philadelphia, PA
Dana-Farber Cancer Center, Boston, MA
Temple University, Philadelphia, PA

The therapeutic efficacy of 5-fluorouracil (5-FU) can be enhanced by the addition of compounds which increase reduced folate pools in tumor cells, thereby increasing the inhibition of thymidylate synthase by 5-FU. *In vitro* studies have suggested that maximal thymidylate synthase inhibition is achieved when the extracellular folate concentration is 10 mmol/L, which can be achieved *in vivo* by intravenous doses of 500 mg/M^2 of body surface area of leucovorin.[1] However, controversy exists concerning the optimal necessary dose of leucovorin, as well as the optimal schedule, when combined with 5-FU. In addition to any theoretical or academic concerns about basing treatment on laboratory-derived, rather than empiric regimens, there are also practical issues involved in choosing an acceptable regimen for clinical practice. In addition to the cost of the leucovorin to the patient, there are also choices to be made concerning the impact of the treatment on nursing facilities, patient travel and patient tolerance.

Based on the earlier cited pharmacologic evidence for the necessary *in vivo* intravenous dose of leucovorin believed to be necessary for maximal thymidylate synthase inhibition, a weekly regimen (RPMI) of 5-FU with high-dose leucovorin was designed: 5-FU 600 mg/M^2 + leucovorin 500 mg/M^2 given weekly for 6 weeks followed by a two-week rest period.[2] Initial studies of this combination in advanced colorectal cancer demonstrated an objective response rate of 38%, with a larger trial from the GITSG documenting a response rate of 30.3% (33/109), which was superior to a control arm of 5-FU alone (12.1%) and to a low-dose leucovorin regimen (18.8%).[2] In this trial, 5-FU alone was given as an intensive regimen of 500 mg/M^2 for 5 days every four weeks, with dose escalation permitted. In this manner, improvements in response rate associated with regimens of 5-FU plus leucovorin could be more fairly attributed to maximization of cytotoxicity by the modulator, rather than simply to the effects of dose intensity. The low-dose leucovorin regimen in this trial used the same dose and schedule of 5-FU, but only 25 mg/M^2 of leucovorin was administered with each infusion. Severe diarrhea was the dose-limiting toxicity of the RPMI regimen, although significant gastrointestinal toxicity was common to all three regimens. Treatment-related toxicity was responsible for the deaths of 5% of patients, with diarrhea in older individuals chiefly responsible for the majority of these treatment-related fatalities. The investigators of this study advocated stricter requirements for dose modifications for diarrhea than is usually recommended for 5-FU based regimens.

Novel Approaches to Selective Treatments of Human Solid Tumors: Laboratory and Clinical Correlation Edited by Y. M. Rustum, Plenum Press, New York, 1993

Other 5-FU + leucovorin regimens have been developed, including 5-day regimens in which leucovorin doses were given at 200 mg/M^2/d based on preclinical rationales, or at an empiric lower dose of 20 mg/M^2/d for potential reduction of cost and toxicity.[3] The 5-day regimen of 5-FU 425 mg/M^2/d + leucovorin 20 mg/M^2/d has been demonstrated by the Mayo Clinic/North Central Cancer Treatment Group (NCCTG) to have a 42% (34/81) objective response rate in advanced colorectal cancer, with survival superiority over 5-FU alone, and with no added benefit to the use of the same 5-FU dose and schedule with the 200 mg/M^2 leucovorin dose.[3,4] These data strongly suggested that an empirically-derived leucovorin dose was as effective as a higher dose based on preclinical laboratory data, with perhaps less toxicity and at lower cost. Although the 5-day regimen of low dose was also associated with diarrhea, mucositis and myelosuppression as dose-limiting toxicities, the mortality appeared lower (1/128) than the 5% treatment-related toxicity reported previously with the high-dose leucovorin RPMI regimen. In further investigation of the low-dose leucovorin regimen (20 mg/M^2) compared to the higher dose regimen (200 mg/M^2), the NCCTG confirmed that the low-dose regimen showed no significant difference in response rate or in survival between the two regimens.[4]

To comparatively assess the overall antitumor activity, toxicity and cost of the RPMI high-dose leucovorin regimen and the NCCTG low-dose leucovorin regimen, a phase III trial was designed and carried out by the Mayo Clinic/NCCTG. The RPMI regimen was given at the original 5-FU/leucovorin doses of 600/500 mg/M^2 weekly for 6 weeks followed by a two week rest, and the NCCTG regimen was given at doses of 5-FU 425 mg/M^2/d x 5 and leucovorin 20 mg/M^2/d x 5 given every 4–5 weeks.

Table 1. Comparison of the RPMI and NCCTG 5-FU plus leucovorin regimen in advanced colorectal cancer.

	RPMI	NCCTG
# pts	153	162
Median Survival	10 mos	10 mos
Rx Mortality	2%	2%
Objective Response Rate	29%	33%
Time in Hospital	436 d	317 d

This comparison suggested no therapeutic difference between the two regimens, either in terms of overall response rate or median survival. There was also no significant difference in treatment mortality between the two regimens. Inpatient management of toxicities, chiefly diarrhea, from the RPMI regimen was longer by one-third (p=.07) than for the NCCTG regimen, and the calculated course of treatment based on the cost of leucovorin was correspondingly higher for the RPMI regimen

INT-0089 is a recently completed comparative trial of four 5-FU-containing adjuvant chemotherapy regimens for Dukes' B$_2$ and C colon cancer. From October, 1989 to July, 1992, 3475 patients were randomized to 4 treatment arms, three of which are based on the RPMI and NCCTG regimens for advanced colorectal cancer:

B [NCCTG] = 5-FU 425 mg/M^2/dx5 + leucovorin 20 mg/M^2/dx5 Q4–5 wks
C [RPMI] = 5-FU 500 mg/M^2 + leucovorin 500 mg/M^2 weekly x 6 Q8 wks
E [Standard] = 5-FU 450 mg/M^2 x5, then weekly for 1 yr + levamisole
F [NCCTG] = arm B + levamisole 150 mg/dx3d Q2 wks

With a median follow-up of less than two years, the data for recurrence and survival are too immature to report. However, toxicity data are available for 2637 patients, and off-study evaluations are complete for 1797 patients. The purpose of this report is to update information concerning the relative toxicities of the RPMI and NCCTG 5-FU plus leucovorin regimens as applied to the adjuvant setting, in a homogeneous population of patients who had recently undergone surgery with curative intent for early stage extrapelvic colon cancer. The RPMI regimen was modified for this trial, based on the actual amount of 5-FU (500 mg/M^2 weekly)administered in the original report[2], and based on the recommendations of the original investigators. The standard treatment regimen in INT-0089 was the levamisole plus 5-FU regimen as originally reported in February of 1990.[6] This treatment was demonstrated to be associated with a 41% reduction in the risk of recurrence and a 33% reduction in the risk of death compared to surgery alone for patients with Dukes' C colon cancer. The purpose of INT-0089 was to determine whether the increased cytotoxicity of 5-FU/leucovorin regimens, as documented in advanced colorectal cancer, would translate into increased benefits compared to 5-FU plus levamisole in the adjuvant setting.

Significant toxicities (grade 3 or worse) for the four treatment arms of INT-0089 are reported in Table 2, expressed as percentages of total patients.

Table 2. INT-0089: Grade 3 or worse toxicities (expressed as grade 3/grade 4 or 5).

	B [NCCTG] (712)	F [NCCTG + lev] (581)	C [RPMI] (726)	E [Standard] (612)
nausea	3.7/-	4.9/-	7.0/0.1	2.6/-
vomiting	2.0/0.6	2.6/0.2	2.8/1.0	1.5/0.2
diarrhea	10.8/7.7	10.6/6.6	14.9/14.0	5.6/2.9
stomatitis	14.2/3.9	15.5/4.2	1.2/0.1	3.1/0.5
leukopenia	8.0/1.8	10.1/3.1	2.5/0.7	6.9/1.3
neutropenia	5.4/11.5	8.0/15.8	1.5/1.7	5.6/8.3
overall worst grade	26.7/21.6 (48.3%)	27.3/26.6 (53.9%)	20.4/17.1 (37.5%)	19.9/14.5 (34.4%)

Overall, the dose-limiting toxicities of the regimens noted in trials of patients with advanced colorectal cancer have been confirmed in the adjuvant setting. The dose-limiting toxicities for the NCCTG regimen are stomatitis, diarrhea and myelosuppression, with half of all patients experiencing at least one severe or worse toxicity. The RPMI regimen is rarely associated with significant stomatitis or myelosuppression, but severe or worse diarrhea is the dose-limiting toxicity, occurring in at least one-quarter of patients. The standard 5-FU + levamisole (arm E) regimen is the least toxic regimen overall by these criteria.

Two other methods of determining tolerability of these regimens is the number of toxic (grade 5 toxicity) deaths and the ability or desire of patients to continue or complete treatment. There have been 21 grade 5 toxicities observed in INT-0089 considered to be attributable to therapy: arm B=6, arm C=4, arm E=6, arm F=5. Of the 1797 patients who have completed all treatment and for whom case evaluations have been completed, treatment outcomes are reported in Table 3.

Although arm E is associated with the fewest severe or worse toxicities, more patients and physicians have been reported to discontinue treatment because of toxicity, perhaps because this regimen is 12 months in duration, compared to 6 months for the other three treatments. The proportion of patients who have completed the regimen may also

Table 3. INT-0089: Treatment outcomes based on toxicity.

	B [NCCTG] (475)	F [NCCTG + lev] (493)	C [RPMI] (460)	E [Standard] (369)
completed all Rx	79.8%	80.3%	69.8%	58.5%
MD d/c'ed, 2° tox.	2.7%	2.8%	4.3%	6.8%
Pt d/c'ed, 2° tox.	7.6%	7.5%	7.6%	10.8%
Pt d/c'ed, other	1.7%	1.4%	4.6%	6.0%
	12.0%	11.7%	16.5%	23.6%

change as more off-study data are received for the 5-FU plus levamisole regimen, which is six months longer in duration. Although a higher proportion of patients on arms B and F completed all treatment as prescribed by protocol, a formal dose-intensity analysis has not been performed. As data from INT-0089 mature for relapse and survival, these toxicity data will be important in judging optimal adjuvant therapy, particularly if therapeutic differences among the regimens are small.

REFERENCES

1. R.M. Evans, J.D. Laskin, and M.T. Hakala: Effect of excess folates and deoxyinosine on the activity and site of action of 5-fluorouracil. *Cancer Res* 41:3283–3295, 1981.

2. N. Petrelli, H.O. Douglass, Jr., H. Lemuel, *et al*: The modulation of fluorouracil with leucovorin in metastatic colorectal carcinoma: A prospective randomized phase III trial. *J Clin Onc* 7:1419–1426, 1989.

3. M.A. Poon, M.J. O'Connell, C.G. Moertel, *et al*: Biochemical modulation of fluorouracil: Evidence of significant improvement of survival and quality of life in patients with advanced colorectal carcinoma. *J Clin Onc* 7:1407–1418, 1989.

4. M.A. Poon, M.J. O'Connell, H.S. Wieand, *et al*: Biochemical modulation of fluorouracil with leucovorin: Confirmatory evidence of improved therapeutic efficacy in advanced colorectal cancer. *J Clin Onc* 9:1967–1972, 1991.

5. J. Gerstner, M.J. O'Connell, H.S. Wieand, *et al*: A prospectively randomized clinical trial comparing 5FU combined with either high- or low-dose leucovorin for the treatment of advanced colorectal cancer (meeting abstract). Proc ASCO; 10:A404, 1991.

6. C.G. Moertel, T.R. Fleming, J.S. Macdonald, *et al*: Levamisole and fluorouracil for adjuvant therapy of resected colon cancer. *N Engl J Med* 322:352–358, 1990.

DISCUSSION OF DR. ALLEGRA'S/DR. MACDONALD'S PRESENTATION

Dr. Petrelli: Jack, in the advanced setting most patients will endure toxicity whether it is stomatitis or diarrhea that is if they get it and there is a dose reduction of the drug they'll go ahead and get back on the regimen. In the adjuvant setting it's a little bit different because you're taking an otherwise healthy patient. Do you have any information between those patients who got severe stomatitis and those patients who got severe diarrhea and the tendency of one or the other group to get on the trial in terms of compliance of the chemotherapy?

Dr. MacDonald: There were no differences. It's interesting. If one looks at the number, the percentage of patients who did not complete the projected course of therapy, there are no differences in the 5-FU/LV arms with or without levamisole. Now, there's a catch here. If you look at 5-FU/levamisole alone, there's a higher dropout rate and we think the reason for that is that the 3 leucovorin arms were all 6 month regimens. The 5-FU/levamisole was a full year but actually the dropout rates were relatively smaller, I think it's in the 5% range.

Dr. Rustum: Dr. Allegra, you have discussed the issue of dose and schedules of leucovorin in the metabolic modulation of FUra. Based on your data and on the available information in literature, what dose and schedule of leucovorin would you recommend?

Dr. Allegra: Well, I think we didn't see any saturation of leucovorin metabolism to the various pools or to polyglutamate. The more you give and the longer you give it the more you're going to expand the pools. There's obvious practical limitations and I think that if given those practical limitations, if one has to choose more drug vs giving a lower dose for a longer period, I guess this data would suggest that giving the doses for a longer time as opposed to higher doses, if you had a choice, it would probably be the more efficient thing.

Dr. MacDonald: I have a question or I guess a comment that is related to Dr.Allegra's presentation and perhaps Dr. Ardalan can address it. Dr. Ardalan's pilot study in Miami is now being examined in a Southwestern Oncology Group which consists of 5-FU/LV and PALA. The schedule 5-FU/LV that Dr. Ardalan used is 2600 mg/m^2 of 5-FU with 500 m/^{2} leucovorin given as a continuous 24 hr infusion weekly schedule. Have you done that without PALA?

Dr. Ardalan: Our initial studies were published in JCO about a couple years ago addressed the issue of 2600 mg of 5-FU with 500 leucovorin that was tolerable and generated good responses.

Dr. MacDonald: That's with 24 hr infusion?

Dr. Ardalan: Yes. Leucovorin dose is 24 hrs. Both 5-FU and leucovorin are given concurrently. PALA was administered 24 hrs before FUra/CF using 250 mg.

Dr. Machover: One question for Dr. Allegra. You were trying to find a better schedule for 5-FU/LV by measuring polyglutamates. Do you think measurement of the total amount of polyglutamates is sufficient? Do you think it would be better to try to identify and quantitate different species of polyglutamates?

Dr. Allegra: I think there are probably others in the audience who can speak on this better than I can, but in studies where people have actually looked or fractionated the folates and looked at the polyglutamate pools, for instance, tetrahydrofolate, I think Dr. Priest is probably better at answering this than I can, but you look at tetrahydrofolate or 5,10-methylene and you separate them and look at the polyglutamate profiles it really is identical to what you find overall in the cells. Is that fair enough Dr. Priest?

Dr. Priest: I agree with you 100% I think what the interconversion of folates themselves is very rapid. I don't think that the pools are all going to have the same polyglutamate status.

EFFECTS OF 5-FLUOROURACIL ON mRNA

Bruce J. Dolnick and Xi-Pu Wu

Department of Experimental Therapeutics
Grace Cancer Drug Center
Roswell Park Cancer Institute
Elm and Carlton Streets
Buffalo, N.Y. 14263

INTRODUCTION

Thymidylate synthase (TS) is the most well studied site of fluorinated pyrimidine action and its inhibition forms the rationale of most clinical protocols which are dependent upon 5-fluorouracil (FU). The basis for this interest rests largely upon the exquisite sensitivity of the enzyme to the antimetabolite 5-fluorodeoxyuridylate, the demonstration of numerous cell culture effects which can be explained by enzyme inhibition, and increased tumor responsiveness when FU activity *in vivo* is modulated by leucovorin. Conversely, while RNA as a site of 5-fluorouracil (FU) action has been indicated by a number of studies, a precise mechanistic basis for RNA related cytotoxicity and its possible contributions to the anticancer action of the drug have not been well defined. This article summarizes some of the data indicating the effects FU can have on mRNA metabolism and function and presents evidence for effects *in vivo*. A discussion of potentially important issues related to mRNA associated effects is presented. Newly available tools which can be used to address previously undefined issues are also described.

DOCUMENTED EFFECTS OF FU ON mRNA *IN VITRO*

It has long been known that incorporation of FU into RNA correlates with its cytotoxic effect in a number of cell lines and can interfere with the maturation of pre-ribosomal RNA (Parker and Cheng, 1990; Weckbecker, 1991; Wilkinson and Pitot, 1973). Effects of FU upon the metabolism of mRNAs and their possible relation to the cytotoxic effects of FU have been hampered by a lack of information as to which mRNAs may be important to the effect of FU and what aspects of mRNA metabolism might be affected, as generally there does not appear to be a major effect of FU on this class of RNA when analyzed *in toto* (Glazer and Hartman, 1981).

Novel Approaches to Selective Treatments of Human Solid Tumors: Laboratory and Clinical Correlation Edited by Y. M. Rustum, Plenum Press, New York, 1993

In the early '80's, it became clear that if effects of FU upon mRNA metabolism were to be understood, a system was required in which steady state substitution of U residues by FU in mRNA was needed and that individual mRNA species should be studied in detail. Dihydrofolate reductase (DHFR) mRNA was chosen as a model system in my laboratory, in large part because of the availability of probes to study this mRNA and because of the relationship of DHFR to TS (Dolnick and Pink, 1983, 1985). A number of early studies demonstrated that under artificial cell culture conditions where FU incorporation into RNA correlated with cytotoxicity, there was a change in the behavior of DHFR prepared from treated cells indicating a likelihood of translational miscoding due to FU incorporation into RNA.

At approximately this point in time information began to accumulate that protein coding genes in eukaryotes were not colinear with mRNAs but instead contained intervening sequences, or introns. As the mechanism for the removal of introns from pre-mRNAs began to be elucidated, it also became clear that a previously identified class of RNAs without a known function, the small nuclear RNAs (i.e. U1, U2, U4, U5, U6) were somehow involved in this splicing process. The fact that these small nuclear RNAs were uracil rich suggested they might be affected by the incorporation of FU in drug-treated cells.

The demonstration by Armstrong et al. (1986) that fluorouridine (FUrd) treatment of murine sarcoma-180 cells resulted in the altered electrophoretic migration of U4 and U6 RNAs on native polyacrylamide gels, while other small nuclear RNA species were qualitatively unaffected suggested possible effects of fluorinated pyrimidines on pre-mRNA splicing. Using an intron specific probe, Will and Dolnick (1986) demonstrated increases in intron containing DHFR RNA in KB cells exposed to FU in the presence of thymidine, further suggesting an effect of FU on pre-mRNA maturation. The implication that pre-mRNA conversion to mRNA might be affected by FU was suggested further by the demonstration that intron-exon probes, specific for splice junctions, also increased in FU-treated KB cells (Will and Dolnick, 1987).

In an attempt to analyze the contribution of incorporation of FU into pre-mRNA on splicing, Doong and Dolnick (1988) investigated the effects of FU incorporation into pre-mRNA on splicing *in vitro* . Using minigene transcripts corresponding to human β-globin, pre-mRNA transcribed in vitro was spliced with HeLa cell nuclear extracts and the products were analyzed. While splicing *per se* was not inhibited with up to 100% FU substitution of U in the pre-mRNA, minor altered splicing products were observed indicating FU incorporation into pre-mRNA could qualitatively alter splicing. Although it was considered possible that some pre-mRNAs might be more sensitive than others to the effects of FU substitution upon splicing, the need for at least 84% substitution of U by FU in pre-mRNA, to observe altered splicing suggested that incorporation of FU into pre-mRNA was not likely to be an important site of FU action *in vivo*. It had been observed that only 2% substitution was found to correlate with 50% growth inhibition in KB cells (Dolnick and Pink, 1985). Conversely, observed changes in the apparent secondary structure of U4 and U6 RNA in FUrd-treated cells (Armstrong et al., 1986), increases in U1 RNA in FU- or FUrd-treated cells (Armstrong et al. 1986; Doong and Dolnick, 1988) and an inability to generate active pre-mRNA splicing extracts from FU-treated HeLa cells (Doong, 1988) suggested small nuclear RNAs might be the site of FU effects upon splicing (Will and Dolnick, 1989).

Two recent studies have shed more light upon FU effects on pre-mRNA splicing. Sierakowska et al. (1989) demonstrated that treatment of HeLa cells with FUrd destabilized U2 RNA and resulted in increased levels of U1 RNA and these changes correlated with the loss of the in vitro splicing activity of nuclear extracts. Will and Dolnick (1989) reported that in KB cells grown in the presence of FU and thymidine, there was no change in the half-lives of DHFR mRNA or pre-mRNA (~11.5 h and 50 min, respectively) but that the rate of conversion of nuclear DHFR RNA to cytoplasmic RNA decreased ~1.8-fold in treated cells, corresponding to the increased ratio of DHFR pre-mRNA/mRNA in the treated cells.

Studies of the effects of fluorinated pyrimidines by a number of laboratories have indicated a variety of effects depending upon the mRNA in question and the cell line employed. However, changes in mRNA levels appear to generally decrease or to decrease relative to pre-mRNA levels. For example Iwata et al. (1986) observed decreased levels of α- or β-globin in MEL (mouse erythroleukemia) cells subsequent to FU exposure, and Heimer and Sartorelli (1990) observed reductions in gamma-globin mRNA levels in K562 (erythroleukemia) cells. However two clonally derived KB cell lines which overproduced DHFR and DHFR mRNA behaved differently with respect to the effect of FU exposure on DHFR mRNA levels. While KB7B cells demonstrated an increase in DHFR mRNA upon FU exposure (Dolnick and Pink, 1983), KB1BT cells responded to FU exposure with a decrease in DHFR mRNA (Will and Dolnick, 1989). Despite the differential responses to FU in the levels of DHFR mRNA, the ratio of DHFR pre-mRNA/mRNA increased in both cell lines (Will and Dolnick, 1989). The increase in the ratio of DHFR pre-mRNA/mRNA suggested splicing of mRNA might be affected by FU incorporation.

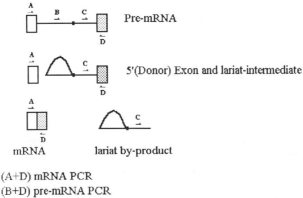

(A+D) mRNA PCR
(B+D) pre-mRNA PCR
(C+D) pre-mRNA + lariat-intermediate PCR

Figure 1. RNA species present throughout the pre-mRNA splicing process and primers and strategy used for quantitative PCR of each. The rightward arrows (A,B,C) indicate relative primer sites for sense strand extensions and the leftward arrows (D) indicate relative primer sites for antisense strand extensions. The closed box where the lariat forms represents the branch point. The levels of the different RNA species obtained are calculated using the various primer sets indicated to determine absolute amounts of the specified RNA species (Wu and Dolnick, manuscript in preparation). Note that the A + D primer set only gives mRNA values and not pre-mRNA values as the primers span a number of introns, preventing pre-mRNA amplification.

Splicing of pre-mRNA occurs as a two step process for each intron, involving cleavage of the 5'-splice donor site with generation of a 5'-exon and 3'-(lariat)intron-3'exon intermediate, followed by ligation of the two exons with release of a lariat-intron (Fig 1 and Padgett et al., 1986). The mechanistic interactions of U1, U2, U4, U5 and U6 in the splicing process have recently been proposed (Wassarman and Steitz, 1992) and the effects of FU upon several of the small nuclear RNAs and *in vitro* splicing suggest that effects upon splicing should be detectable in drug-treated cells. Recently, my laboratory has developed a quantitative polymerase chain reaction (PCR) assay which can be used to measure the levels of a DHFR pre-mRNA, a splicing intermediate and mature mRNA in RNA from cells treated with FU (Wu and Dolnick, 1993). The relative positions of the oligonucleotide primers and the species they prime during reverse transcription of RNA and subsequent PCR, are presented in Fig 1. When this assay was employed in the quantitation of the three different species present at the different stages of DHFR mRNA splicing in FU-treated KB1BT cells (a KB cell variant which overproduces DHFR and its mRNA approximately 250-fold, Will and Dolnick, 1989), a decrease in the level of splicing intermediate and mature mRNA was observed at 1 μM FU, while the level of DHFR pre-mRNA was unaffected. Addition of methotrexate (MTX) to the cells prior to the addition of FU, resulted in a slight enhancement of the decrease in the DHFR splicing intermediate and mature mRNA and correlated with an enhanced incorporation of FU into RNA (Wu and Dolnick, 1993). This (and other) data suggest that while FU incorporation into RNA does not affect pre-mRNA synthesis (Will and Dolnick, 1989), steps distal to the first cleavage reaction (at the 5'-intron/exon junction) of the splicing process may be inhibited by FU.

EFFECTS OF FU ON mRNA *IN VIVO*

Clinically relevant documentation of FU-related effects on mRNA are limited. This relates to the lack of well founded rationales to investigate mRNAs with existing clinical protocols, the general inability to accurately quantitate mRNA species from small tumor samples and the unavailability of suitable tumor samples for analysis. The development of competitive template-based PCR assays to quantitate mRNA has altered the ability to address questions of the effects of drugs on mRNA in clinically derived specimens. While the PCR assay can quantitate TS mRNA in the amol (i.e. 10^{-18} mol) range, the level of TS protein in the same samples are only accurate to within three-fold. While this level of accuracy may preclude predictions of FU response based upon TS directed therapy, the sensitivity should allow for the collection of data with other mRNAs which may be more diagnostic of RNA effects. This assay, which exploits the ability to add various known amounts of an essentially identical, *in vitro* prepared RNA to RNA prepared from cells allows for the accurate quantitation of both relative changes and absolute amounts of mRNA levels (Becker-Andrè and Hahlbrock, 1989, Gilliland et al.,1990, Dolnick et al., 1992). The application of this PCR technique to the quantitation of DHFR and TS mRNAs in patients, before and after treatment with FU and leucovorin revealed rapid and dramatic changes in the levels of TS mRNA, but no significant effects on DHFR mRNA in tumor samples (Dolnick et al., 1992). As reported by Dolnick et. al. (1992), the level of TS mRNA increased approximately an order of magnitude at 4 and 24 h in colorectal tumors of two treated patients. Of the samples analyzed for both TS mRNA and enzyme levels, the two treated patients were the only ones in which the ratio of TS/TS-mRNA was found to deviate significantly from a linear relationship (see Table 1). It is worthwhile noting that in virtually all the samples analyzed from cell culture or from untreated patient specimens, that the ratio of TS protein to TS mRNA was relatively constant, at approximaely 200 molecules TS protein per molecule mRNA.

SUMMARY

Currently, there are a number of studies which suggest that FU can have pronounced effects on mRNA and its metabolism. However, the relevance of these changes to the antitumor effect of FU are still not clear. Generally, the mRNAs which have been studied to date involve those genes which are associated with the TS-directed effects of FU and have generally been limited to the changes in mRNA levels. The recent development of PCR methodology to investigate changes in pre-mRNA and splicing provides the tool to study a number of RNA effects of FU simultaneously. The major question is which mRNAs are important for study.

DHFR mRNA has a half life of 11.5 in KB1BT cells (Will and Dolnick, 1989) and is thus, on a kinetic basis alone, unlikely to provide a significant RNA target for RNA-directed effects of FU. There is a greater likelihood that shorter lived mRNAs which not only turnover rapidly, but are important to cell proliferation will eventually be shown to be key targets for the effects of FU at the RNA level. Interestingly, many of the growth factors are encoded by short-lived and tightly regulated mRNAs (e.g. GM-CSF, Shaw and Kamen,1986). In fact the half-lives of some of these mRNAs are regulated by U-rich sequences in their 3'-noncoding regions. The presence of U-rich sequences in these growth factor mRNAs and the small nuclear RNAs suggests these are worthwhile targets for studies, which could now be performed on clinical samples. Laboratory data which shows alterations in the small nuclear RNAs, under conditions which only provide for very low-level substitution of U residues by FU also suggest that RNA effects of FU may be a much more tightly related to cytotoxicity *in vivo* than previously thought.

Table 1. Levels of TS mRNA and TS in various cell lines and tumor specimens. (Adapted from Dolnick et al., 1992). Values have been rounded off to whole numbers. ND, not determined.

Cell line or Tumor Specimen	TS mRNA amol/µg RNA	TS fmol/mg
KB	90	ND
KB1BT	133	ND
HCT8	15	1520
K562	32	2850
MCF7	3	179
SE	4	273
COLORECTAL 1	15	944
COLORECTAL 2	5	264
COLORECTAL 3 (Pretreatment)	1	160
COLORECTAL 3 (4 h post FU + CF)	14	12
COLORECTAL 4 (Pretreatment)	4	17
COLORECTAL 4 (24 h post FU + CF)	40	9

ACKNOWLEDGEMENTS

Supported in part by PHS grant CA34306 awarded to B.J. Dolnick and CORE grant CA16056.

REFERENCES

Armstrong, R.D., Takimoto, C.H., and Cadman, E.C., 1986, Fluoropyrimidine-mediated changes in small nuclear RNA, *J. Biol. Chem.* 261:21.

Becker-Andrè, M., and Hahlbrock, K., 1989, Absolute mRNA quantitation using the polymerase chain reaction. A novel approach by a PCR aided transcript titration assay. *Nucl. Acids Res.* 17:9437.

Dolnick, B.J. and Pink, J.J., 1983, 5-Fluorouracil modulation of dihydrofolate reductase RNA levels in methotrexate-resistant KB cells. *J. Biol. Chem.* 258:13299.

Dolnick, B.J. and Pink, J.J., 1985, Effects of 5-fluorouracil on dihydrofolate reductase and dihydrofolate reductase mRNA from methotrexate-resistant KB cells. *J. Biol. Chem.* 260:3006.

Dolnick, B.J., Zhang, Z.G., Hines, J. D., and Rustum, Y.M., 1992, Quantitation of dihydrofolate reductase and thymidylate synthase mRNAs in vivo and in vitro by polymerase chain reaction, *Oncol. Res.* 4:65.

Doong, S.L., 1988, Effect of 5-fluorouracil incorporation into pre-mRNA on RNA splicing *in vitro*, Ph.D. Thesis, University of Wisconsin.

Doong, S.L. and Dolnick, B.J., 1988, 5-Fluorouracil substitution alters pre-mRNA splicing *in vitro*, *J. Biol. Chem.* 263:4467.

Gilliland, G., Perrin, S., Blanchard, K., and Bunn, H.F., 1990, Analysis of cytokine mRNA and DNA: detection and quantitation by competitive polymerase chain reaction, *Proc. Natl. Acad. Sci. USA* 87:2725.

Glazer, R.I. and Hartman, K.D., 1981, Analysis of the effect of 5-fluorouracil on the synthesis and translation of polysomal poly(A)RNA from Ehrlich ascites cells. *Molec. Pharmacol.* 19:117.

Heimer, R. and Sartorelli, A.C., 1990, Reductions in γ-globin mRNA levels restricted to the cytoplasm of 5-fluorouridine treated K-562 human erythroleukemia cells, *Cancer Comm.* 2:45.

Iwata, T., Watanabe, T., and Kufe, D.W., 1986, Effects of 5-fluorouracil on globin mRNA synthesis in murine erythroleukemia cells, *Biochemistry* 25:2703.

Padgett, R.A., Grabowski, P.J., Konarska, M.M., Seiler, S., and Sharp, P.A., 1986, Splicing of messenger RNA precursors, in: *Methods in Enzymology* 55:1119, C.C. Richardson, P.D. Boyer, I.B. Dawid and A. Meister, eds. Academic Reviews Inc, Palo Alto.

Parker, W.B. and Cheng, Y.C., 1990, Metabolism and mechanism of action of 5-fluorouracil, *Pharmac. Ther.* 48:381.

Shaw, G. and Kamen, R., 1986, A conserved AU sequence from the 3'untranslated region of GM-CSF mRNA mediates selective mRNA degradation, *Cell* 46:659.

Sierakowska, H., Shukla, R.R., Dominski, Z., and Kole, R., 1989, Inhibition of pre-mRNA splicing by 5-fluoro, 5-chloro- and 5-bromouridine, *J. Biol. Chem.* 264:1989.

Wang, A.M., Doyle, M.V., and Mark, D.F., 1989, Quantitation of mRNA by the polymerase chain reaction, *Proc. Natl. Acad. Sci. USA* 86:9717.

Wassarman, D.A. and Steitz, J.A., 1992, Interactions of small nuclear RNA's with precursor messenger RNA during in vitro splicing, *Science* 257:1918.

Weckbecker, G., 1991, Biochemical pharmacology and analysis of fluoropyrimidines alone and in combination with modulators, *Pharmac. Ther.* 50:367.

Wilkinson, D.S. and Pitot, H.C., 1973, Inhibition of riosomal ribonucleic acid maturation in Novikoff hepatoma cells by 5-fluorouracil and 5-fluorouridine. *J. Biol. Chem.* 248:63.

Will, C.L. and Dolnick, B.J., 1987, 5-Fluorouracil augmentation of dihydrofolate reductase gene transcripts containing intervening sequences in methotrexate-resistant KB cells, *Mol. Pharm.* 29:643.

Will, C.L. and Dolnick, B.J., 1987, 5-Fluorouracil augmentation of dihydrofolate reductase RNA containing contiguous exon and intron sequences in KB7B cells, *J. Biol. Chem.* 262:5433.

Will, C.L. and Dolnick, B.J., 1989, 5-Fluorouracil inhibits dihydrofolate reductase precursor mRNA processing and/or nuclear mRNA stability in methotrexate-resistant KB cells, *J. Biol. Chem.* 264:21413.

DISCUSSION OF DR. DOLNICK'S PRESENTATION

Dr. Moran: First, these types of studies that you have been doing and a few others have been doing are really facinating. Everytime I get in a discussion on this topic with somebody they bring up the question, well how do you know it's a direct effect of FU into these species and it's not due to synchronization of cells?

Dr. Dolnick: That's a good question Rick. I don't know whether these species are cell cyle regulated I think they're spliced in the process and they go throughout the cell cycles so they may not be regulated. But the other point you raised about how do you know it's a direct effect is real appropriate and I think the answer is we don't know. I know that FU has a lot of indirect effects on other messenger RNA's I didn't mention here. I think it's probably generally not known because the guy who does the work isn't interested in fluorouracil per se, believe it or not, but found that if you treat cells with fluorodeoxyuridine for about 30 min some histone m-RNA's get degraded. It's probably not due to incorporation it's an indirect effect. There are indirect effects no question about it. What amazes me is how little we really know about RNA effects.

Dr. Peters: Dr. Dolnick, have you analyzed more patients of m-RNA thymidylate synthase?

Dr. Dolnick: If I understand the question you asked, if we've analyzed more than we've shown. These are the only two samples where we have before and after. So the answer is no.

Dr. Peters: Collaborates with Peter Danenberg's using PCR methods we have analyzed about 30 patients and we didn't find any relation between the expression of TS and the enzyme activity.

Dr. Dolnick: I'm sorry. I'm having a hard time understanding. You're saying he did get an increase in message but didn't get a correlation between message and enzyme?

Dr. Peters: There's is no correlation between the message and enzyme activity.

Dr. Dolnick: Is he getting a decrease in enzyme activity?

Dr. Peters: Enzyme activity was decreased but so we looked both at the inhibited activity and the total activity afterward.

GENETIC VARIATION IN THYMIDYLATE SYNTHASE CONFERS RESISTANCE TO 5-FLUORODEOXYURIDINE

C. Todd Hughey, *Karen W. Barbour, *Franklin G. Berger, and Sondra H. Berger

Departments of Basic Pharmaceutical Sciences and *Biological Sciences
University of South Carolina
Columbia, SC   29208

ABSTRACT

The human colorectal tumor cell line HCT 116 was resistant to the cytotoxic effects of 5-fluorodeoxyuridine (FdUrd). The response to FdUrd was increased only slightly by the presence of 10 µM folinic acid (CF). HCT 116 formed FdUMP and $CH_2H_4PteGlu$ polyglutamates after exposure to FdUrd and CF. The sensitivity to FdUrd correlated well with the extent of TS inhibition. The role of TS in the resistance of the cells to FdUrd was examined. HCT 116 expresses two TS enzymes, which differ in pI. The more basic TS has been detected in only HCT 116 cells. The other TS is identical in pI to the enzymes detected in other human cells. The variant TS differs from the common by His replacement of Tyr at residue 33. The variant TS exhibited a 3-fold lower affinity for FdUMP than the common TS. The enzymes co-expressed in HCT 116 exhibited an FdUMP binding constant similar to that of the variant TS. TS-deficient cells were transfected with cDNAs encoding the two TS polypeptides. Transfectants expressing the variant TS were more resistant to FdUrd cytotoxicity than cells expressing the common TS. Thus, the structural variation in TS reduced enzyme affinity for FdUMP and conferred resistance to FdUrd.

INTRODUCTION

5-Fluoropyrimidine drugs such as 5-fluorouracil (FUra) and 5-fluorodeoxyuridine (FdUrd) are utilized in the therapy of cancers of the breast, gastrointestinal tract, pancreas, and head and neck. A major mechanism of action underlying the cytotoxicity of these drugs is inhibition of the enzyme, thymidylate synthase (TS). TS catalyzes the formation of thymidylate (TMP) from the substrates, deoxyuridylate (dUMP) and 5,10-methylenetetrahydrofolate ($CH_2H_4PteGlu$). The fluoropyrimidine metabolite, 5-fluorodeoxyuridylate (FdUMP), a substrate analog of dUMP, binds tightly to the enzyme in the presence of the folate substrate, $CH_2H_4PteGlu$. A ternary complex is formed, resulting in the loss of enzyme activity and depletion of TMP that is required for DNA biosynthesis.

*Novel Approaches to Selective Treatments of Human Solid Tumors: Laboratory
and Clinical Correlation* Edited by Y. M. Rustum, Plenum Press, New York, 1993

That inhibition of TS by FdUMP underlies the antitumor activity of the flouropyrimidines is suggested by clinical studies utilizing protocols that are designed to increase the TS-directed actions of fluoropyrimidine agents. An increased objective response has been observed in patients receiving a fluoropyrimidine agent in combination with calcium leucovorin (citrovorum factor, CF) (reviewed in 1). The inclusion of CF is thought to increase the action of the fluoropyrimidine at TS by providing a source of $CH_2H_4PteGlu$ required for the tight binding of FdUMP to TS. While clinical response to fluoropyrimidines is increased by CF, the majority of patients receiving the combination have no demonstrable increase in tumor response. Furthermore, patients that respond to the combination have no significant increase in survival relative to nonresponders. These observations suggest that innate and acquired resistance mechanisms are barriers to the effective use of fluoropyrimidines in the clinic. Since TS is a primary target of fluoropyrimidine-CF therapy, variation in enzyme levels or affinity for the ligands involved in inhibition may underlie clinical resistance.

Regulation of mammalian TS expression is thought to occur at the transcriptional, post-transcriptional, and translational levels (2,3). Studies of the relationship between TS levels and response to FdUrd in human gastrointestinal tumor cells revealed that, in general, cells with higher TS expression are more resistant to FdUrd (4,5). This has clinical relevance since TS levels vary significantly in breast and colon tumors (6,7). Human gastrointestinal and pharyngeal tumor cells have been isolated that have acquired resistance to high levels of FdUrd. In these cells, TS is expressed at high levels due to amplification of the TS gene (8,9). TS gene amplification was identified in a human colorectal tumor that exhibited progression during FUra-CF chemotherapy (10). These studies, in total, demonstrate that variation in TS gene copy number or in the regulation of TS expression can affect the response of tumor cells to fluoropyrimidines.

The affinity of TS for ligands involved in enzyme inhibition may be altered by TS structural gene variation or by post-translational modification of the TS polypeptide. TS that is altered in FdUMP binding was isolated from tumor cells selected for resistance to FdUrd in culture and in the mouse (11,12). Variation in FdUMP binding has also been observed in TS isolated from human colon tumors (13). Structural variation in TS has been identified in cell line HCT 116 derived from a human colorectal tumor not previously exposed to 5-fluoropyrimidines (5). HCT 116 is more resistant to the cytotoxic effects of FdUrd than six other human colorectal tumor cell lines (5). Two TS polypeptides are expressed in HCT 116 cells, as detected by isoelectric focusing (5). The more basic TS, designated as the variant TS, has been detected only in HCT 116 cells. The other TS, designated as the common TS, is identical in charge to the enzymes detected in other human cells. The genes encoding the TS polypeptides differ by a single base change that results in the replacement of evolutionarily-conserved Tyr33 by a histidine residue in the gene encoding the variant TS (14). The role of the structural variation in the resistance of HCT 116 to 5-fluoropyrimidines and the effect of the structural variation on enzyme affinity for ligands involved in inhibition have been investigated. The data, presented in this report, indicate that the structural variation alters the affinity of the TS polypeptide for FdUMP and confers resistance to 5-fluoropyrimidines in cells expressing the variant polypeptide.

METHODS

Cell Culture and Growth Conditions

The human colorectal tumor cell line HCT 116 was maintained in RPMI 1640 medium supplemented with 5% fetal bovine serum. Cells were depleted of folates by growth for 12 days in folate-free RPMI 1640 medium supplemented with 5% charcoal-stripped fetal bovine serum and hypoxanthine, thymidine, and glycine as described previously (15). In all studies with HCT 116, the cells were folate-depleted. A subline of HCT 116 (HCT 116/200) that is resistant to 200 nM FdUrd by overexpression of TS was isolated by adaptation to progressively increasing concentrations of FdUrd (9). Cloning of the HCT 116/200 population led to the isolation of HCT 116/200-clone 10, which overexpresses the common TS, and HCT 116/200-clone 11, which overexpresses the variant TS (9). HCT 116/200 clones were maintained in RPMI 1640 medium supplemented with 10% fetal bovine serum, 100 nM FdUrd, and 10 μM CF. The clones were grown for 12-14 days in drug-free medium before TS isolation. The TS-deficient subline of V79 Chinese hamster lung (CHL) cells (kindly provided by Robert L. Nussbaum, University of Pennsylvania School of Medicine) was maintained in Dulbecco's modified Eagle medium supplemented with 10% fetal bovine serum and 10 μM thymidine (16).

For determination of growth response to FdUrd, HCT 116 cells were exposed to varying concentrations of CF for 24 hr, then to CF and varying concentrations of FdUrd for 3 hr. The cells were then grown in CF-supplemented medium for 5-6 cell generations, after which cell growth was determined by protein analysis. TS-deficient CHL cells transfected with cDNAs encoding human TS (17) were exposed to varying concentrations of FdUrd continuously for 3 cell generations, after which growth was determined by protein analysis.

Analysis of FdUMP and $CH_2H_4PteGlu$

For analysis of FdUMP pools, HCT 116 cells were exposed to either 30 nM or 10 μM CF for 24 hr, then to CF and varying concentrations of FdUrd and CF for 3 hr. The acid-soluble nucleotides were extracted from the cells by 5% trichloroacetic acid and quantitated as described previously (18).

For analysis of $CH_2H_4PteGlu$, HCT 116 cells were exposed for 24 hr to varying concentrations of CF. Folates were extracted from the cells and quantitated by a ligand binding assay as described previously (15). The glutamyl chain-length distribution of $CH_2H_4PteGlu$ derivatives was determined by denaturing isoelectric focusing gel electrophoresis of ternary complexes formed among extracted folates, $[^{32}P]$ FdUMP (20 Ci/mmol), and human HEp-2/500 TS as described previously (15).

FdUMP Binding Constants for TS

TS was partially purified from HCT 116 cells by ammonium sulfate fractionation (19). TS from HCT 116/200 clones was purified to apparent homogeneity by successive ammonium sulfate fractionation and Affigel blue-agarose, 10-formylfolate-Sepharose, and DEAE-cellulose chromatography by established procedures (19-21). The apparent K_D value for FdUMP binding to partially purified TS was determined by modification of a previously described procedure (15). TS (3.0 nM FdUMP binding sites) was incubated with 0.3-300 nM $[6-^3H]$ FdUMP and 150 μM (6RS) $CH_2H_4PteGlu$ in a reaction supplemented with 100 mM NaF and 15 mM CMP (22). For determination of apparent K_D values for FdUMP binding to purified TS, 1.7 nM FdUMP binding sites were incubated with 0.5-32 nM $[6-^3H]$ FdUMP and 150 μM (6RS) $CH_2H_4PteGlu$ as described previously (23). Protein-bound FdUMP was determined after adsorption of unbound radiolabel by charcoal as described previously (18). Apparent K_D values were determined by computer-assisted analysis of data graphed according to the Scatchard equation (24).

TS Activity and Levels

TS activity in situ was determined by modification of a previously described procedure (25). Cells in monolayer were incubated with medium supplemented with 1 μM

[5-H] dUrd (2.5 Ci/mmol) for 2 hr. Reactions were terminated by trichloroacetic acid (final concentration, 0.2 N) and unreacted radiolabel adsorbed by charcoal as described previously (18). The data were expressed as dpm ^3H_2O formed per min per mg total cell protein.

TS levels were determined by utilizing [6-^{3}H] FdUMP and $CH_2H_4PteGlu$ as described previously (5). The data are based on the assumption that 1.7 moles of FdUMP are bound per mole of TS.

RESULTS

The effect of CF on the response of HCT 116 cells to FdUrd is shown in Table 1. A 300-fold increase in CF concentration increased the response to FdUrd only 1.4-fold. At 10 μM CF, HCT 116 cells were 5-fold more resistant to FdUrd than two other human colorectal tumor cell lines (15). The basis for the resistance of HCT 116 to FdUrd at high CF concentrations was examined by determining the levels of intracellular metabolites derived from CF and FdUrd that are involved in TS inhibition and the effect of CF on TS inhibition. The levels of $CH_2H_4PteGlu$ derived from CF are shown in Table 1. The levels of $CH_2H_4PteGlu$ increased in cells exposed to increasing concentrations of CF. The glutamyl chain-length distribution of $CH_2H_4PteGlu$ derivatives was dependent on CF concentration; at 30 nM CF, the predominant derivative was the hexaglutamate, while at 10 μM CF, the majority of derivatives were lower in chain-length (data not shown). The pools of free FdUMP after FdUrd and either 30 nM or 10 μM CF are shown in Figure 1. FdUMP levels increased with increasing FdUrd. The pools of FdUMP were lower in cells exposed to 30 nM CF and 300 nM FdUrd than in cells exposed to 10 μM CF and 300 nM.

Table 1. Growth sensitivity, intracellular $CH_2H_4PteGlu$ pools, and TS inhibition after FdUrd and CF in HCT 116

CF Concentration (μM)	[a]ID$_{50}$ Growth (nM)	[b]$CH_2H_4PteGlu$ (pmol/mg prot)	[a]ID$_{50}$ TS (nM)
0.03	200	0.8 ± 0.1	4.3
10	140	2.1 ± 0.4	2.1

[a]Folate-depleted cells were exposed to CF for 24 hr and FdUrd and CF for 3 hr. Cell growth and residual TS activity were determined as described in Methods. The ID$_{50}$ is the concentration of FdUrd required to inhibit either cell growth or TS activity by 50% relative to untreated controls. The growth data are the average of 2 separate determinations each carried out in triplicate. TS inhibition was determined in 3 separate experiments.
[b]Folates were extracted from folate-depleted cells exposed to CF for 24 hr. $CH_2H_4PteGlu$ was quantitated as described in Methods. The data are the mean ± S.D. of 3 separate determinations. FdUrd; however, the pools of FdUMP at the ID$_{50}$ for FdUrd were similar, regardless of CF concentration (designated by arrows, Figure 1). The effect of CF on TS inhibition is shown in Table 1. TS inhibition was determined by measuring the endogenous activity remaining after exposure to FdUrd and CF. The concentration of FdUrd required for 50% inhibition of endogenous TS activity decreased by 2-fold between 30 nM and 10 μM CF.

The affinity of TS for FdUMP may play a role in the resistance to FdUrd cytotoxicity. The apparent K_D value for FdUMP binding to TS partially purified from HCT 116 cells was 3.3 x 10^{-10} M (Figure 2). A single class of binding sites was observed for FdUMP that were saturable under the conditions of the experiment. Since two structural

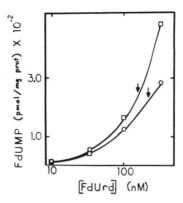

Figure 1. Pools of free FdUMP after FdUrd and CF in HCT 116. Folate-depleted cells were exposed to 30 nM (o) or 10 μM (□) CF for 24 hr, then to FdUrd for 3 hr in CF-supplemented medium. After drug removal, free FdUMP pools were determined as described in Methods. Free FdUMP pools are expressed as pmoles of FdUMP per mg protein. The data are the mean of 3 separate determinations.

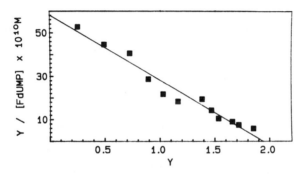

Figure 2. Scatchard analysis of FdUMP binding to TS from HCT 116. Partially purified TS (3 nM) was incubated with 0.3 - 300 nM [6-^{3}H] FdUMP and 150 μM (6RS)-CH$_2$H$_4$PteGlu as described in Methods. The data are the mean of 3 separate determinations. K$_D$ values were derived by linear regression analysis of Scatchard plots.

forms of TS are expressed in HCT 116 cells, the affinity of each structural form for FdUMP was determined. Sublines of HCT 116 were utilized that overexpress each TS form independently of the other (Figure 3). HCT 116/200 clone 10 overexpresses the common TS form observed in most human cell lines, while HCT 116/200 clone 11 overexpresses the variant TS form observed in only HCT 116 parental cells. TS was purified to apparent homogeneity from the clones. The K$_D$ values for FdUMP for the two enzymes were determined by equilibrium binding studies. The values, estimated by Scatchard analysis, were 1.1 x 10^{-10} and 3.1 x 10^{-10} M, for the common and variant TS, respectively.

The presence of a variant TS with a reduced affinity for FdUMP, relative to the common TS, may contribute to the resistance of HCT 116 to FdUrd. TS-deficient CHL cells were transfected with TS cDNA constructs encoding the common and variant TS. TS activity in situ and TS levels were measured in the transfectants prior to determination of FdUrd growth sensitivity. TS-deficient CHL cells had no detectable TS activity (Figure 4). The TS activity was slightly lower in the transfectants than in CHL parental cells. No significant difference in TS activity was observed between transfectants expressing the

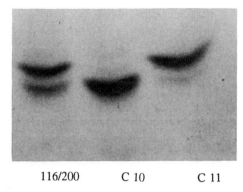

116/200   C 10   C 11

Figure 3. Isoelectric focusing gel electrophoresis of TS ternary complexes. Cell extracts of HCT 116/200 parental cells and clonal derivatives 10 and 11 were incubated with [^{32}P] FdUMP and $CH_2H_4PteGlu$ as described previously (26). The resulting ternary complexes were separated by isoelectric focusing electrophoresis and detected by autoradiography as described previously (26). Reproduced by permission from Plenum Press (26).

Table 2. Relationship between TS concentration and FdUrd sensitivity

[a]Cell Line	[b]TS Concentration (pmol/mg prot)	[c]ID$_{50}$ FdUrd (nM)
CHL-hTSY33 (I)	0.14 ± 0.02	1.2
CHL-hTSH33 (I)	0.59 ± 0.10	19
CHL-hTSY33 (II)	0.17	1.4
CHL-hTSH33 (II)	0.15	6.3

[a]CHL TS-deficient transfectants expressing the common (CHL-hTSY33) or variant TS (CHL-hTSH33) were isolated in two separate selections (I, II)
[b]TS concentration was determined by FdUMP binding as described in Methods. The data are the mean of 2-4 separate determinations.
[c]FdUrd sensitivity was determined in cells in monolayer exposed to FdUrd continuously for 3 days as described in Methods. The ID$_{50}$ is the concentration of FdUrd required to inhibit cell growth by 50% relative to untreated controls. The data is the mean of 3 separate determinations.

common and variant TS. The levels of TS in the transfectants, as determined by FdUMP binding, are shown in Table 2 (designated by I). Since transfectants with similar TS activity differed in TS levels, additional transfectants were isolated that exhibit similar TS levels (II, Table 2). The cytotoxicity of FdUrd to the four cell lines is shown in Table 2.

DISCUSSION

HCT 116 cells are highly resistant to the cytotoxic effects of FdUrd (5). The cells are also resistant to the cytotoxic effects of FdUrd-10 μM CF. The basis for the resistance to FdUrd-10 μM CF was investigated by examination of the intracellular levels of $CH_2H_4PteGlu$ and FdUMP formed from CF and FdUrd, respectively. The intracellular

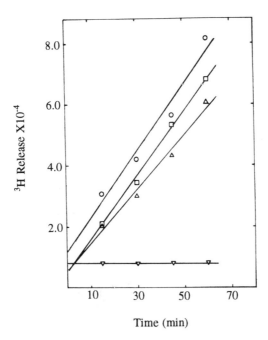

Figure 4. TS activity in situ in CHL cells. Cells in monolayer were incubated with 1 μM [5-^{3}H] dUrd as described in Methods. The amount of [^{3}H] H_2O released into the medium was determined as described in Methods. The rate of [^{3}H] H_2O formation in CHL parental cells (o), CHL TS-deficient cells (∇), and CHL TS-deficient transfectants expressing the common ($\square$) or variant (Δ) TS polypeptide is shown. The data are the mean of two separate experiments.

levels of FdUMP and $CH_2H_4PteGlu$ increased with increasing concentration of FdUrd and CF, respectively. At all concentrations of FdUrd, the levels of free FdUMP were higher in HCT 116 than in the human tumor cell line, HEp-2 (27). Since the response of HEp-2 cells to FdUrd is increased by 10-fold by 10 μM CF, the data suggested that the pools of FdUMP in HCT 116 were adequate for modulation of FdUrd cytotoxicity by 10 μM CF (28). In fact, at 10 nM FdUrd, the pools of free FdUMP in HCT 116 were 12-fold higher than the concentration of FdUMP binding sites in the cells (5). The levels of $CH_2H_4PteGlu$ at 10 μM CF were similar in HCT 116 and in two human colorectal tumor cells that are 5-fold more sensitive to FdUrd at this CF concentration. Moreover, the distribution of $CH_2H_4PteGlu$ polyglutamates in HCT 116 cells was similar to that in two human colorectal tumor cells that are sensitive to FdUrd at 10 μM CF (15). The glutamyl chain-length distribution of $CH_2H_4PteGlu$ was analyzed in the cells since TS exhibits a higher affinity for higher chain-length derivatives of $CH_2H_4PteGlu$ and ternary complexes comprised of higher chain-length derivatives are more stable (20,29). Thus, the resistance to FdUrd-10 μM CF is not due to lack of $CH_2H_4PteGlu$ formation or $CH_2H_4PteGlu$ polyglutamation.

In an effort to determine whether the resistance to FdUrd-10 μM CF was related to the extent of TS inhibition, TS activity remaining after exposure of cells to FdUrd and CF was measured. Increasing CF over 2.5 orders of magnitude increased TS inhibition by 2-fold. Over this CF concentration range, the response to FdUrd increased by 1.4-fold. The close correlation between extent of TS inhibition and FdUrd sensitivity suggested that TS is a primary determinant in the resistance of HCT 116 to FdUrd.

Mechanisms involving TS that are associated with resistance to FdUrd include elevation of TS levels and reduction in TS affinity for ligands involved in inhibition. Previous studies revealed that HCT 116 cells have TS levels similar to that of cells that are more sensitive to FdUrd (5). These studies also revealed that HCT 116 expresses two structurally distinct forms of TS. Since structural variation could underlie functional variation in TS, the affinity of the two TS forms for FdUMP was determined. A 3-fold difference in affinity was observed, with the variant TS having the lower affinity for FdUMP. The binding constant obtained for the variant TS was similar in value to the constant obtained for the two enzymes co-expressed in HCT 116 cells (Figure 2). In fact, a single class of binding sites was observed for the enzyme in HCT 116, which is a mixture of both forms. This result was unexpected based on the data obtained for the separate enzymes. The lack of resolution of two classes of binding sites may be due to the formation of TS heterodimers in cells expressing both TS polypeptides. In such a case, three different enzyme species in a ratio of 1:2:1 would be expected. Resolution of distinct binding classes in an enzyme population with an overall difference in binding constants of 3-fold would be unlikely.

The binding studies revealed that the variant TS has a lower affinity for FdUMP than the common TS. The effect of the functional variation on the response to FdUrd was examined in cells transfected with cDNAs encoding the common or variant TS. The growth studies were conducted in transfectants expressing similar TS activity. The transfectants differed, however, in the levels of TS, with cells expressing the variant TS having 4-fold higher enzyme levels. This is an important consideration, given the relationship between TS levels and FdUrd response. In transfectants with similar TS activity, cells expressing the common TS were 16-fold more sensitive to FdUrd than those expressing the variant TS. In transfectants expressing similar levels of TS, cells expressing the common TS were 4.5-fold more sensitive to FdUrd than those expressing the variant TS. Interestingly, HCT 116 200-clone 10, which overexpresses the common TS, was 4-fold more sensitive to FdUrd-10 μM CF than HCT 116/200-clone 11, which overexpresses the variant TS. TS levels were similar in the two clonal sublines (9). Thus, the substitution of Tyr33 by a histidine residue in human TS conferred resistance to FdUrd. The HCT 116 cell line was derived from the tumor of a patient with no previous exposure to 5-fluoropyrimidines. Whether TS variation, such as that identified in HCT 116, exists in human tumors is unknown. Evidence for TS variation in human tumors has been accumulating (7,13). The existence of variation in human TS, whether in the germ-line or in tumors, will impact upon the effective use of TS-directed chemotherapy.

REFERENCES

1.   Mini, E., Trave, F., Rustum, Y.M., and Bertino, J.R. Enhancement of the antitumor effects of 5-fluorouracil by folinic acid. Pharmac. Ther. 47:1-19 (1990).

2.   Jenh, C.-H., Geyer, P.K., and Johnson, L.F. Control of thymidylate synthase mRNA content and gene transcription in an overproducing mouse cell line. Mol. Cell. Biol. 5:2527-2532 (1985).

3.   Chu, E., Koeller, D.M., Casey, J.L., Drake, J.C., Chabner, B.A., Elwood, P.C., Zinn, S., and Allegra, C.J. Autoregulation of human thymidylate synthase messenger RNA translation by thymidylate synthase. Proc. Natl. Acad. Sci. USA 88:8977-8981 (1991).

4.   Washtien, W.L. Thymidylate synthetase levels as a factor in 5-fluorodeoxyuridine and methotrexate cytotoxicity in gastrointestinal tumor cells. Mol. Pharmacol. 21:723-238 (1982).

5.   Berger, S.H. and Berger, F.G. Thymidylate synthase as a determinant of 5-fluoro-2'-deoxyuridine response in human colonic tumor cell lines. Mol. Pharmacol. 34:474-479 (1988).

6.   Spears, C.P., Gustavsson, B.G., Berne, M., Frosing, R., Bernstein, L., and Hayes, A.A. Mechanisms of innate resistance to thymidylate synthase inhibition after 5-fluorouracil. Cancer Res. 48:5894-5900 (1988).

7.   Peters, G.J., van Groeningen, C.J., van der Wilt, C.L., Meijer, S., Smid, K., Laurensse, E., and Pinedo, H.M. Time course of inhibition of thymidylate synthase in patients treated with fluorouracil and leucovorin. Sem. Oncol. 19:26-35 (1992).

8.   Berger, S.H., Jenh, C.-H., Johnson, L.F., and Berger, F.G. Thymidylate synthase overproduction and gene amplification in fluorodeoxyuridine-resistant human cells. Mol. Pharmacol. 28:461-467 (1985).

9.   Berger, S.H., Barbour, K.W., and Berger, F.G. A naturally occurring variation in thymidylate synthase is associated with a reduced response to 5-fluoro-2'-deoxyuridine in a human colon tumor cell line. Mol. Pharmacol. 34:480-484 (1988).

10.   Clark, J.L., Berger, S.H., Mittleman, A., and Berger, F.G. Thymidylate synthase gene amplification n a colon tumor resistant to fluoropyrimidine chemotherapy. Cancer Treat. Rep. 71:261-265 (1987).

11.   Bapat, A.R., Zarow, C., and Danenberg, P.V. Human leukemic cells resistant to 5-fluoro-2'-deoxyuridine contain a thymidylate synthetase with lower affinity for nucleotides. J. Biol. Chem. 258:4130-4136 (1983).

12.   Jastreboff, M.M., Kedzierska, B., and Rode, W. Altered thymidylate synthetase in 5-fluorodeoxyuridine-resistant Ehrlich ascites carcinoma cells. Biochem. Pharmacol. 32:2259-2267 (1983).

13.   Danenberg, P.V. and Bapat, A.R. Thymidylate synthases isolated from human colon tumors have varied affinity towards 5-fluoro-2'-deoxyuridylate. Reg. Cancer Treat. 2:1-4 (1989).

14.   Barbour, K.W., Berger, S.H., and Berger, F.G. Single amino acid substitution defines a naturally occurring genetic variant of human thymidylate synthase. Mol. Pharmacol. 37:515-518 (1990).

15.   Davis, S.T. and Berger, S.H. Modulation of 5-fluoro-2'-deoxyuridine response by folinic acid in human colonic tumor cell lines: the role of thymidylate synthase. Mol. Pharmacol. 35:422-427 (1989).

16.   Nussbaum, R.L., Walmsley, R.M., Lesko, J.G., Airhart, S.D., and Ledbetter, D.H. Thymidylate synthase-deficient Chinese hamster cells: a selection system for human chromosome 18 and experimental system for the study of thymidylate synthase regulation and fragile X expression. Am. J. Hum. Genet. 37:1192-1205 (1985).

17.   Barbour, K.W., Hoganson, D.K., Berger, S.H., and Berger, F.G. A naturally-occurring tyrosine histidine replacement at residue 33 of human thymidylate synthase confers resistance to 5-fluoro-2'-deoxyuridine in mammalian and bacterial cells. Mol. Pharmacol. 42:242-248 (1992).

18.   Moran, R.G., Spears, C.P., and Heidelberger, C. Biochemical determinants of tumor sensitivity to 5-fluorouracil: ultrasensitive methods for the determination of 5-fluoro-2'-deoxyuridylate, 2'-deoxyuridylate, and thymidylate synthetase. Proc. Natl. Acad. Sci. USA 76:1456-1460 (1979).

19.   Dolnick, B.J. and Cheng, Y.-C. Human thymidylate synthetase derived from blast cells of patients with acute myelocytic leukemia. J. Biol. Chem. 252:7697-7703 (1977).

20.   Radparvar, S., Houghton, P.J., and Houghton, J.A. Characteristics of thymidylate synthase purified from a human adenocarcinoma. Arch. Biochem. Biophys. 260:342-350 (1988).

21.   Banerjee, C.K., Bennett, L.L., Jr., Brockman, R.W., Sani, B.P., and Temple, C., Jr. A convenient procedure for purification of thymidylate synthase from L1210 cells. Anal. Biochem. 72:248-254 (1982).

22.   Spears, C.P., Shahinian, A.H., Moran, R.G., Heidelberger, C., and Corbett, T.H. In vivo kinetics of thymidylate synthetase inhibition in 5-fluorouracil-sensitive and -resistant murine colon adenocarcinomas. Cancer Res. 42:450-456 (1982).

23.   Lockshin, A. and Danenberg, P.V. Biochemical factors affecting the tightness of 5-fluorodeoxyuridylate binding to human thymidylate synthetase. Biochem. Pharmacol. 30:247-257 (1981).

24.   Scatchard, G. The attractions of proteins for small molecules and ions. Ann. N.Y. Acad. Sci. 51:660-672 (1940).

25.   Yalowich, J.C. and Kalman, T.I. Rapid determination of thymidylate synthase activity and its inhibition in intact L1210 leukemic cells in vitro. Biochem. Pharmacol. 34:2319-2324 (1985).

26.   Berger, S.H., Davis, S.T., Barbour, K.W., and Berger, F.G. The role of thymidylate synthase in the response to fluoropyrimidine-folinic acid conbinations. Adv. Exptl. Med. Biol. 244:59-69 (1988).

27.   Berger, S.H. Biochemical factors which influence the action of 5-fluoropyrimidines on thymidylate synthetase. Ph.D. Thesis, State University of New York at Buffalo (1982).

28.   Evans, R.M., Laskin, J.D., and Hakala, M.T. Effect of excess folates and deoxyinosine on the activity and site of action of 5-fluorouracil. Cancer Res. 41: 3288-3295 (1981).

29.   Priest, D.G. and Mangum, M. Relative affinity of 5,10-methylenetetrahydro-folylpolyglutamates for the Lactobacillus casei thymidylate synthetase-5-fluorodeoxyuridylate binary complex. Arch. Biochem. Biophys. 210:118-123 (1981).

EXPERIENCE WITH 5FU + L-LEUCOVORIN

C. Erlichman[1], S. Fine[2], I. Kerr[3], W. Hoffman[4], C. Gorg[5], H-J. Schmoll[6], P. Preusser[7], H-J. Senn[8], B. Gustavsson[9]

[1] Princess Margaret Hospital, Toronto, Canada
[2] Credit Valley Hospital, Mississauga, Canada
[3] Sunnybrook Medical Centre, Toronto, Canada
[4] City Hospital Leverkusen, Leverkusen, Germany
[5] Phillipps University, Marburg, Germany
[6] Hannover Medical University, Hannover, Germany
[7] University Hospital, Munster German
[8] Kantonsspital, St. Gallen, Switzerland
[9] East Hospital, Gothenburg, Sweden

INTRODUCTION

The mainstay of treatment for patients with metastatic colorectal cancer is chemotherapy with the combination of 5-Fluorouracil (5FU) and Leucovorin (LV)[1]. This treatment has resulted in a response rate of 23 % compared to 11% for 5FU in nine randomized trials of patients with previously untreated metastatic colorectal cancer[2]. When compared to 5FU the odds ratio for response was 0.45 favouring 5FU + LV. The clinical modulation of 5FU antitumor effects supported the experimental studies in which the addition of LV in vitro led to increased cytotoxicity. This was related to stabilization of the thymidylate synthase (TS) folate and fluorodeoxyuridine monophosphate (FdUMP) complex and increased TS inhibition. Many questions of regarding the optimal dose of 5FU and LV and schedule of adminstration remain unresolved at present. The importance of the l-LV in the antitumor effect of 5FU and the potential for interference of d-LV in the action of l-LV must also be addressed.

The clinical formulation of LV commonly available is a racemic mixture of the biologically active l-LV and the chemical byproduct d-LV which constitutes approximately 50% of the total drug. The relative contribution of the d-LV in the clinical preparation is unclear. On a pharmacological basis d-LV could interfere with l-LV disposition at the level of l-LV distribution, metabolism or excretion. Furthermore,

Novel Approaches to Selective Treatments of Human Solid Tumors: Laboratory and Clinical Correlation Edited by Y. M. Rustum, Plenum Press, New York, 1993

the d-LV may interfere with l-LV transport into cells, polyglutamation and ultimately in the level of intracellular cofactor for binding to TS. The potential consequences of these interactions might include decreased antitumor effect of the combination of 5FU + LV or increased normal tissue toxicity. Although experimental studies have indicated that the d-LV does not interfere with l-LV at the cellular level clinical trials are necessary to determine whether there is a significant clinal impact.

METHODS AND RESULTS

We undertook a multicentre phase II trial of 5FU + l-LV in previously untreated patients with measurable metastatic colorectal cancer to determine the response rate, time to response, duration of overall response, time to progression, survival and toxicity spectrum. Toxicity was evaluated using WHO toxicity criteria. Patients eligible for study were treated with 5FU 370 mg/m^2/day and l-LV 100 mg/m^2/day x 5 every 28 days. The l-LV dose was selected on the assumption that the d-form in the standard clinical preparation was inert.

One hundred and twenty-six patients from 9 centres in Canada and Europe were entered on trial from July 1989 to July 1990. One hundred and nineteen patients were eligible and evaluable.

Stomatitis, diarrhoea, nausea and granulocytopenia were the most common toxicities.

The overall response rate was 22/119 (18.5%, 95% confidence limits 12.0 - 26.6).

DISCUSSION

The use of d,l-LV in trials ofthe combination of 5FU + LV has raised the possibility that the d-LV may interfere with the l-LV effect. This could lead to decreased antitumour effects or increased toxicity if the d-LV interferes with binding to TS or if it affects the drug disposition of l-LV. Thus this phase II study was designed to determine the clinical efficacy and toxicity in patients with metastatic colorectal cancer.

The results of our phase II trial indicates that l-LV toxicity is similar in pattern and severity as that of the d,l racemic mixture suggesting that the d-form is inert when considering side effects. The overall response rate is lower than that previously reported[1] for the racemic mixture in the same dose and schedule. However the confidence limits for the current study overlaps those of the previous trial. Furthermore the results of a recent meta-analysis[2] reported that the overall response rate was 23% which is consistent with the response rate seen in this study. The survival of patients entered in this trial was similar to that observed in the other trials. In conclusion, the combination of 5FU + l-LV at half the dose of d,l-LV has comparable antitumour effects to 5FU + LV with no significant difference in toxicity. Whether a higher dose of l - LV can increase the clinical efficacy of the 5FU + LV combination will require further study.

Machover et al[1] has recently reported the results of a phase I-II trial. The toxicity pattern was similar to that which we observed with respect to diarrhea and stomatitis but no grade 4 toxicity was reported. Interestingly, there was little neutropenia and no grade 4 toxicity observed with doses of 5FU which were higher than that used in this trial. The response rate of 52% is higher that what we observed. This may be due to differences in the patient population, the small sample size, the higher doses of 5FU administered to some patients in this dose seeking trial or the ability to administer the therapy every 21 days. Each of these factors can explain the differences between the results in our respective trials.

ACKNOWLEDGEMENTS

Supported by a grant from Lederle Cyanamid International Inc.

REFERENCES

1. Erlichman C, Fine S, Wong A, Elhakim T. A randomized trial of fluorouracil and folinic acid in patients with metastatic colorectal carcinoma. J Clin Oncol 1988; 6:469-75.

2. The advanced colorectal cancer meta-analysis project. Modulation of fluorouracil by leucovorin in patients with advanced colorectal cancer: Evidence in terms of response rate. J Clin Oncol 1992; 10:896-903.

3. Machover D, Grison X, Goldschmidt E, et al. Fluorouracil combined with the pure (6S)-stereoisomer of folinic acid in high doses for treatment of patients with advanced colorectal carcinoma - A phase-I-II study. J Nat Cancer Inst 1992; 84:321-327.

5-FLUOROURACIL COMBINED WITH THE PURE [6S]-STEREOISOMER OF FOLINIC ACID IN HIGH DOSES FOR TREATMENT OF PATIENTS WITH ADVANCED COLORECTAL CARCINOMA: A PHASE I-II STUDY OF TWO CONSECUTIVE REGIMENS

David Machover[1], Xavier Grison[1], Emma Goldschmidt[2],
Jacqueline Zittoun[3], Jean-Pierre Lotz[1], Gerard Metzger[2],
Jocelyne Richaud[4], Laurent Hannoun[5], Jeanine Marquet[3],
Thierry Guillot[6], Mia Bardon[6], Rémy Salmon[7], Alain Sezeur[8],
Serge Mauban[1], Rolland Parc[6], and Victor Izrael[1]

[1] Department of Oncology, Hospital Tenon, Paris; [2] Service of Hematology and Oncology, Hospital Paul Brousse, Villejuif; [3] Service of Hematology and Immunology, Hospital Henri Mondor, Créteil; [4] Service of Radiology, Hospital Tenon, Paris; [5] Service of Surgery, Hospital Saint Antoine, Paris; [6] Lederle Laboratories, Rungis; [7] Service of Surgery, Institut Curie, Paris; and [8] Service of Surgery, Hospital Rothschild, Paris, France

Folinic acid ([6R,S]-5-CHO-FH4) given in concentrations greatly exceeding that required for optimal cell growth, increases the cytotoxic action of 5-fluorouracil (5-FU) and fluorodeoxyuridine (FUdR)] *in vitro* (1,2,3). Potentiation of the antitumor activity of 5-FU by folinic acid has been demonstrated in patients with gastrointestinal carcinomas (4-10); this has resulted in effective palliative treatment for patients with advanced colorectal adenocarcinoma (6-7).

The cytotoxicity of the fluoropyrimidines has been found to be associated with the extent and duration of the inhibition of thymidylate synthase (TS) (2,11,12). The anabolite FdUMP binds to TS, leading, in the presence of the cofactor methylene tetrahydrofolate ($5,10\text{-}CH2\text{-}FH4$), to the formation of a ternary complex with concomitant enzyme inactivation. The time for dissociation of the ternary complex increases with increasing

Novel Approaches to Selective Treatments of Human Solid Tumors: Laboratory and Clinical Correlation Edited by Y. M. Rustum, Plenum Press, New York, 1993

81

concentrations of 5,10-CH2-FH4 (13). However, the maximal intracellular amount of 5,10-CH2-FH4 which can be attained after administration of its precursor, folinic acid, differs in various tumors, as demonstrated by experimental results in human cell lines (14). This may account, in part, for the variation in the antitumor activity observed in clinical trials of combined fluoropyrimidines and folinic acid (5-10,15,16).

The expansion of the cellular pools of folates involved in thymidylate (dTMP) synthesis could be limited by several mechanisms resulting from the pharmacologic properties of the clinical form of folinic acid available at present. Folinic acid consists of a mixture of equal parts of two stereoisomers differing in chirality at the C6 carbon of the pteridine ring. Only the levorotatory [6S]-5-CHO-FH4 is transformed into active folate cofactors. However, the [6R]-form is not inert; it has been shown to compete with the active [6S]-stereoisomer for uptake by cells (17-19). It was also reported to be an inhibitor and a substrate for mouse folylpolyglutamate synthetase (FPGS) (20), an enzyme that plays a critical role in the folate-induced modulation of the fluoropyrimidines (21,22). Furthermore, after IV administration of folinic acid, the [6R]-form accumulates in plasma at concentrations highly exceeding that of the [6S]-folinic acid (23,24).

Lack of interference of [6R]-5-CHO-FH4 with the enhancement of the cytotoxic effect of the fluoropyrimidines induced by the natural stereoisomer was reported in the human cell-lines CCRF-CEM (19) and HCT-8 (25), *in vitro*. Moreover, absence of interaction of the unnatural compound with rat and human FPGS has been recently reported (26). However, the demonstrated action of [6R]-5-CHO-FH4 at the cellular level of various experimental models (17,18,20) supports the possibility of a deleterious effect of the unnatural stereoisomer on the modulation of 5-FU and FUdR.

We conducted two consecutive phase I-II studies of 5-FU combined with high doses of [6S]-5-CHO-FH4 for treatment of patients with colorectal carcinoma in advanced stages. The 2 regimens of therapy described herein (*i.e.* Regimen I and Regimen II) differed by the dose and the mode of administration of the [6S]-folinic acid. The trial was designed to overcome the possible limitations of the mixture of the [6S] and [6R] stereoisomers of folinic acid in potentiating the antitumor activity of the fluoropyrimidines.

MATERIALS AND METHODS

PATIENTS (Table 1)

To be included in these 2 consecutive studies, each patient was required to have a previously resected colorectal carcinoma with visceral metastases which could be measured in two dimensions by CT scan. Eligibility criteria were those usually required for phase II studies and have already been reported (27).

The trials were designed for accrual of 25 eligible patients in each study who could be assessed for response. Twenty-six patients were entered in the first study (27) One patient was later excluded; she had cerebral metastases which had not been diagnosed because of an error in the interpretation of the initial CT scan. Twenty-five patients were evaluated for antitumor response, but all 26 patients entered were evaluated for toxicity.

Twenty-nine patients were entered in the second study. The planned accrual was modified during the study because 4 patients who were entered were initially thought to be non-assessable for response. After review of the cases, only 2 patients were later excluded (one with cerebral metastases, and one patient who died of hemorrhage due to gastric ulcer before the second course of therapy was initiated). Therefore, 27 patients entered in the second study were assessable for response.

TREATMENT PROTOCOLS

Therapy consisted of 5-day courses of [6S]-CHO-FH4 as calcium salt (Lederle Laboratories, Rungis, France) and 5-FU (Roche Laboratories, Neuilly sur Seine, France) repeated every 21 days.

In the first study (Regimen I), [6S]-Folinic acid was administered in a dose of 100 $mg/m^2/d$ by IV rapid injection. Immediately afterward, 5-FU was administered initially at a dose of 350 $mg/m^2/d$ by IV infusion for 2 hours. This dose was given to the first 18 patients entered in the trial. For the remaining patients, we chose to start with 375 $mg/m^2/d$ x 5d. In the subsequent study (Regimen II) [6S]-CHO-FH4 was administered daily in a dose of 100 mg/m^2 by IV rapid injection, followed by 250 mg/m^2 given as a 2-hour IV infusion Therefore, the total daily dose of [6S]-CHO-FH4 administered to patients treated with Regimen II was 350 mg/m^2. 5-Fluorouracil was administered to all patients treated with Regimen II at the initial dose of 375 mg/m^2/day. In both, Regimens I and II, the daily dose of 5-FU was raised stepwise by 25 mg/m^2 for each course if toxicity was either absent or mild at the previous dose level. The maximal daily dose of 5-FU was fixed at 550 mg/m^2.

The daily dose of 5-FU was reduced by 25 mg/m^2 in cases of World Health Organization (WHO) grades $\geq$ 3 oral mucositis, diarrhea, or dermatitis (28). Courses were repeated until treatment failure became evident in non-responding patients. In responding and in stable patients, cycles of treatment were repeated until massive tumor growth developed.

The [6S] form of folinic acid was obtained by crystallization from [6R,S]-5-CHO-FH4. This procedure provides [6S]-5-CHO-FH4 with less than 0.5% of the unnatural stereoisomer (Dr. C. Hancock, Cyanamid Lederle, personal communication).

TREATMENT EVALUATION

Patients were examined and monitored for antitumor response at regular intervals as previously described (27).

Objective responses were categorized as complete (CR), partial (PR), no change (NC), or progressive disease (PD), according to the WHO criteria (28). The times to disease progression were calculated from the date of initiation of therapy to the date when PD was first observed. The duration of response was calculated from the date when the response was

TABLE 1.PATIENT CHARACTERISTICS

CHARACTERISTIC	No. OF PATIENTS (%)	
	REGIMEN I	REGIMEN II
Entered	26	29
Eligible	25	27
Age in yrs (median; range)	(62.5; 42-82)	(61; 42-82)
42-49	3 (12)	2 (7)
50-69	17 (68)	21 (78)
70-82	5 (20)	4 (15)
Sex		
Male	13 (52)	14 (52)
Female	12 (48)	13 (48)
Performance status (Karnofsky)		
80-100	14 (56)	22 (81)
50-70	8 (32)	5 (18)
30-40	3 (12)	0
Site of primary		
Colon	18 (72)	17 (63)
Rectum	7 (28)	10 (37)
Disease-free interval (mos)		
0	12 (42)	16 (59)
2-12	5 (10)	4 (15)
>12	7 (28)	7 (26)
unknown	1	0
Plasma LDH level		
≤N	7 (28)	16 (59)
abnormal, ≤4xN	16 (64)	9 (33)
>4xN	2 (8)	1 (3)
unknown	0	1
Sites of tumor involvement		
Liver only[1]	16 (64)	12 (44)
Liver and other sites[1,2]	5 (20)	12 (44)
Other sites[3]	4 (16)	3 (11)

[1] The numbers of detectable liver metastases were: Regimen I: 1 in 3 patients (14%), 2 to 3 in 3 patients (14%), and ≥ 4 in 15 patients (71%); Regimen II: 1 in 5 patients (21%), 2 to 3 in 8 patients (33%) and ≥4 in 11 patients (46%). For patients treated with Regimen I one lobe was involved in 3 patients (14%) and 2 lobes in 18 (86%); for patients treated with Regimen II, one lobe was involved in 7 patints ((29%) and 2 lobes in 17 (71%).

[2] Including lung, bone, retroperitoneum, mediastinum and lymph nodes.

[3] Including lung, ovary, mediastinum, and lymph nodes.

first recorded. Survival times were calculated from the start of therapy and survival analysis was performed according to the method of Kaplan and Meier.

Patients were evaluable for assessment of improvement of performance status if their pretreatment Karnofsky PS was 80 or less. They were evaluable for gain in body weight if they had a loss of $\geq 5\%$ of their usual body mass. Patients were evaluable for symptomatic improvement if they had pain caused by the tumor. These abnormalities were considered improved if there was (a) an increase in Karnofsky PS by at least 20, (b) a weight gain of $\geq$ 5% compared to the pretreatment value, and (c) disappearance of pain recorded during the follow-up period.

PLASMA PHARMACOKINETICS OF FOLATES

Eight subjects with normal hepatic function, normal creatinine clearance, and no diagnosis of visceral failure were selected for study. They had had no prior folate therapy. Four patients were given [6S]-folinic acid at a dose of 100 mg/m^2 as an IV rapid injection, and 4 patients received the drug at a dose of 100 mg/m^2 by IV rapid injection followed by 250 mg/m^2 as an IV infusion given over 2 hours. Blood samples were drawn before drug administration and at 5, 10, 15, 20, and 30 minutes and 1, 2, 4, 8, 12, and 24 hours after the IV injection. Blood was collected in heparinized tubes containing ascorbic acid (1 mg/mL of blood). The plasma was stored at -20°C.

Assay for folates

The quantity of folates was measured on two bacterial strains as previously described (23). *Pediococcus cerevisiae* was used for the measurement of [6S]-5-CHO-FH4, and *Lactobacillus casei* for all [6S] folates. The detection limit of the method was 5 x 10^{-10} mol/L. The plasma concentration of the total amount of folates resulting from the metabolism of [6S]-5-CHO-FH4 was calculated as the difference between the measured concentrations of all folate forms and those of [6S]-5-CHO-FH4.

Data analysis

The data on the plasma concentration *versus* time (t) for [6S]-folinic acid were fitted to the equation $C(t) = Ae^{-\alpha t} + Be^{-\beta t}$ by the method of least squares to yield the elimination rate constants (α and β) and the half-lives (t 1/2) for each subject. Areas under the curve (AUC) were calculated from the observed values at each point using the linear trapezoidal method.

RESULTS

TOXICITY

REGIMEN I
The 26 patients treated with Regimen I received 351 courses of therapy (range, 5 to 21

courses per patient; median, 14 courses) which were evaluated for toxicity (Table 2). Dose-limiting toxic effects were grade 3 diarrhea, dermatitis, and oral mucositis.

Nineteen patients (73%) had at least one episode of diarrhea. The overall incidence of this toxic effect increased at increasing daily doses of 5-FU. Grade 3 diarrhea was observed in 8 patients (31%). Dermatitis was observed in 42% of patients; its overall incidence increased with increasing daily doses of 5-FU. Severe dermatitis occurred in 2 patients (8%); it appeared for doses of 5-FU $\geq$ 425 mg/m^2/d x 5 d. Twelve patients (46%) experienced at least one episode of stomatitis. Grade 3 stomatitis occurred in 4 patients (15%). We did not observe any trend toward an increase in the overall incidence of stomatitis with increases in the daily dose of 5-FU.

Grade 4 toxicity did not occur. Severe toxic effects required reduction of the dose of 5-FU by 25 mg/m^2/d x 5 d. In most cases, this resulted in the disappearance of the toxic effect, or in a decrease of the toxicity grade to acceptable levels in further courses.

The maximal doses of 5-FU which did not produce any dose-limiting toxic effect were explored in 23 patients. The numbers of patients who received at least 1 course of therapy at the maximal dose which did not produce dose-limiting toxic effects were: 10 patients (43%) at 550 mg/m^2/d x 5 d, 3 (13%) at 525 mg/m^2/d x 5 d, 5 (22%) at 500 mg/m^2/d x 5 d, 3 (13%) at 425 mg/m^2/d x 5 d, one (3%) at 400 mg/m^2/d x 5 d, and one patient (3%) at 350 mg/m^2/d x 5 d.

Moderate lacrimation occurred in 2 patients (8%). The incidence of this toxic effect increased at increasing daily doses of 5-FU and was often accompanied by mild rhinitis. Neurologic and cardiac toxicity was not observed. Mild nausea was common.

Myeloid toxicity was studied in 21 patients who had peripheral-blood cell counts each week at each of the dose levels which they received. The cell numbers measured on days 1, 8, and 15 from the start of each course at the 9 dose levels of 5-FU combined were [mean (range)] 4.72 (1.6-23.4), 4.43 (1.7-24), and 4.75 (1.8-34.1) x 10^9 cells/L and 304 (143-727), 298 (145-623), and 298 (170-647) x 10^9 cells/L for polymorphonuclears (PMN) and for platelets, respectively. Variance analysis did not disclose any significant decrease in the mean PMN numbers (F=0.81; df=2; p=0.44), nor in the mean platelet numbers (F= 0.48; df=2; p=0.61) which were measured each week in the 21 patients at each of the 9 dose levels explored in the present study.

REGIMEN II

The 29 patients treated with Regimen II received 298 courses of therapy which were evaluated for toxicity (Table 3). Dose-limiting toxic effects were grade 3 and grade 4 diarrhea, and grade 3 oral mucositis. Four patients (14%) had typical angina pectoris-like pain which reappeared at each course of therapy requiring cessation of treatment.

Diarrhea was observed in 45% of patients who had at least one episode of this toxic effect. Nine patients (31%) experienced mucositis, and 6 (20%) had dermatitis. One episode of grade 4 diarrhea occurred in one patient. We did not observe any trend toward an increased incidence or severity of these toxic effects with increasing daily doses of 5-FU.

The maximal doses of 5-FU which did not produce any dose-limiting toxic effect could be explored in 20 patients who were treated with Regimen II. The numbers of patients who received at least 1 course of therapy at the maximal dose which did not produce dose-limiting toxic effects were: 14 patients (70%) at 550 mg/m^2/d x 5 d, 2 (10%) at 525 mg/m^2/d x 5 d, 1 (5%) at 475 mg/m^2/d x 5 d, one (5%) at 450 mg/m^2/d x 5 d, one (5%) at 425 mg/m^2, and one patient (5%) at 375 mg/m^2/d x 5 d.

RESPONSE TO THERAPY

REGIMEN I

The median follow-up time for the 25 patients was 9 months (range, 3.5 - 15.2 months) at the time of evaluation of the study.

Objective response and survival (Table 4). Of the 25 patients, 3 (12%) attained CRs, and 10 patients (40%) had PRs. The overall response rate was 52% (95% confidence interval, 0.32 to 0.72), and the median duration of response was 5.6 months. Times to disease progression for responding patients ranged from 5.9 months to 15+ months (median, 9.2 months). The median time required for a response from the start of treatment was 2.8 months (range, 1.6 to 5.6 months).

The estimated probability of survival at 12 months was 73% (95% confidence interval, 0.53 to 0.93).

Palliative effect resulting from treatment is shown in Table 5.

REGIMEN II

The median follow-up time for the 27 patients was 15.5 months (range, 4 - 26 months) at the time of evaluation of the study.

Objective response and survival (Table 4). Of the 27 patients, 2 (7%) attained CRs, and 8 patients (30%) had PRs. The overall response rate was 37% (95% confidence interval, 0.19 to 0.55), and the median duration of response was 7 months. Times to disease progression for responding patients ranged from 6 to 15+ months (median, 8.9 months). The median time required for a response from the start of treatment was 4 months (range, 0.5 to 5 months).

The estimated probability of survival at 12 months was 67%.

Palliative effect resulting from treatment is shown in Table 5.

PLASMA PHARMACOKINETICS OF FOLATES (Figure 1)

[6S]-FOLINIC ACID AT THE DOSE OF 100 mg/m^2 ADMINISTERED AS A SINGLE IV RAPID INJECTION

[6S]-5-CHO-FH4 reached a maximal concentration of 52 ± 13.3 µmol/L. It was cleared from the plasma with t 1/2 α and t 1/2 β values of 7.2 ± 1.8 minutes and 126 ± 6.5 minutes, respectively. Concentrations of [6S]-5-CHO-FH4 above 10 µmol/L were maintained during 75 minutes from the time of the injection; the plasma levels were 5.8 ± 2.0 µmol/L and 0.05 ± 0.02 µmol/L 2 hours and 12 hours after the injection, respectively. Large amounts

TABLE 2. TOXIC EFFECTS. REGIMEN I

No. of Patients With Toxic Effects (%)

Toxic effect and Degree	Total [1,2]	Dose of 5-FU in mg/m2/d x 5 d [3] [Total No. of Patients per Dose Level]								
		350 [18]	375 [25]	400 [24]	425 [23]	450 [23]	475 [21]	500 [20]	525 [18]	550 [10]
Diarrhea [4]	19 (73)									
1		1 (6)	2 (8)	3 (13)	2 (9)	4 (17)	6 (29)	5 (25)	3 (17)	2 (20)
2		1 (6)	2 (8)	1 (4)	3 (13)	3 (13)	3 (14)	6 (30)	3 (17)	2 (20)
3		-	1 (4)	2 (8)	2 (9)	-	1 (5)	1 (5)	3 (17)	-
Oral Mucositis [5]	12 (46)									
1		1 (6)	2 (8)	1 (4)	5 (22)	2 (9)	-	2 (10)	2 (11)	1 (10)
2		1 (6)	-	1 (4)	-	-	2 (10)	1 (5)	1 (6)	1 (10)
3		-	1 (4)	-	1 (4)	2 (9)	-	-	-	-
Dermatitis [6]	11 (42)									
1		-	-	-	2 (9)	-	-	5 (25)	4 (22)	3 (30)
2		1 (6)	3 (12)	1 (4)	-	-	-	1 (5)	-	-
3		-	-	-	1 (4)	-	2 (10)	-	-	-
Lacrimation	13 (50)									
Mild		-	2 (8)	1 (4)	4 (17)	3 (13)	3 (14)	5 (25)	2 (11)	3 (30)
Moderate		-	-	-	-	-	-	1 (5)	2 (11)	-

[1] The 26 patients were given 351 courses of therapy; all were evaluated for toxicity.
[2] The table includes patients who experienced at least 1 episode of toxicity of any degree at all of the dose levels which they received.
[3] The table includes patients with the highest grade of toxicity experienced after all of the courses which they received at the indicated dose level.
[4] WHO grades: 1, transient, < 2 days; 2, tolerable, > 2 days; 3, intolerable, requires therapy; 4, dehydration.
[5] WHO grades: 1, soreness; 2, ulcers, can eat solids; 3, ulcers, requires liquid diet; 4, alimentation not possible.
[6] WHO grades: 1, erythema; 2, dry desquamation; 3, moist desquamation, ulceration; 4, exfoliative dermatitis.

TABLE 3. TOXIC EFFECTS. REGIMEN II

No. of Patients With Toxic Effects (%)

Toxic effect and Degree	Total [1,2]	Dose of 5-FU in mg/m2/d x 5 d [3] [Total No. of Patients per Dose Level]							
		375 [10]	400 [22]	425 [28]	450 [19]	475 [23]	500 [14]	525 [17]	550 [16]
Diarrhea [4]	13 (45)								
1		1 (10)	4 (18)	2 (7)	3 (15)	3 (13)	2 (14)	2 (12)	2 (12)
2		1 (10)	2 (9)	2 (7)	1 (6)	1 (5)	3 (22)	2 (12)	2 (12)
3		-	-	1 (4)	1 (6)	-	-	-	-
4		-	1 (5)	-	-	-	-	-	-
Oral Mucositis [5]	9 (31)								
1		1 (10)	1 (5)	1 (4)	1 (6)	2 (8)	3 (22)	4 (23)	1 (6)
2		-	-	1 (4)	-	-	1 (7)	-	1 (6)
3		-	1 (5)	-	1 (6)	1 (5)	-	1 (7)	1 (6)
Dermatitis [6]	6 (20)								
1		-	1 (5)	1 (4)	-	1 (5)	1 (7)	2 (12)	2 (12)
2		1 (10)	1 (5)	1 (4)	-	-	-	-	-
Lacrimation	8 (27)								
Mild		-	1 (5)	3 (11)	2 (12)	2 (8)	4 (29)	3 (18)	3 (19)
Thoracic pain[7]	4 (14)								

[1] The 29 patients were given 298 courses of therapy; all were evaluated for toxicity.
[2,3,4,5,6] See footnotes on Table 2
[7] Angina pectoris-like pain.

TABLE 4. RESPONSE TO THERAPY

RESPONSE TO THERAPY	NO. OF PATIENTS (%)	DURATION (mos)
REGIMEN I [1]		
CR	3 (12)	(3.3, 7.6, 11.5)
PR	10 (40)	(median, 5.2, range, 3.2+ -15.2)
NC + PD	12 (48)	
Total	25 (100)	
REGIMEN II [1]		
CR	2 (7)	(4, 10+)
PR	8 (30)	(median, 7, range, 1.5+ -9.5)
NC + PD	17 (63)	
Total	27 (100)	
OVERALL		
CR + PR	23 (44)	
Total	52 (100)	

[1] For patients treated with Regimen I, the median follow-up at the time of evaluation was 9 mos. (range, 3.5-15.2 mos), and that for patients treated with Regimen II was 15.5 months, (range, 4-26 months).

TABLE 5. PALLIATIVE EFFECT OF TREATMENT

TYPE OF EFFECT	NO. OF PATIENTS (%)	
	REGIMEN I (Total NO, 25)	REGIMEN II (Total NO, 27)
Improvement in PS by ≥ 20		
Evaluable	14	9
Yes	13 (93)	6 (67)
No	1 (7)	3 (33)
Weight gain > 5%		
Evaluable	17	6
Yes	16 (94)	5 (83)
No	1 (6)	1 (17)
Relief of pain		
Evaluable	13	7
Yes	12 (92)	4 (57)
No	1 (8)	3 (43)

of folate metabolites appeared rapidly, reaching a mean maximal concentration of 15 μmol/L 10 minutes after injection; at 12 hours, their plasma level was 1.31 ± 0.26 μmol/L. Folate metabolites consist mainly of methyl tetrahydrofolate, as demonstrated in previous studies (23,24). AUCs were 40.3 ± 11.7 μmol/L x h, and 51.7 ± 1.7 μmol/L x h for [6S]-5-CHO-FH4 and for folate metabolites, respectively.

[6S]-FOLINIC ACID AT THE DOSE OF 100 mg/m^2 ADMINISTERED AS A RAPID IV INJECTION FOLLOWED BY A 2-HOUR INFUSION OF 250 mg/m^2

[6S]-5-CHO-FH4 reached a maximal concentration of 58 ± 13.5 μmol/L.10 minutes after start of the injection Concentrations of [6S]-5-CHO-FH4 above 10 μmol/L were maintained during approximately 6 hours from the start of the injection; the plasma levels were 57.5 ± 16.6 μmol/L and 3.57 ± 0.7 μmol/L 2 hours and 12 hours after the injection, respectively. Folate metabolites reached a mean maximal concentration of 30.1 μmol/L 60 minutes after injection; at 12 hours, their plasma level was 1.93 μmol/L. AUCs were 261.6 μmol/L x h, and 136.9 μmol/L x h for [6S]-5-CHO-FH4 and for folate metabolites, respectively.

DISCUSSION

Numerous phase II (5,15) and phase III studies (3,6-10,16) of 5-FU given in combination with [6R,S]-5-CHO-FH4 for treatment of advanced colorectal carcinoma have been conducted in the past. These trials, in which the doses of both compounds and their schedules and modalities of administration were varied, produced response rates ranging from 15% to 54%. Up to now, it has not been possible to define the regimen that yields optimal antitumor activity.

We previously reported on a therapeutic scheme with 5-FU, 340 to 400 mg/m^2/d by IV infusion for 15 minutes, and [6R,S]-folinic acid, 200 mg/m^2/d by IV bolus for 5 consecutive days, repeated every 26 days (4,23). We are now reporting the results of two consecutive phase I-II studies which differ by the dose of the pure [6S]-folinic acid administered to patients. Regimen I comprised a dose of the [6S]-stereoisomer equivalent to that given in our initial trial in which we used the mixture of the two stereoisomers of folinic acid. It differed, however, in a slightly shorter time between courses, and a longer duration of the daily infusions of 5-FU (27) .Regimen II comprised [6S]-folinic acid at a dose 3.5-fold higher than that used in Regimen I; it was administered as a 2-hour infusion preceded by a loading dose, with the aim to achieve constant plasma concentrations of [6S]-CHO-FH4 greater than 10^{-5} mol/L for at least 2 hours from the time of start of the infusion (*i.e.* the duration of the infusion of 5-FU given concomitantly).

The plasma pharmacokinetic data obtained with [6S]-CHO-FH4 used in Regimen I are similar to those previously reported for [6S]-5-CHO-FH4 and for folate metabolites after rapid IV injection of [6R,S]-5-CHO-FH4 at a dose of 200 mg/m^2 (23); the reported *t* 1/2 β for [6S]-5-CHO-FH4 was 122 ± 20 minutes, and the mean plasma level of folate metabolites 12 hours after the injection was 1.7 μmol/L. The present plasma pharmacokinetic studies showed that [6S]-5-CHO-FH4 given as a single rapid IV injection at 100 mg/m^2, and as an IV

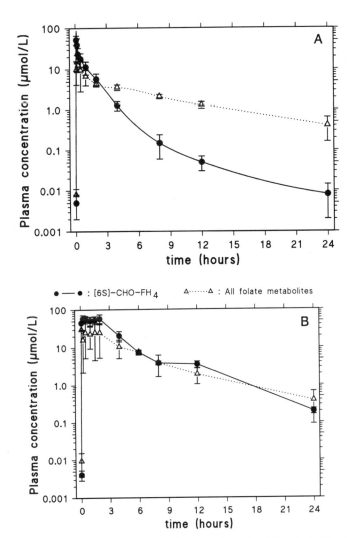

Figure 1. Plasma concentration of folates (mean ± SD) *versus* time after (A) a single IV injection of folinic acid at a dose of 100 mg/m² and (B) a rapid IV injection at 100 mg/m2 followed by an IV infusion at a dose of 250 mg/m2. Each study was performed in 4 subjects. Dark circles indicate [6S]-5-CHO-FH4, and open triangles indicate all folate metabolites which resulted from the metabolism of folinic acid.

injection of 100 mg/m^2 followed by a 2-hour infusion at 250 mg/m^2 produces plasma concentrations of the unchanged compound of $\geq 10^{-5}$ mol/L for 75 minutes, and for 6 hours after the start of the injection, respectively. These levels of folinic acid are within the concentration range required for maximal potentiation of the fluoropyrimidines *in vitro* (1,2,11,25,29). We considered the plasma levels of [6S]-CHO-FH4, and the times during which these levels are maintained, important for trials of fluoropyrimidines and folinic acid because these parameters play a role in both the expansion and the retention of the intracellular folate pools involved in dTMP synthesis (14,30,31). Moreover, experiments in which human colorectal and bladder carcinoma cell lines were incubated with both 5-FU and [6R,S]-5-CHO-FH4 at varying durations of exposure have demonstrated that the more extensive the exposure to high concentrations of folinic acid, the greater is the cytotoxicity of a continuously present concentration of 5-FU (29).

It was noticeable from the plasma pharmacokinetic data reported here, that the ratio of the AUC of [6S]-CHO-FH4 to the AUC of the folate compounds resulting from its metabolism was lower when the folate was given according to the scheme of administration used in Regimen I than when it was given at 100 mg/m2 followed by a 2-hour infusion of 250 mg/m2. This finding suggests that saturation of the metabolic conversion of folinic acid occurs when large doses of [6S]-CHO-FH4 are administered.

The overall incidence of toxicity in our patients was high (Tables 2 and 3). However, the degree of toxicity was moderate and could be controlled by slight modifications in the daily doses of 5-FU. It was possible to give large amounts of 5-FU to most patients. Diarrhea, mucositis, dermatitis, and lacrimation were less frequent and less severe (except for 1 single episode of grade 4 diarrhea) in patients treated with Regimen II than in patients who received Regimen I. However, angina pectoris-like pain was observed in 4 patients who were treated with Regimen II. The reasons for these differences in toxicity are not known.

The incidence and severity of toxic effects observed in the present studies were less frequent and less severe than that reported in a previous study in which 5-FU was given as a 15-minute IV infusion in combination with [6R,S]-5-CHO-FH4, when the same daily doses of fluoropyrimidine are compared (4,23). Additional studies will be necessary for determining the cause of these differences in toxicity. However, previously reported data (32) suggest that the observed altered toxicity pattern might be due to the greater duration of the infusion of 5-FU used in the present study. The reduced toxicity rates produced by the treatment described here justify the administration of 5-FU by IV infusion for 2 hours in combination with [6S]-5-CHO-FH4.

The response rates observed in these studies were 52% (CR, 12%; PR, 40%) and 37% (CR, 7%; PR, 30%) for Regimen I and for Regimen II, respectively. These results are within the range obtained in previous studies of 5-FU combined with [6R,S]-5-CHO-FH4 for treatment of patients with advanced colorectal carcinoma. In these earlier studies, the mean response rates were 31% (range, 15% - 54%) for phase-II (5-15) and 29% (range, 15.5%-48%) for 6 reported phase-III trials (6-10,16). In the phase III studies, the mean response rate attained by patients treated with 5-FU as a single agent was 11.5% (range, 7%-18.4%).

The response rates achieved by patients treated with Regimen I and Regimen II were considered similar because their 95% confience intervals overlap. Therefore, we can not recommend to augment the daily dose of [6S]-CHO-FH4 above 100 mg/m2 given as a single rapid IV injection for additional potentiation of the antitumor activity of 5-FU.

Our results suggest that the [6S]-stereoisomer of folinic acid employed in the present study potentiates the cytotoxic effect of 5-FU in patients with colorectal carcinoma. However, differences in antitumor activity obtained with 5-FU given in combination with each of the two clinical formulations of folinic acid can be demonstrated only in adequate randomized studies.

ACKNOWLEDGEMENT

Sponsored by Lederle Laboratories, Rungis, France.

REFERENCES

1 ULLMAN B, LEE M, MARTIN DW Jr, et al: Cytotoxicity of 5-fluoro-2'-deoxyuridine: Requirement for reduced folate cofactors and antagonism by methotrexate. Proc Natl Acad Sci USA 75:980-983, 1978

2 KEYOMARSI K, MORAN RG: Mechanism of the cytotoxic synergism of fluoropyrimidines and folinic acid in mouse leukemic cells. J Biol Chem 263:14402-14409, 1988

3 PIEDBOIS P, BUYSE M, RUSTUM Y, et al, for the Advanced Colorectal Cancer Meta-Analysis Project: Modulation of 5-fluorouracil by leucovorin in patients with advanced colorectal cancer: Evidence in terms of response rate. J Clin Oncol 10:896-903, 1992

4 MACHOVER D, SCHWARZENBERG L, GOLDSCHMIDT E, et al: Treatment of advanced colorectal and gastric carcinomas with 5-FU combined with high-dose folinic acid: A pilot study. Cancer Treat Rep 66:1803-1807, 1982

5 ARBUCK SG: Overview of clinical trials using 5-fluorouracil and leucovorin for the treatment of colorectal cancer. Cancer 63:1036-1044, 1989

6 ERLICHMAN C, FINE S, WONG A, et al: A randomized trial of fluorouracil and folinic acid in patients with metastatic colorectal carcinoma. J Clin Oncol 6:469-475, 1988

7 POON MA, O'CONNELL MJ, MOERTEL CG, et al: Biochemical modulation of fluorouracil: Evidence of significant improvement of survival and quality of life in patients with advanced colorectal carcinoma. J Clin Oncol 7:1407-1417, 1989

8 PETRELLI N, HERRERA L, RUSTUM Y, et al: A prospective randomized trial of 5-fluorouracil and high-dose leucovorin versus 5-fluorouracil and methotrexate in previously untreated patients with advanced colorectal carcinoma. J Clin Oncol 5:1559-1565, 1987

9 PETRELLI N, DOUGLASS HO, Jr, HERRERA L, et al: The modulation of 5-fluorouracil with leucovorin in metastatic colorectal carcinoma: A prospective randomized phase III trial. J Clin Oncol 7:1419-1426, 1989

10. DOROSHOW JH, MULTHAUF P, LEONG L, et al: Prospective randomized comparison of fluorouracil versus fluorouracil and high-dose continuous infusion leucovorin calcium for treatment of advanced measurable colorectal cancer in patients previously unexposed to chemotherapy. J Clin Oncol 8:491-501, 1990

11. EVANS RM, LASKIN JD, HAKALA MT: Effect of excess folates and deoxyinosine on the activity and site of action of 5-fluorouracil. Cancer Res 41:3288-3295, 1981

12. SWAIN SM, LIPPMAN ME, EGAN EF, et al: Fluorouracil and high-dose leucovorin in previously treated patients with metastatic breast cancer. J Clin Oncol 7:890-899, 1989

12. LOCKSHIN A, DANENBERG PV: Biochemical factors affecting the tightness of 5-fluorodeoxyuridylate binding to human thymidylate synthetase. Biochem Pharmacol 30: 247-257, 1981

14. HOUGHTON JA, WILLIAMS LG, CHESHIRE PJ, et al: Influence of dose of [6RS] leucovorin on reduced folate pools and 5-fluorouracil-mediated thymidylate synthase inhibition in human colon adenocarcinoma xenografts. Cancer Res 50:3940-3946, 1990

15. MACHOVER D: Potentiation of the antitumor activity of the fluoropyrimidines by leucovorin: Rationale and clinical data. In: Pinedo HM, Rustum YM, eds. Leucovorin modulation of fluoropyrimidines: A new frontier in cancer chemotherapy. International congress and symposium series number 158. London - New York: Royal Society of Medicine Services, 1989: 1-9

16. VALONE FH, FRIEDMAN MA, WITTLINGER PS, et al: Treatment of patients with advanced colorectal carcinomas with 5-fluorouracil alone, high-dose leucovorin plus 5-fluorouracil, or sequential methotrexate, fluorouracil, and leucovorin: A randomized trial of the Northern California Oncology Group. J Clin Oncol 7:1427-1436, 1989

17. WHITE JC, BAILEY BD, GOLDMAN ID: Lack of stereospecificity at carbon 6 of methyltetrahydrofolate transport in Ehrlich ascites tumor cells. Carrier-mediated transport of both stereoisomers. J Biol Chem 253:242-245, 1978

18. SIROTNAK FM, CHELLO PL, MOCCIO DM, et al: Stereospecificity at carbon 6 of formyltetrahydrofolate as a competitive inhibitor of transport and cytotoxicity of methotrexate *in vitro.* Biochem Pharmacol 28:2993-2997, 1979

19. BERTRAND R, JOLIVET J: Lack of interference by the unnatural isomer of 5-formyltetrahydrofolate with the effects of the natural isomer in leucovorin preparations. J Natl Cancer Inst 81:1175-1178, 1989

20. SATO JK, MORAN RG: Interaction of methotrexate and citrovorum factor at folyl polyglutamate synthetase. Proc Am Assoc Cancer Res 3:312, 1984 (abstr)

21. ROMANINI A, LIN JT, NIEDZWIECKI D, et al: Role of polyglutamates in biochemical modulation of fluoropyrimidines by leucovorin. Cancer Res 51: 789-793, 1991

22. RADVADPAR S, HOUGHTON PJ, HOUGHTON JA: Effect of polyglutamylation of 5,10-methylenetetrahydrofolate on the binding of 5-fluoro-2'-deoxyuridylate to thymidylate synthase purified from a human colon adenocarcinoma xenograft. Biochem Pharmacol 38:335-342, 1989

23. MACHOVER D, GOLDSCHMIDT E, CHOLLET P, et al: Treatment of advanced colorectal and gastric adenocarcinomas with 5-fluorouracil and high-dose folinic acid. J Clin Oncol 4:685-696, 1986

24. NEWMAN EM, STRAW JA, DOROSHOW JH: Pharmacokinetics of diastereoisomers of [6R,S]-folinic acid (leucovorin) in humans during constant high-dose intravenous infusion. Cancer Res 49:5755-5760, 1989

25. ZHANG ZG, RUSTUM YM: Effects of diastereoisomers of 5-formyltetrahydrofolate on cellular growth, sensitivity to 5-fluoro-2'-deoxyuridine, and methylenetetrahydrofolate polyglutamate levels in HCT-8 cells. Cancer Res 51:3476-3481, 1991

26. McGUIRE JJ, RUSSELL CA. Biological and biochemical properties of the natural (6S) and the unnatural (6R) isomers of leucovorin and their racemic (6R,S) mixture. J Cell Pharmacol 2:317-323, 1991

27. MACHOVER D, GRISON X, GOLDSCHMIDT E et al. 5-Fluorouracil combined with the pure [6S]-stereoisomer of folinic acid in high doses for treatment of patients with advanced colorectal carcinoma. A phase I-II study. J Natl Cancer Inst 84: 321-327, 1992

28. WHO Handbook for reporting results of cancer treatment. Geneva, World Health Organization, 1979

29. MORAN RG, SCANLON KL: Schedule-dependent enhancement of the cytotoxicity of fluoropyrimidines to human carcinoma cells in the presence of folinic acid. Cancer Res 51:4618-4623, 1991

30. WRIGHT JE, DREYFUSS A, EL-MAGHARBEL I, et al: Selective expansion of 5,10-methylenetetrahydrofolate pools and modulation of 5-fluorouracil antitumor activity by leucovorin *in vivo.* Cancer Res 49:2592-2596,1989

31. HOUGHTON JA, WILLIAMS LG, de GRAAF SSN, et al: Relationship between dose rate of [6RS]-leucovorin administration, plasma concentrations of reduced folates, and pools of 5,10-methylene tetrahydrofolates and tetrahydrofolates in human adenocarcinoma xenografts. Cancer Res 50:3493-3502, 1990

32. LOKICH JJ, AHLGREN JD, GULLO JJ, et al: A prospective randomized comparison of continuous infusion fluorouracil with a conventional bolus schedule in metastatic colorectal carcinoma: A Mid-Atlantic Oncology Program study. J Clin Oncol 7:425-432, 1989

DISCUSSION OF DR. ERLICHMAN'S/DR. MACHOVER'S PRESENTATION

Dr. Sorensen: I have a question for both presenters regarding the future desirability of doing randomized studies with 6R vs 6S leucovorin. It may be that 6R is totally inert and everything that you have presented, both toxicity and response, seems to indicate that 6S and 6RS leucovorin give basically the same result except that 6RS was given double of 6S. Is there really any need for a randomized study? Why not just substitute 6S for 6RS leucovorin?

Dr. Erlichman: Well based on our data, the results would suggest that they're similar and if you wanted to do randomized trial you're really going to be looking at an equivalency study. My own feeling is that that's not the direction to go and I would accept that they're comparable based on the data that is available in terms of our own experience and the experience of Dr. Machover.

Audience: Dr. Machover you and Dr. Erlichman and other people in the audience have been advocates of stratifying patients in advanced disease studies according to the extent of hepatic resection and whether they have hepatic alone, hepatic with extra, hepatic intraabdominal disease. Dr. Erlichman is your trial overloaded with people with 50,60, 70% of hepatic involvement with extrahepatic disease which may effect response in the overall survival?

Dr. Machover: I think it should be done but I don't think with those small numbers of patients would address that problem. Whether they're overloaded or not in terms of comparing to other trials is hard to answer. I think what I can say is that the population we have is representative of the source of patients that one sees. We had patients on this trial that had extensive hepatic metastases and very few hepatic metastases and also patients that had no metastases to the liver as I showed you. The whole issue of how much liver disease is there is a valid one that has to be considered in the design of any Phase III trial and should be included. I guess my problem with that whole issue how do you define 50% of liver, vs 10% of liver? It's probably simpler at this point in time to say you know isolated to one lobe vs the other lobe vs both lobes. That's about as best as we can do right now. The techniques are being developed to try to quantify liver involvement but I don't think they're at a stage where we can use it on a routine basis.

Dr. Sobrero: Dr. Erlichman's trial all the patients had to be clearly progressive to be eligible for treatment. Did Dr. Machover's trial have the same requirement, because that may account for the difference in the response rate.

Dr. Machover: Of progressive disease?

Dr. Sobrero: Yes. Eligibility criteria. Do they include that the patient had to be clearly progressive?

Dr. Machover: Not really. We didn't wait a certain time to see if they progressed but they were metastatic all of them with disease progression.

Audience: What would be the future of 6S leucovorin, Dr. Machover?

Dr. Machover: Well, I don't think we can say at this time. I don't think that the randomized studies, studying the two isomers of folinic acid will bring new information because if the difference exists it will be small.

5-FLUOROURACIL MODULATION IN COLORECTAL CARCINOMA

EXPERIENCE OF GERMAN INVESTIGATORS

Claus-Henning Kohne-Wompner and Hans-Joachim Schmoll

Department of Hematology and Oncology
Hannover Medical School
Konstanty-Gutschow-Strasse 8
3000 Hannover 61
Germany

INTRODUCTION

5-Fluorouracil (FU) is the most active drug in the treatment of colorectal carcinoma. Treatment results have mainly improved by biochemical modulation of FU. Among the modulating agents folinic acid (FA) has been proven to increase response rates, while its impact on patients survival is still questionable[1]. Nevertheless FU in combination with FA is considered by most oncologists as standard treatment in advanced stages of colorectal cancer. Its biochemical rational is based on the observation that 5,10-methylene-tetrathydrofolate is necessary to stabilize the ternary complex between 5-fluoro-deoxy-uridine-monohposphate (FdUMP) and thymidilate synthase a key enzyme for thymidine incorporation into DNA[2].

Another approach that has gained interest is the use of interferon in combination with FU. The high response rates obtained by Wadler and colleagues in their phase II trials[3,4] has inspired investigators to study various schedules and dosages of both drugs.

The intracellular mechanisms for this drug combination may involve a direct effect on thymidylate snythase[5], reduction of the cellular uptake of thymidine[6], interfering with the enzyme thymidine kinase[7]. Interferons also produce changes in the pharmacokinetics of FU leading to a higher area under the concentration time curve (AUC)[8].

Resistance to FU is diverse[9]. It has been suggested that preformed extracellular nucleosides like thymidine may enter tumor cells by facilitated transport mechanisms[10] and thereby by-passing the FU induced depletion of thymidine triphosphate. The nucleoside transport inhibitor dipyridamole has been shown in preclinical models to interfere with the cellular uptake of nucleic acid precursors[11]. In tumor cells, in which the inhibition of thymidylate synthase is critical, dipyridamole results in depletion of thymidine triphosphate pools. Studies by Grem and Fischer[12-14] suggest a different mechanism. Dipyridamole in combination with FU potently inhibits the efflux of flyorodeoxy-uridine leading to an increased retention of intracellular FdUMP.

Novel Approaches to Selective Treatments of Human Solid Tumors: Laboratory and Clinical Correlation Edited by Y. M. Rustum, Plenum Press, New York, 1993

Hereby we summarize the results of trials conducted at the Medizinische Hochschule Hannover and report the observations of other German investigators in the treatment of advanced colorectal cancer.

Modulation of FU with folinic acid and dipyridamole

Within a period of 18 months 181 patients have been randomized to the following regimens:

Arm A: Folinic acid 300mg/m^2 as 10 minute infusion
      50 minutes later
      5-Fluorouracil 600mg/m^2 by i.v. push
      on three consecutive day repeated on day 22-29 for 6 cycles

Arm B: Folinic acid 300mg/m^2 as 10 minute infusion
      50 minutes later
      5-Fluorouracil 600mg/m^2 by i.v. push
      on three consecutive days
      plus
      Dipyridamole 3x75mg p.o. on day 0-4

All patients had histologically confirmed colorectal cancer and measurable disease that has shown tumor progression within a 8 weeks period. All patients were untreated prior to chemotherapy and had a Karnofsky performance status of at least 60%. Age was restricted to 75 years or less. Major endpoints of this randomized multicenter phase II trial were toxicity, response rate and progression free interval.

Due to protocol violations, 164 patients were evaluable for toxicity (Arm A: 86 patients, Arm B: 78 patients). Because of patient withdrawal after the first cycle, 164 patients could be evaluated for response (Arm A: 84 patients, Arm B: 73 patients).

The median age was 60 years in both treatment arms and the Karnofsky performance status (KPS) was equally distributed. 81% of patients had a KPS of 80% or above. The tumor burden did not differ in both groups with the exception of a higher rate liver metastases in the dipyridamole arm (75% vs. 88%, p=0.04).

The reqponse rate observed in both groups did not differ significantly as shown in table 1.

Table 1. Response rate in FU/FA vs. FU/FA/Dipyridamole

	FU/FA n=84	FU/FA/Dipyridamole n=73
CR	1%	3%
PR	16%	12%
MR	14%	8%
NC	51%	49%
CR/PR	17%	15%
PD	18%	27%

The median response duration for the responding patients in arm A was 4.1 months (range 2.5-5.1) and 7.2 months (range 3.8-8.6) with no statistical difference. The progression free interval reached a median of 8.1 months in both treatment arms.

Table 2. Overall toxicity in FU/FA vs. FU/FA/Dipyridamole

WHO Grade	FU/FA (n=86)			FU/FA/Dipyridamole (n=78)		
	2	3	4	2	3	4
Leucopenia	28%	12%	1%	27%	10%	4%
Mucositis		23%	11%		21%	5%
Diarrhea		26%	1%		14%	4%
Nausea/Vomitus		12%	4%		14%	4%

The maximum observed toxicity per patient (Table 2) was equal in both treatment arms and covered the range, that is expected with FU/FA. In arm B, headache was unique and lead to the denial of treatment in 3 patients after the first cycle.

We adminstered 384 cycles for patients treated without dipyridamole and 320 cycles for patients with dipyridamole.

The toxicity per cycle did show some difference for both treatment arms. The overall rate of leucopenia (grade 1-4 WHO) was 55% for arm A and 44% for arm B (p=0.005). Mucositis of grade 2-4 WHO was experienced in 19% of patients treated in arm A and in 11% of patients receiving the dipyridamole combination (p<0.01). We did not observe such a difference in respect to diarrhea.

The median survival time was 12.7 months (range 8.3 to 19.4 months) for all patients and did not differ significantly in both groups.

Modulation of 5-Fluorouracil with folinic acid and interferon

Our group has conducted two consecutive phase I-II trials for the combination of FU/FA plus interferon alpha-2b (IFN). In these trials we used the following schedules that differed in their FU dose:

Folinic acid	200mg/m^2 i.v. as 10 minute infusion d1-5
Alpha-2b Interferon	5 Mio IE/m^2 s.c. d1-5

Trial 1
5-Fluorouracil 500mg/m^2 d1-5 as 2 hour infusion or
600mg/m^2 d1-5 as 2 hour infusion

Trial 2
5-Fluorouracil 350mg/m^2 d1-5 i.v. push

In both trials we performed an individual dose escalation of FU in steps of 100mg/m^2 for trial 1 and steps of 50mg/m^2 in steps of 50mg/m^2 if in the previous cycle patients did not experience mucositis or diarrhea grade 2 WHO, leucopenia grade 3 WHO or platelet levels of grade 2 WHO. Maximal tolerated dose (MTD) was defined, if any of the above levels of toxicity occurred in a patient. In case of any toxicity above MTD, a FU dose reduction was performed.

All patients were previously untreated by chemo- or immunotherapy. they had histologically confirmed colorectal cancer and measurable disease with documented disease progression prior to therapy. A KPS of at least 60% and an age less than 75 years was required.

Major goals of this two trials was to determine toxicity and response rate for this three drug combination and to gain experience for the FU concentration suitable for further investigation.

Results of trial 1

43 Patients entered trial 1 and were evaluable for toxicity. Due to various reasons, 37 were evaluable for tumor response. The median age was 59 years (range 35-70 years) and 67% of patients were males. The majority (88%) of patients had a KPS of 80% or above. The liver (74%) was the major tumor site and only 27% of patients had only one tumor site involved.

27 Patients were started with an FU dose of 500mg/m^2 as 2h infusion and 16 patients began with FU 600mg/m^2 as 2h infusion.

The toxicity for the first cycle of the 27 patients started with FU 500mg/m^2 and for the 16 patients started on FU 600mg/m^2 is listed in table 3. Mainly gastrointestinal toxicity was observed but was more severe in the second starting dose level with pronounced mucositis, diarrhea and leucopenia. One patient died of severe diarrhea, mucositis and septicemia.

Table 3. Toxicity of the first cycle of patients starting on FU 500mg/m^2 (N=27) or 600mg/m^2 (n=6).

| | FU-starting dose | | | | | |
| | 500mg/m^2 (n=27) | | | 600mg/m^2 (n=16) | | |
WHO Grade	2	3	4	2	3	4
Leucopenia	7%	–	–	13%	6%	6%
Mucositis	19%	4%	–	25%	–	13%
Diarrhea	41%	–	–	19%	6%	6%
Nausea/Vomitus	15%	7%	–	19%	13%	–

The maximum observed toxicity is listed in table 4. Grade 3 and 4 (WHO) toxicities were mainly due to the toxicity experienced within the first cycle. Fever and flu like syndrome was a complaint of 84% of patients but no severe neurological side occurred. One female patient developed hyperthyroidism's during treatment.

Table 4. Maximum observed toxicity for all patients (n=43)

WHO Grade	2	3	4
Leucopenia	21%	14%	2%
Mucositis	44%	12%	5%
Diarrhea	51%	5%	2%
Nausea/Vomitus	26%	9%	–

3 of 27 patients (11%), who started on FU 500mg/m^2, experienced grade 3 or 4 (WHO) toxicity in contrast to 5 of 16 patients (31%), who started on FU 600mg/m^2. In this group FU dose reductions had to be performed more often.

37 patients were evaluable for tumor response. the response rate achieved with this schedule does not seem to be superior to FU/FA combinations alone (Table 5).

Table 5. Response rate with FU 2h infusion FA/INF

PR	8/37	22%
MR/NC	20/37	54%
PD	9/37	24%

Median time to progression was 4.3 months and median survival time was 11.3 months.

The results of this trial may be summarized as follows: the recommended FU-dose for further trials is 500 mg/m^2 as 2h infusion when combined with FA 200 mg/m^2 and alpha-2b interferon 9 Mio IE/m^2 as a d1-5 schedule. The response rate observed does not warrant further investigation with this schedule.

Results of Trial 2

Thirty patients entered trial 2 and were evaluable for toxicity. The median age was 57 years (range 34-70 years) and 66% of patients had a KPS of at least 80%. The majority of patients (71%) had liver involvement and only 32% of patients had only one tumor site.

The toxicity observed after the first cycle was substantial (Table 6) and was mainly gastrointestinal. Grade 3 and 4 (WHO) toxicity was seen in 16/31 (52%) of patients after the first cycle. Dose reduction for FU had to be performed within these patients. The majority tolerated an FU dose of 300 mg/m^2 as i.v. push.

Tumor response has been observed in 6 of 30 evaluable patients (20%) and does not suggest superiority over FU/FA alone (Table 7).

Table 6. Toxicity after the first cycle.

WHO Grade	2	3	4
Leucopenia	14%	–	–
Mucositis	10%	30%	–
Diarrhea	21%	18%	–

Table 7. Response rate observed with FU i.v. push FA/IFN

PR	6/30	20%
MR/NC	20/30	67%
PD	4/30	13%

Median time to progression after initiation of chemotherapy was 4.7 months and median survival 9.9 months.

The results of this trial indicate that when interferon alpha-2b is added to FU/FA in a d1-5 schedule, FU has to be reduced to 300 mg/m^2. This three drug combination increases toxicity by not efficacy and does not seem to be superior to other schedules containing FU/FA alone.

DISCUSSION

In contrast to other investigators, we constantly observe a lower response rate for FU/FA combination therapy. This is true for the dipyridamole study as well as for the FU/FA/IFN trials. today weekly high dose folinic acid plus bolus FU[15] or low dose folinic acid plus bolus FU as d1-5 schedule[16] is considered as standard treatment for patients with advanced colorectal cancer. Response rate achieved with either regimen are around 30-40% in randomized trials. These response rates are mainly reported by investigators from the United States, while European oncologists repeatedly found a lower rate of objective tumor regression (16-23%)[16-20] in randomized trials. The reason for this difference is unclear. Our patients differ from other trials. We only treat patients with documented disease progression prior to therapy. This is based on the clinical observation, that a substantial number of patients do not show any disease progression over a long period of time without treatment[21]. As on the other hand, chemotherapy may seldom induce complete remissions and partial responses may doubtfully have any impact on survival, we believe that no change without therapy is most beneficial for our patients. If patients exhibit disease progression prior to therapy, no change or minor remission may be considered as treatment success. In our patients tumor stabilization is achieved in approximately 80% of cases. Synchronizing patients to disease progression prior to therapy may represent an unfavourable subgroup of patients and may explain the low response rate observed in our trials. It seems doubtful that the three day schedule used in our dipyridamole trial is responsible for the low response rate. Loffler et al.[19] conducted a randomized trial of FU alone vs. FU/FA. They used a d1-5 schedule with FU 400 mg/m^2 plus or minus FA 100 mg/m^2 d1-5 qd29. An identical patient group (disease progression prior to therapy) as in our trials entered this study. Interestingly the objective response rate was 16% for both treatment arms (with or without FA) but patient survival was superior to FU/FA combination treatment. This was mainly due to the lower rate of patients that continued to have disease progression under chemotherapy. The survival time observed in our trials indicates that waiting for disease progression did not compromise patients survival. Although not randomized against a d1-5 schedule, we believe that our 3 day regimen may be an alternative to conventional 5 day schedules.

The results of our dipyridamole trial are truly negative. Dipyridamole in this dose and schedule did not improve response rates, time to progression or patient survival when compared to FU/FA alone. The toxicity per cycle was more pronounced for FU/FA although the cumulative dose intensity was higher for FU/FA/Dipyridamole (data not shown). A possible explanation for this observation may be that dipyridamole rather modulated FU pharmacology than the intracellular metabolism of FU. Remick et al.[22] observed a higher FU clearance and lower steady state when dipyridamole was present. This could explain the higher cumulative FU dose intensity despite a lower toxicity profile. Furthermore, in vitro dipyridamole concentrations used were above 0.5-5 mol of free dipyridamole[14]. Dipyridamole is highly bound to plasma proteins especially alpha-1-acid-glycoprotein and serum albumin[23]. Therefore the in vivo concentration of free dipyridamole is much lower than the total dipyridamole. Conventional oral dipyridamole with 75-100 mg four times daily may result in plasma levels of 3-5 mol equivalent to 0.05-0.15 mol in tissue cultures[23]. This concentration is substantially lower than the concentrations used in in vitro models with effects on FU cytotoxicity.

Our interferon studies demonstrated increased toxicity compared to FU/FA alone but an equal response rate when compared with FU/FA combinations. This experience has been made by other investigators[24-34]. It remains unclear whether interferon in this combination simply results in higher FU serum concentration or whether a truly enhancement of intracellular active FU metabolites occurs. As dipyridamole and interferon both modulate the pharmacology and intracellular metabolism of FU, it seems important to gain knowledge, which of these effects is superior in patients. Higher serum FU concentrations are simple achieved with a higher FU dose and may not need a modulator. At this point, it may be important to mention that pharmacological modulation of FU by folinic acid has not been described.

Treatment results for patients with advanced colorectal cancer are still to be improved. New approaches are warranted. Our group has just finished a phase II study with FU/methotrexate plus PALA. Inspired by the data reported by Ardalan et al.[35,36] and Loffler et al.[37], we currently conducted a 3-armed randomized phase II trial using a weekly schedule of FU as 24 h infusion modulated with FA or interferon or both modulators.

REFERENCES

1. Modulation of fluorouracil by leucovoroin in patients with advanced colorectal cancer: evidence in terms of response rate. Advanced Colorectal Cancer Meta-Analysis Project. J. Clin. Oncol. 10:896-903 (1992).
2. Keyomarski, K. and Moran, R.G. Folinic acid augmentation of the effects of fluoropyrimidines on murine and human leukemic cells. Cancer Res. 46:5529-5253 (1985).
3. Wadler, S., Lembersky, B., Kirkwood, J., Atkins, M. and Petrelli, N. Phase II trial of fluorouracil (5FU) and recombinant alpha-2 interferon (IFN) in patients (pts) with advanced colorectal cancer: An Eastern Cooperative Oncology Group (ECOG) study. Proc. Am. Soc. Clin. Oncol. 10:136 (1991).
4. Wadler, S., Schwartz, E.L., Goldman, M., et al. Fluorouracil and recombinant alfa-2a-interferon: an active regimen against colorectal carcinoma (see comments). J. Clin. Oncol. 7:1769-1775 (1989).
5. Chu, E., Zinn, S., Boarman, D. and Allegra, C.J. Interaction of gamma interferon and 5-fluorouracil in the H630 human colon carcinoma cell line. Cancer Res. 50:5834-5840 (1990).
6. Gewert, D.R., Moore, G., Clemens and M.J. Inhibition of cell division by interferons. The relationship between changes in utilization of thymidine for DNA synthesis and control of proliferation in Daudi cells. Biochem. J. 214:983-990 (1983).

7. Gewert, D.R., Shah, S. and Clemns, M.J. Inhibition of cell division by interferons. Changes in the transport and intracellular metabolism of thymidine in human lymphoblastoid (Daudi) cells. Eur. J. Biochem. 116:487-492 (1981).

8. Grem, J.L., Chu, E., Boarman, D., et al. Biochemical modulation of fluorouracil with leucovorin and interferon: preclinical and clinical investigations. Semin. Oncol. 19:36-44 (1992).

9. Peters, G.J. and van-Groeningen, C.J. Clinical relevance of biochemical modulation of 5-fluorouracil. ann. Oncol. 2:469-480 (1991).

10. Schwartz, J. Alberts, D., Einspahr, J., Peng, Y.M. and Spears, P. Dipyridamole (D) potentiation of FUDR activity against human colon cancer in vitro and in patients. Proc. Am. Soc. Clin. Oncol. 6:83 (1987).

11. Gati, W.P., Belt, J.A., Jakobs, E.S., Young, J.D., Jarvis, S.M. and Paterson, A.R. Photoaffinity labelling of a nitrobenzylthioinosine-binding polypeptide from cultured Novikoff hepatoma cells. Biochem. J. 236:665-670 (1986).

12. Grem, J.L. and Fischer, P.H. Alteration of fluorouracil metabolism in human colon cancer cells by dipyridamole with selective increase in fluorodeoxyuridine monophosphate levels. Cancer Res. 46:6191-6199 (1986).

13. Grem, J.L. and Fischer, P.H. Augmentation of 5-fluorouracil cyto-toxicity in human colon cancer cells by dipyridamole. Cancer Res. 45:2967-2972 (1985).

14. Grem, J.L. and Fischer, P.H. Enhancement of 5-fluorouracil's anticancer activity by dipyridamole. Pharmacol. Ther. 40:349-371 (1989).

15. Petrelli, N.J., Madajewicz, S., Herrera, L., et al. Biologic modulation of 5-fluorouracil with high-dose leucovorin and combination chemotherapy of 5-fluorouracil and cisplatin in metastatic colorectal adenocarcinoma. NCI Monogr. 189-192 (1987).

16. Poon, M.A.,O'Connel, M.J., Wieand, H.S., et al. Biochemical modulation of fluorouracil with leucovorin: Confirmatory evidence of improved therapeutic efficacy in advanced colorectal cancer. J. Clin. Oncol. 9:1967-1972 (1991).

17. Labianca, R., Pancera, G., Aitini, E., et al. Folinic acid + 5-fluoro-uracil (5-FU) versus equidose 5-FU in advanced colorectal cancer. Phase III study of "GISCAD" (Italian Group for the Study of Digestive Tract Cancer). Ann. Oncol. 2:673-679 (1991).

18. Nobile, M.T., Rosso, R., Sertoli, M.R., et al. Randomized comparison of weekly bolus 5-fluorouracil with or without leucovorin in metastatic colorectal carcinoma. Eur. J. Cancer 28A:1823-1827 (1992).

19. Loffler, T.M., Korsten, F.W., Reis, H.E., et al. Fluorouracil as mono-therapy or combined with folinic acid in the treatment of metastasizing colorectal carcinoma. Dtsch. Med. Wochenschr 117:1007-1013 (1992).

20. Di-Costanzo, F., Bartolucci, R., Calabresi, F., et al. Fluorouracil-alone versus high-dose folinic acid and fluorouracil in advanced colorectal cancer: a randomized trial of the Italian Oncology Group for Clinical Research (GOIRC). Ann. Oncol. 3:371-376 (1992).

21. Moertel, C.G., Fleming, T.R., Creagan, E.T., Rubin, J., O'Connell, M.J. and Ames, M.M. High-dose vitamin C versus placebo in the treatment of patients with advanced cancer who have had no prior chemotherapy. A randomized double-blind comparison. N. Engl. J. Med. 312:137-141 (1985).

22. Remick, S.C., Grem, J.L., Fischer, P.H., et al. Phase I trial of 5-fluorouracil and dipyridamole administered by seventy-two hour concurrent continuous infusion. Cancer Res. 50:2667-2672 (1990).

23. Szebeni, J. and Weinstein, J.N. Dipyridamole binding to proteins in human plasma and tissue culture media. J. Lab. Clin. Med. 117:485-492 (1991).

24. Inoshita, G., Yalavarthi, P., Murthy, S., et al. Phase I trial of 5FU, leucovorin (LV) and rHuIFN-A2a in metastatic colorectal cancer (CR Ca). Proc. Am. Soc. Clin. Oncol. 10:152 (1991).
25. Labianca, R., Pancera, G., Tedeschi, L., Dallavalle, G., Luporini, A. and Luporini, G. High dose alpha-2b interferon + folinic acid in the modulation of 5-fluorouracil. A phase II study in advanced colorectal cancer with evidence of an unfavourable cost/benefit ratio. Tumori 78:32-34 (1992).
26. Labianca, R., Pancera, Luporini, A., et al. Double modulation of 5-fluorouracil (5FU) with A2b interferon (IFN) and folinic acid (FA) in advanced colorectal cancer.
27. Punt, C.J.A., de Mulder, P.H.M., Burghouts, J.T.M. and Wagener, D.J.T. A phase I study of A-interferon (AIfN) in combination with 5fU and leucovorin (LV) in colorectal cancer patients (pts). Ann. Oncol. 1 (Suppl):92 (1990).
28. Punt, C.J.A., de Mulder, P.H.M. and Burghouts, J.T.M. A phase I-II study of high dose 5-fluorouracil (5FU), leucovorin (LV) and A-interferon (AIFN) in patients with advanced colorectal cancer. Proc. Am. Soc. Clin. Oncol. 10:150 (1991).
29. Kreuser, E.D., Hilgenfeld, R.U., Matthias, M., et al. A phase II trial of interferon alpha-2b with folinic acid and 5-fluorouracil administered by 4-hour infusion in metastatic colorectal carcinoma. Semin. Oncol. 19:57-62 (1992).
30. Bukowski, R.M., Inoshita, G., Yalavarthi, P., et al. A phase I trial of 5-fluorouracil, folinic acid, and alpha-2a-interferon in patients with metastatic colorectal carcinoma. Cancer 69:889-892 (1992).
31. Punt, C.J., de Mulder, P.H.M., Burghouts, J.T.M. and Wagener, D.J.T. Fluorouracil continuous infusion plus alfa interferon plus oral folinic acid in advanced colorectal cancer. Semin. Oncol. 19:208-210 (1992).
32. Weh, H.J., Platz, D., Braumann, D., et al. Phase II trial of 5-fluorouracil and recombinant interferon alfa-2B in metastatic colorectal carcinoma. Eur. J. Cancer 28A:1820-1823 (1992).
33. Sobrero, A., Nobile, M.T., Guglielmi, A., et al. Phase II study of 5-fluorouracil plus leucovorin and interferon alpha 2b in advanced colorectal cancer. Eur. J. Cancer 28A:850-852 (1992).
34. Cascinu, S., Fedeli, A., Fedli, S.L. and Catalano, G. Double biochemical modulation of 5-fluorouracil by leucovorin and cyclic low dose interferon alpha 2b in advanced colorectal cancer patients. Ann. Oncol. 3:489-491 (1992).
35. Ardalan, B., Singh, G. and Silberman, H. A randomized phase I and II study of short-term infusion of high-dose fluorouracil with or without N-(phosphonacetyl)-L-aspartic acid in patients with advanced pancreatic and colorectal cancers. J. Clin. Oncol. 6:1053-1058 (1988).
36. Ardalan, B., Chua, L., Tian, E.M. et al. A phase II study of weekly 24-hour infusion with high-dose fluorouracil with leucovorin in colorectal carcinoma. J. Clin. Oncol. 9:625-630 (1991).
37. Loffler, T.M., Weber, F.W., and Hausamen, T.U. Double modulation of 5-fluorouracil (FU) with leucovorin (LV) and interferon-alpha-2b in metastatic colorectal cnacer. Results of a pilot study. Onkologie 14 (suppl.):25 (1991).

AN OVERVIEW OF ADJUVANT TREATMENT OF COLON CANCER

Sheldon Fine

Credit Valley Medical Associates
Mississauga, Ontario
LSM 2VB

INTRODUCTION

Colorectal cancer ranks as a major cause of morbidity and mortality in North America. It is estimated that in excess of 175,000 incident cases and 50,000 deaths will occcur this year[1]. Although surgical resection has been the mainstay of curative therapy approximately 25% of patients with serosal penetration (T3 in the TNM classification/B2 in the Astler-Coller modification of Duke's) and 60% of those with regional nodal involvement will ultimately relapse and die. Although refinements in risk assessment appear to be possible using newer technologies (in particular DNA analysis as it relates to ploidy and 'S' phase content[2]) the underlying problem still remains, that is, to develop more effective strategies to prevent systemic relapse.

In this review I will summarize the previous experience presented in the literature as it relates to systemic adjuvant treatment and will outline current strategies that are being studied with a particular emphasis on pharmacological modulation.

Single Agent Trials

Although radiation had been shown to be an effective modality in cancer treatment, the patterns of relapse seen in colon cancer would generally preclude its importance. Five studies have been reported on the literature as of 1991 encompassing 2068 patients[3,4,5,6,7]. In these studies local recurrence accounted for a minority of first relapses (3.9% to 12.2%) whereas distant disease was seen in 11% to 30.8% of patients as their first evidence of failure (excluding combined local and distant relapses). With this information and the recognition that systemic chemotherapy may play an important role in the management of some solid tumors attempts have been made to use these agents in an adjuvant setting. The first non-randomized trials in colon cancer date back over 20 years and employed the use of nitrogen mustard given as an intraluminal injection following isolation of the bowel segment but without ligation of the venous or arterial supply. Following intraluminal injection systemic treatment with the same agent was given for two consecutive days. Rousselot and colleagues entered 122 patients between 1960 and 1967 using

Novel Approaches to Selective Treatments of Human Solid Tumors: Laboratory
and Clinical Correlation Edited by Y. M. Rustum, Plenum Press, New York, 1993

109

nitrogen mustard in the first 41 patients and 5-FU in the remaining 81[8]. The 5-year overall survival in node positive patients was 56% compared with 32% in historical controls. Lawrence et al. conducted a randomized trial of intraluminal and systemic treatment in 241 patients between 1968 and 1973 in an attempt to reproduce this observed benefit[9]. Their trial differed in several components; firstly, the systemic treatment component, 5-FU, was given orally for a period of one year and secondly almost one third of patients were excluded from the analysis following randomization primarily related to unresectability of the primary tumor. Nevertheless, in spite of these qualifications, this study proved to be negative in terms of demonstrating any improvement in disease free or overall survival. Subset analysis did not show any benefit in the node positive patients as suggested in the Rousselot paper. Since this time this approach to adjuvant treatment has been abandoned.

Prospective, controlled randomized trials of adjuvant treatment began in 1957 with the Surgical Adjuvant Colorectal Cancer Chemotherapy Study (SACCCS)[10] and the Veteran's Administration[11] both studying the role of thiotepa. This agent was chosen on the basis of animal studies and was given via the portal vein (in the SACCCS study) as well as intraperitoneally, and subsequently intravenously on the first two post operative days. A total of 1757 patients were studied and no advantage to therapy could be demonstrated either in terms of disease free survival or overall survival with follow-up exceeding 10 years.

Subsequent trials in North America concentrated on evaluating the efficacy of the fluoropyrimidines, either 5-FU or FUDR. Four trials were conducted between 1964 and 1976[10,11,12,13]. One thousand six hundred and seven patients were enrolled with essentially no benefit observed regardless of treatment dose, schedule or duration. A recent metaanalysis published by Buyse[4] in 1988 has confirmed this finding with a meager 3.4% 5-year survival "advantage" for 5-FU as compared to controls.

Do these results entirely negate the possible benefit of systemic chemotherapy? A careful examination of the trial designs employed would suggest that "optimal" use of either 5-FU or FUDR may not have been employed. In the case of the VA study of FUDR, only two cycles of treatment were given, the first, started on the first post operative day and the second repeated approximately 40 days later (note that 51% of patients did not receive a second course). In their follow-up study of 5-FU, once again only two courses of chemotherapy were delivered (dose in both courses 12 mg/kg, daily for five days with 6 weeks between cycles) due to a concern, in part, of increased post operative morbidity related to systemic chemotherapy. In hindsight, this problem proved to be an unfounded with 5.1% and 6.8% of treated and control patients, respectively, dying within the first three months. The VA trial of Prolonged Intermittent Infusion of 5-FU attempted to address the issue of long versus short treatment duration, but it used a different selection criteria for "high" risk patients and did not include a concurrent control arm of short duration treatment. Interestingly, only the Central Oncology Group attempted to evaluate systemic treatment using a trial design similar to those currently employed and in their study a trend to improved disease free and overall survival was seen. Subset analysis confirmed that the majority of benefit was related to an advantage in Duke's C patients.

Combination trials

Nonetheless, it was obvious that any improvement that might be achieved would require not only better trial design and dose scheduling but rather a fundamental improvement in the systemic treatment being used. Methyl-CCNU was incorporated into several second generation trials based on activity reported in a number of phase II trials as well as the results of the large (294 patients) SWOG trial[15] which compared 5-FU to 5-FU and Me-CCNU in the treatment of metastatic gastrointestinal cancer and demonstrated a response rate of 31.6% for the combination as compared to 9.5% for single agent 5-FU. In addition, BCG or its methanol extracted residue (MER) was added in several trials either as a separate arm or in combination with one of the chemotherapy regimens. The rational for its inclusion was based on limited human data published by Moertel[16] showing a 4% response rate in advanced colorectal cancer and the presence of an additive antitumor effect when BCG(MER) was added to chemotherapy in an animal system[17].

Once again, these trials did not show any significant advantage to treatment as compared to control patients when taken as a group. Even the NSABP C-01 trial[18] which initially demonstrated a small benefit to treatment has now been updated and at ten years of follow-up there has been a convergence of the survival curves such that statistical significance has disappeared. Somewhat more soberingly, however, with prolonged follow-up, it now appears that second malignancies, in particular blood dyscrasias are increased in the treatment arms which include a nitrosurea. Estimates from Boice's review place the relative risk at 12.4 (95% confidence limits 1.7 to 250), making this approach even less palatable[19].

Levamisole in the Adjuvant Setting

Following these generally negative results, the next group of protocols initiated looked at the potential merit of the "immune stimulant" levamisole. This agent had been used previously in veterinary practice as an antihelminthic[20] but was brought into clinical trials in man on the basis of laboratory data demonstrating a broad range of immunomodulatory effects including the enhancement of antibody production, augmentation of a variety of cellular immune responses, augmentation of chemotaxis and increases in delayed-type hypersensitivity reactions in humans[21,22,23,24]. Initial studies in advanced disease failed to demonstrate any specific anti-tumor effect when levamisole was given alone although one trial from Wisconsin suggested a prolongation of survival when levamisole as combined with 5-FU in the treatment of patients with advanced disease. These results, interestingly, have not been duplicated[25].

In the adjuvant setting, Verhaegen first reported a possible beneficial effect to Levamisole[26]. His study was a historically controlled trial comparing oral Levamisole to matched control patients with either colon or rectal primaries. The 5-year overall survival was 69% compared to 37% in the controls. Subset analysis suggested that the benefit was confined to colon patients only, with a striking difference in survival of 75% versus 15%. The obvious concerns relating to trial design, sample size, subset analysis and the poor outcome in the control patients are self-evident. In 1972 the Western Cancer Study Group[27] initiated a prospective, randomized trial of Levamisole versus a surgery only control arm. Levamisole was given weekly for a period of 18 months using a dose/schedule of 2.5 mg/kg per day orally on two consecutive days. Seventy eight patients were randomized in in a 2:1 ratio. Five year data demonstrates no difference in survival (controls 78%, treatment 68%). The EORTC has similarly reported the mature results of a similar trial encompassing 289 patients[28]. The 5-year overall survival is 51% versus 39%, treatment/control; p = 0.35. Of note, the disease free survivals are virtually identical; treatment arm 38%, control arm 35%.

Based on these results, or perhaps in spite of them, two randomized trials were undertaken to evaluate the relative merits of Levamisole with or without concomitant chemotherapy. Windle and colleagues[29] reported in the British Journal of Surgery on a three arm trial comparing control patients to those treated with 5-FU alone or a combination of 5-FU and Levamisole. Levamisole was given orally on three consecutive days in a dose of 150 mg/day. 5-FU was administered as an IV bolus on the first two post operative days in a dose of 1 gram and subsequently per os on a weekly basis for 6 months. A total of 131 patients were analyzed and a significant difference in the 5-year overall survival was seen in the combination arm (68% versus 55%). Chemotherapy alone did no better than control although the sample size, and route of administration of 5-FU have been put forward as possible criticisms. In 1989, the Mayo Clinic reported the results of their initial trial of Levamisole[30]. Once again a three arm trial design was employed (control, Levamisole, Levamisole and 5-FU) and in this program 5-FU was given with an initial IV bolus followed by weekly IV treatment. The schedule of Levamisole remained similar to the British trial, with the drug given in a dose of 50 mg TID for three consecutive days every two weeks. Treatment continued for a total of one year. Although a difference in 5-year overall survival was not seen for the entire group, in the subset of Duke's C patients a borderline advantage was achieved for those randomized to the combination (p = 0.05 log rank). On this basis, a large confirmatory study was launched by the NCI through the NCCTG/Intergroup. Results of this trial were first published in the New England Journal of Medicine in 1990 and subsequently updated at the American Society of Clinical Oncology annual meeting in 1992[31,32]. In this large study, two distinct groups were treated. With the absence of any benefit in the previous Mayo trial of Levamisole alone in the treatment of Duke's B2 tumors, 318 patients were randomized to either control or the combination of 5-FU and Levamisole. In the Duke's C patients, a third arm of Levamisole alone was added to clarify the effects of this agent. In this component of the study 929 patients were randomized. The most recent results confirm the advantage of the combination of 5-FU and Levamisole in preventing relapse and in prolonging survival in the subset of Duke's C patients. At present, with a median follow-up of 5 years, there have been 168 recurrence in the control arm, 162 in the Levamisole arm and 112 in the combination arm. The relative reduction in recurrence/cancer related death/and overall death rate are 39%, 32%, and 31%, respectively. Unfortunately patients with Duke's B tumors have shown no effect from the adjuvant treatment employed. These results formed the basis of a NCI clinical alert in 1990, and have resulted in a recommendation for adjuvant treatment with 5-FU and Levamisole for all patients with Duke's C tumors not enrolling in a clinical trial.

Portal Vein Infusion

In parallel with ongoing trials evaluating systemic chemotherapy, several protocols were initiated studying the merits of portal vein infusion. The rational of this approach was based on the preponderance of hepatic metastases seen in patients who ultimately recurred, the sense that the portal system and the liver itself might act as a "first station" for subsequent distant spread and the hope that higher doses of drug could be used to advantage in this peri-operative setting. Taylor and his colleagues[33] reported the final results of his provocative trial in 1985 after a 7 year hiatus from the initial report. This study randomized 244 patients to either surgery alone or surgery followed by a one week portal vein infusion of 5-FU and heparin (doses: 5-FU 1 gram/day, heparin 5,000 units/day). With more than 4 years of median follow-up, the overall survival of treatment versus control patient is 78% versus 58%, respectively. To further support the hypothesis, the relative recurrence rates in liver were examined and found to be significantly different (control 17.3%, treatment 4.2%). Although all curative stages of colorectal cancer were included only 20 Duke's A patients are represented. In a subset analysis the greatest benefit appeared to be in those patients with either Duke's B colon or Duke's C rectal cancer. Four confirmatory trials have subsequently been conducted and reported. Conflicting results abound. In the multi-institutional Dutch trial[34], portal vein infusion of 5-FU and heparin was found to decrease the incidence of hepatic metastases compared to their "control" arm of urokinase, but overall survival was no different. The NCCTG/Mayo compared treatment with 50% of the dose of 5-FU as used in the Taylor trial to no additional post operative treatment and found no difference in overall survival or hepatic recurrence rates[35]. The Swiss Group for Clinical Cancer Research[36] reported on improvement in 5-year overall survival using an infusion of 5-FU and Mitomycin (71% versus 57%) and finally the NSABP in a study duplicating the Taylor arms has recently found a statistically significant overall survival advantage to treatment (77% versus 71%) with 65.7 months of median follow-up[37]. In this study initial hepatic recurrence was not reduced as a result of treatment (9.6% treatment versus 8.1% controls) and the authors have speculated that the effect seen may simply be related to the systemic effect of the 5-FU. Nonetheless, at the present time, portal vein infusion remains an interesting area for further research, but not a standard treatment recommendation.

5-FU Modulation and Its Role in the Adjuvant Setting

Over a decade ago, Houghton[38] and others began to formally characterize the pathways of 5-FU activation and the determinates which affected its cytotoxicity. Although it cannot be completely quantified, it is clear that 5-FU cytotoxicity mediated through the binding of FdUMP to the enzyme thymidilate synthase is an important component of the drug's anti-tumor effect. Laboratory work confirmed that endogeneous folates were required to stabilize the binding of FdUMP to its target enzyme and that in the absence of sufficient substrate exogeneously supplied drug could enhance or restore responsiveness. Machover and his colleagues[39] reported significant enhancement in response rates using leucovorin to modulate the activity of 5-FU in patients with colon and gastric cancer and subsequent prospective randomized trials have confirmed this finding in advanced colorectal cancer. Studies evaluating the potential role of leucovorin modulated 5-FU in the adjuvant setting were started in 1987. In Canada, the NCI initiated a trial comparing 5-FU and Leucovorin, using a daily times 5 schedule, to no additional therapy in patients with T3NXMO and TXN1-2MO (Duke's B2 and C) cancers of the colon. This study accrued 370 patients in awaiting analysis. Because of the similarity in design the NCI(C) trial data will be pooled with that of the Instituto "Mario Negri" in Milan, as well as the Foundation Francaise de Cancerologie Digestive in Dijon. In the U.S.A., the NSABP has completed a study of 5-FU and Leucovorin, given on a weekly basis compared to MOF (their previous "standard"). This trial accrued 1081 patients as of April 14, 1989; preliminary results are pending. In order to evaluate the relative importance of leucovorin and levamisole both the Intergroup and the NSABP have conducted trials of complementary design comparing single arms of either 5-FU and leucovorin/levamisole to combinations of both. The NCCTG in collaboration with the NCI of Canada has recently completed a 4 arm trial studying both the significance of the addition of leucovorin to their standard of 5-FU and levamisole as well as addressing the issue of length of treatment. This trial may provide interesting pharmacological as well as financial insights as the dose of leucovorin is reduced to 20 mg in all arms. Moving beyond leucovorin as the sole modulator being examined in the adjuvant setting, the NSABP has recently initiated a 3 arm trial CO-5 which will attempt to integrate interferon into the combination.

FUTURE DIRECTIONS

Clearly, further improvement in our ability to reduce mortality in these tumors will depend in large part on the identification of increasingly more active regimens in the advanced disease setting. Although primary prevention through dietary modification is being studied, neither this nor current screening techniques is likely to have any immediate impact. Work is in progress studying additional means to modulate the activity of the fluoropyrimidines with hydroxurea[40], PALA[41], and dipyridamole[42]. Some of these trials appear encouraging at this time. In addition, alteration in the scheduling of treatment either with short term infusions of 5-FU +/- Leucovorin[43] appear to have some merit in increasing response rates and perhaps rescuing some patients who have been previously treated. Along similar lines, studies have been recently presented looking at the chronobiologic timing of chemotherapy with encouraging results[44].

The next decade is likely to see significant changes in the way we treat colon cancer. Whereas 15 years ago there was virtually no optimiism either in the palliative treatment of these patients or in the ability to offer effective adjuvant treatment, soon we may be asked to choose among several effective strategies. As a health care professional, I look forward to the challenge and the dilemma.

REFERENCES

1. C.C. Boring, T.S. Squires and T. Tong. Cancer Statistics CA 41(1): 19-36 (1991).
2. D.B. Moertel, L.L. Loprinzi, T.E. Witig, et al. The dilemma of B2 colon cancer. Is adjuvant therapy justified? A Mayo/North Central Cancer Therapy Group Study Proc. Am. Soc. Clin. Oncol. 9: 108 (1990).
3. E. Pihl, S.R. Hughes, F.T. McDermott, et al. Disease free survival and recurrence after resection of colorectal carcinoma. J. Surg. Oncol. 16: 333-341 (1981).
4. C. Willett, J.E. Tepper, A. Cohen, et al. Local failure following curative resection of colonic adenocarcinoma. Int. J. Radiation Oncology Biol. Phys. 10: 645-651 (1984).
5. A.H. Russell, D. Tong, L.E. Dawson, et al. Adenocarcinoma of the proximal colon. Sites of initial dissemination and patterns of recurrence following surgery alone. Cancer 53: 360-367 (1984).
6. N. Wolmark, B. Fisher, H. Rockette, et al. Postoperative adjuvant chemotherapy or BCG for colon cancer. Results from NSABP Protocol C-01. J. Natl. Cancer Inst. 80: 30-36 (1988).
7. M. Marangolo, G. Pezzuoli, E. Marubini, et al. Adjuvant chemotherapy with fluorouracil and CCNU in colon cancer. Results of a multicenter randomized study. Tumori 75: 269-276 (1989).
8. L.M. Rousselot, D.R. Cole, C.E. Grossi, et al. Adjuvant chemotherapy with 5-fluorouracil in surgery for colorectal cancer. Eight year progress report. Dis. Colon Rectum 15: 169-174 (1972).

9. W. Lawrence, Jr., J.J. Terz, S. Horsley, et al. Chemotherapy as an adjuvant to surgery for colorectal cancer. Ann. Surg. 181: 616-623 (1975).

10. W.J. Dixon, W.P. Longmire, Jr., and Holden, W.D. Use of triethylene-thiophosphoramide as an adjuvant to the surgical treatment of gastric and colorectal carcinoma. Ten-year follow-up. Ann. Surg. 173: 26-39 (1971).

11. Veterans Administrataion Adjuvant Cancer Chemotherapy Cooperative Group: The use of 5-fluorodeoxyuridine (FUDR) as a surgical adjuvant in carcinoma of the stomach and colorectum. Arch. Surg 86: 926-931 (1963).

12. G.A. Higgins, R.W. Dwight, J.V. Smith, et al. Fluorouracil as an adjuvant to surgery in carcinoma of the colon. Arch. Surg. 102: 339-343, (1971).

13. G.A. Higgins, R.C. Donaldson, C.W. Humpharcy, et al. Adjuvant therapy for large bowel cancer. Update of Veterans Administration surgial oncology group trials. Surg. Clin. North. Am. 61: 1311-1320 (1981).

14. M. Buyse, A. Zeleniuch-Jacquotte and T.C. Chalmers. Adjuvant therapy of colorectal cancer. Why we still don't know. JAMA 259: 3571-3578 (1988).

15. L.H. Baker, R.W. Talley, R. Matter, et al. Phase III comparison of the treatment of advanced gastrointestinal cancer with bolus weekly 5-FU vs. methyl-CCNU plus bolus weekly 5-FU. A Southwest Oncology Group Study. Cancer 38: 1-7, (1976).

16. C.G. Moertel, R.E. Ritts, Jr., A.J. Schutt, et al. Clinical studies of methanol extraction residue of Bacillus CalmetteGuerin as an immunostimulant in patients with advanced cancer. Cancer Res.

17. I. Yron, D.W. Weiss, E. Robinson, et al. Immunotherapeutic studies in mice with methanol-extraction (MER) fraction of BCG: Solid tumors. Natl. Cancer Inst. Monograph 39: 33-54 (1973).

18. NSABP Progress Report, Spring Meeting, April 12-15, 1992.

19. J.D. Boice, M.H. Green, J.Y. Killen, et al. Leukemia and preleukemia after adjuvant treatment of gastrointestinal cancer with semustine (Methyl-CCNU). N. Engl. J. Med. 309: 1079-1084 (1983).

20. A.H. Raeymaikers, F.T.N. Allewijn, J. Vandenberk, et al. Novel and broad spectrum anthelmintic tetramisole and related derivatives of 6-arylimidzole (2,1-b) thiazole. J. Med. Chem. 9: 545 (1988).

21. D.Tripodi, L.C. Parks, and J. Brugmans. Drug-induced restoration of cutaneous delayed hypersensitivity in anergic patients with cancer. N. Engl. J. Med. 289: 354-357, (1973).

22. U. Lewinski, G. Mavligit, and __ Hershe. Cellular immune modulation after a single high dose of levamisole in patients with carcinoma. Cancer 46: 2185-2194 (1980).

23. K. Meretey, G. Roo and R.N. Maini. Effect of histamine on the mitogenic response of human lymphocytes in its modification by cimetidine and levamisole. Agents Actions 11: 84-92, 1981.

24. G.S. DelGiacco, S. Tognella, A.L. Leone, et al. Interference of levamisole with inhibition of E-rosette formation by Hodgkin's disease and systemic lupus erythematous cytotoxic serum. Blood 53: 1002-1006 (1979).

25. E.C. Borden, T.E. Davis, J.J. Crowley, J.J., et al. Interim analysis of a trial of levamisole and 5-fluorouracil in metastatic colorectal carcinoma. In W.D. Terry, S.A. Rosenberg (eds): Immunotherapy of Human Cancer. New York, NY, Excerpta Medica, pp 231-235 (1982).

26. H. Verhaegen. Postoperative levamisole in colorectal cancer. Symposium on immunotherapy of malignant diseases. Vienna, Austria, 1977.

27. R.T. Chlebowski, S. Nystrom, R. Reynolds, et al. Long-term survival following levamisole or placebo adjuvant treatment of colorectal cancer: A Western Cancer Study Group Trial. Oncology 45: 141-143, (1988).

28. J.P. Arnaud, M. Buyse, B. Nordlinger, et al. Adjuvant therapy of poor prognosis colon cancer with levamisole. Results of an EORTC double-blind randomized clinical trial. Br. J. Surg. 76: 284-289, 1989.

29. R. Windle, P.R.F. Bell and D. Shaw. Five year results of a randomized trial of adjuvant 5-fluorouracil and levamisole in colorectal cancer. Br. J. Surg 74: 569-572 (1987).

30. J.A. Laurie, C.G. Moertel, T.R. Flemining, et al. Surgical adjuvant therapy of large-bowel carcinoma: An evaluation of Levamisole and the combination of Levamisole and Fluorouracil. J. Clin. Oncol. 7: 1447-1456 (1989).

31. C.G. Moertel, T.R. Fleming, J.S. MacDonald, et al. Levamisole and Fluorouracil for adjuvant therapy of resected colon carcinoma. N. Engl. J. Med. 322: 352-358 (1990).

32. C.G. Moertel, T. Fleming, J. MacDonald, et al. The Intergroup Study of Fluorouracil (5-FU) plus Levamisole (LEV) and Levamisole alone as adjuvant therapy for Stage C colon cancer. Abstract 457, p. 161 ASCO, Vol. 11, March 1992.

33. I. Taylor, D. Machin, M. Mullee, et al. A randomized controlled trial of adjuvant portal vein cytotoxic perfusion in colon cancer. Br. J. Surg. 72: 359-363, 1985.

34. J.C.J. Wereldsma, E.D.M. Bruggink, W.S. Meijer, et al. Adjuvant portal liver infusion in colorectal cancer with 5-fluorouracil/ heparin versus urokinase versus control. Cancer 65: 425-432 (1990).

35. R.W. Beart, C.G. Moertel, H.S. Wieand, et al. Adjuvant therapy for respectable colorectal carcinoma with fluorouracil administered by portal vein infusion. Arch. Surg. 125: 897-901 (1990).

36. R.J. Mayer and D.M. Stablein. Adjuvant colon cancer trials of the Gastrointestinal Tumor Study Group. In J.M. Hamilton, J.M. Elliott (eds.). NIH Consensus Development of Conference Adjuvant Therapy for Patients with Colon and Rectum Cancer. Program and Abstracts, Bethesda, MD, National Institutes of Health, 1990.

37. NSABP Progress Report, Spring Meeting, April 12-15, 1992.

38. J. Houghton, C. Schmidt and P.J. Houghton. The effect of derivatives of folic acid on the fluorodeoxyuridylate thymidylate synthetase covalent complex in human colon xenografts. Eur. J. Cancer Clin. Oncol. 18: 347-354 (1982).

39. D. Machover, E. Goldschmidt, P., Chollet et al. Treatment of advanced colorectal and gastric adenocarcinomas with 5-fluorouracil and high dose folinic acid. J. Clin. Oncol. 4: 685-696 (1986).

40. F. DiCostanzo, R. Bartolucci, L. Piccinini, et al. High dose folinic acid (FA) and 5FU alone or combined with Hydroxyurea (HU) in advaned colorectal cancer (CRC): A randomized trial of the Italian Oncology Group for Clinical Research (GOIRC). Abstract 463, p. 162, ASCO Vol 11, March 1992.

41. P.J. O'Dwyer, A.R. Paul, R. Peter, et al. Biochemical modulation of 5-fluorouracil (5-FU) by Pala: Phase II study in colorectal cancer. Proc. Am. Soc. Clin. Oncol. 8: 107, 1989 (abstract).

42. J.L. Grem. Biohemical modulation of fluorouracil by dipyidamole: Preclinical and clinical experience. Seminars in Oncology, Vol. 19, No. 2, Suppl. 3 (April), pp. 56-65 (1992).

43. B. Ardalan, L. Chua, E. Tian, et al. A Phase II study of weekly 24-hour infusion with high-dose fluorouracil with leucovorin in colorectal carcinoma. J. Clin. Oncol 9: 625-630 (1991).

44. G. Bjarnasson. Personal communication, 1992.

DISCUSSION OF DR. PETRELLI'S/DR. FINE'S PRESENTATION

Audience: Just a few quick couple of comments, questions. In regard to the GI toxicity of the RPMI regimen, it's interesting now looking at Dr. Petrelli's analysis of the NASP data if you look at our analysis of the intergroup study we have 28% grade 3 and 4 diarrhea you have about 25%. We put together the absolute numbers on that group of studies, we're talking about over 5000 patients being treated in real time. Probably half of them have received 5-FU/leucovorin so we really have I think a very significant powerful assessment of what the toxicity really is. It was very interesting in the NCI/Canada study which was predominantly a Dukes B2 study. I don't know whether you are beginning to look at flow cytometry or to determine if aneuploidy is a prognostic indicator. We've begun to do that in the Southwestern Oncology group studies. We've done over 200 Southwestern Oncology group patients who were on the original 5-FU/levamisol study. We find that about 60% of the patients did had aneuploid tumors and now we are in the process of analyzing that and are you going to be able to look at aneuploidy?

Dr. Petrelli: We will be able to look at aneuploidy and as I mentioned the trial was not designed to be predominantly B2 but these are how things were.

Audience: Just one other quick comment. Dr. Petrelli eluded to the issue of 5-FU/leucovorin combined with radiation. I quess this is sort of a toxicity weak. There is another study out there that's been ongoing now for almost precisely a year and that's our adjuvant gastric study, our national intergroup gastric study which randomizes patients between gastric resection vs 5-FU/leucovorin using the NCCTG schedule followed by 5000 rads of radiation with 5-FU/leucovorin being used in radiosensitizing doses followed by 2 more cycles of 5-FU/leucovorin in the NCCTG scheduling. We now have 66 patients all in the first year and we have taken a look at the toxicity and it's interesting that are no grade 4 diarrhea's at all. There are 2 patients of the 20 patients who have completed all therapy, there are 2 patients who have had grade 4 granulocytopenia but the GI toxicity is surprisingly well tolerated.

Dr. Petrelli: I know you're aware of Bruce Minsky's data at Memorial for the treatment of advanced rectal carcinomas where he's combining radiation with the modified Machover regimen of the 200 mg leucovorin and that seems effective. The diarrhea is very low also.

Audience: May I ask you a question regarding radiotherapy? You're using post-operative radiotherapy.

Dr. Petrelli: Yes. The RO2 is post-operative the intergroup is post-operative most of the trials in this country adjuvantly are post-operative. However, there is the potential for RO3 in discussions of having a pre-operative <u>vs</u> post-operative radiotherapy with 5-FU/leucovorin that is being considered at the momemt. But RO2 is post-operative and the intergroup is post-operative.

DOSE-DEPENDENT INHIBITION OF ASPARTATE CARBAMOYLTRANSFERASE IN PERIPHERAL BLOOD MONONUCLEAR CELLS IN PATIENTS RECEIVING N-(PHOSPHONACETYL)-L-ASPARTATE

Jean L. Grem,[1] Nanette McAtee,[2] James C. Drake,[1]
Seth Steinberg,[3] and Carmen J. Allegra[1]

National Cancer Institute
Navy Medical Oncology Branch[1]
National Naval Medical Center
Bldg. 8, Room 5101
Bethesda, MD 20889-5105

Cancer Nursing Service,[2] Clinical Center
and Biostatistics Branch,[3] Clinical Oncology Program
Division of Cancer Treatment, National Cancer Institute
National Institutes of Health
Bethesda, MD 20892

INTRODUCTION

N-(Phosphonacetyl)-L-aspartate (PALA) inhibits aspartate carbamoyltransferase (ACTase), the second step in *de novo* pyrimidine biosynthesis, resulting in a decrease in uridine and cytidine nucleotide pools and accumulation of phosphoribosylpyrophosphate.[1,2] Preclinical studies suggest that the biochemical effects of PALA may increase the metabolism of 5-fluorouracil (5-FU) and enhance its cytotoxicity through both RNA- and DNA-directed mechanisms.[2-6] Further, promising clinical activity has been reported with low dose PALA, 250 mg/m^2, given 24 hours prior to high-dose infusional 5-FU on a weekly schedule.[7,8]

Preclinical and clinical studies have shown that the addition of leucovorin to 5-FU enhances its efficacy.[9,10] Because preclinical studies suggest that extending the duration of 5-FU exposure improves the anticancer activity,[11,12] we first planned to determine the maximally tolerated dose of 5-FU given with high-dose leucovorin as a concurrent 72 hour infusion. We then planned to determine the maximally tolerated dose of PALA given 24 hours prior to the start of the highest tolerable dose of 5-FU/leucovorin. We wished to examine the biochemical effects of PALA by using a direct assay of ACTase activity in peripheral blood lymphocytes with each patient serving as his own control.

Novel Approaches to Selective Treatments of Human Solid Tumors: Laboratory and Clinical Correlation Edited by Y. M. Rustum, Plenum Press, New York, 1993

RESULTS

Clinical Toxicity

In the initial part of the study, cohorts of patients were entered at escalating dose levels of 5-FU starting at 1150 mg/m^2/d. The patients received a loading dose of leucovorin, 500 mg/m^2 followed by a concurrent 72 hr infusion of 5-FU with high-dose leucovorin (500 mg/m^2/d). Each individual was allowed to escalate to his/her own 5-FU tolerance, then PALA at 250 mg/m^2 was added the next cycle 24 hours prior to the start of 5-FU/leucovorin. Dose-limiting mucositis and myelosuppression occurred in 3 of 5 patients entered at 2300 mg/m^2/d of 5-FU. Therefore, the 2000 mg/m^2/d dose of 5-FU was selected for the remainder of the study. The dose of PALA was then escalated in 50% increments in separate patient cohorts. Dose-limiting toxicity was not observed the initial cycle until the 2848 mg/m^2 PALA dose level. Severe and life-threatening mucositis occurred in 2 of 3 patients; the latter patient also developed grade 4 pancytopenia and died on day 19.

The incidence of dose-limiting granulocyte toxicity did not appear to be related to PALA dose; overall, a granulocyte nadir below 500 cells/mm^3 eventually occurred in 29% of patients. Serious mucositis, diarrhea and skin rash occurred in 30% or fewer patients treated at or below 1266 mg/m^2 PALA. With 1899 mg/m^2 PALA, however, dose-limiting mucositis and skin rash ultimately occurred in 4 of 5 patients who received more than 3 cycles of therapy. CNS toxicity in the form of confusion and seizures occurred sporadically.

For patients entered at or above 1750 mg/m^2/d 5-FU, the delivered 5-FU dose intensity was similar over the range of 250 to 1266 mg/m^2 PALA. There was, however, a trend for lower 5-FU dose-intensity at the two highest PALA doses, 1899 and 2848 mg/m^2.

Biochemical Studies

To measure ACTase activity, we developed a sensitive, direct HPLC assay using [^{14}C]carbamoyl phosphate and excess cold aspartate. The product of the reaction, [^{14}C]carbamoyl aspartate, could be readily separated from the substrate as well as distal metabolites by anion exchange high performance liquid chromatography with an on-line liquid scinitillation detector. In preliminary experiments, we determined the optimal conditions for this cytosolic assay. The apparent K$_m$ of carbamoyl phosphate was 50 μM. Because PALA is a competitive inhibitor of ACTase with respect to carbamoyl phosphate, we selected 50 μM as the substrate concentration to increase our ability to detect inhibition of ACTase in patient samples. Peripheral blood mononuclear cells were isolated from patients pretreatment, and 24 and 96 hours after PALA. The cell pellets were reconstituted in 50 μl of 50 mM Tris HCl (pH 8.0); 30 μl of the supernatant was then added to a final reaction volume of 40 μl containing 5 μl of 16 mM aspartate (final concentration 2 mM) in 200 mM Tris HCl (pH 8.0), and 5 μl of [^{14}C]carbamoyl phosphate (approximately 80,000 dpm, sp. act. 17.6 μCi/μmol). The reactants were driven together by acceleration in a microcentrifuge for 10 seconds, then incubated at 37°C. Aliquots were taken at intervals up to 10 minutes and the reaction was quenched on ice by the addition of 500 μl of 0.001 M ammonium phosphate (pH 3.0). The sample was frozen on dry ice until the time of HPLC analysis.

Fig. 1 shows ACTase activity in cytosol from peripheral blood mononuclear cells obtained at baseline and 24 hours following PALA in 32 matched patient cycles as determined by the HPLC assay. The variation in the baseline ACTase activity was not statistically significant, but emphasizes the importance of comparing post-treatment enzyme activity to each patient's own baseline. ACTase activity was similar at baseline and 24 hours in patients treated with 250 mg/m^2 of PALA. A dose-dependent decrease in ACTase activity at 24 hours was apparent. The trend was significant ($P_2 = 0.004$, Jonckheere's Test for trend), and a meaningful decrease from baseline was seen at or above the 1266 mg/m^2 dose of PALA.

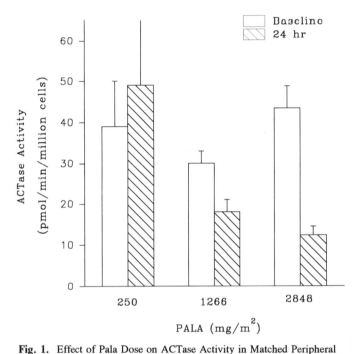

Fig. 1. Effect of Pala Dose on ACTase Activity in Matched Peripheral Blood Mononuclear Cell Samples.
ACTase activity was determined by analyzing the conversion of [^{14}C]carbamoyl phosphate to [^{14}C]carbamoyl aspartate by anion exchange HPLC with an on-line liquid scintillation detector. Within a matched set, the baseline and post-treatment samples were drawn at the same time of day. The data reflect paired samples obtained at 0 and 24 hours. The number of cycles at each PALA dose level (mg/m^2) is as follows: 250, 6; 1266, 21; 2848, 5.

Table 1 presents the percentage of cycles in which enzyme activity was inhibited by 50% or more at 24 hours compared to each patient's baseline value. With 250 mg/m^2 PALA, ACTase was inhibited by at least 50% in only one-third of the cycles. With 1266 PALA, ACTase was inhibited by 50% or more in about 60% of the patient cycles. With the 2848 mg/m^2 dose of PALA, each cycle had pronounced inhibition of ACTase. The trend was significant with a P_2 value of 0.01 by the Mantel test. In contrast, ACTase activity 96 hours after PALA was not significantly different from baseline even with the higher doses of PALA.

Table 1. Percentage of Cycles in Which ACTase Activity was Inhibited by at Least 50% at 24 Hours.

	PALA (mg/m²)		
	250	1266	2848
# Cycles (# Pts.)	7 (3)	23 (10)	5 (3)
% 0 h ACTase act: median	66%	49%	28%
range	35%-189%	13%-366%	20%-35%
> 50% decrease	29%	52%	100%

ACTase activity was determined in cytosol isolated from peripheral blood mononuclear cells obtained pretreatment (0 hours) and 24 hours by HPLC analysis. Within a matched set, all samples were drawn at the same time of day. In 4 cases in which cell counts were not available, ACTase activity was expressed in the baseline and post-treatment sample as pmol/min/mg protein, and the % baseline was then calculated.

SUMMARY

Forty-eight patients with adenocarcinoma of the gastrointestinal tract were treated on this trial. The MTD of 5-FU given as a 72 hour infusion with high-dose leucovorin was initially determined to be 2000 mg/m²/d. Patients were treated at PALA dose levels ranging from 250 to 2848 mg/m². Biochemical assessment of target enzyme activity was performed at each PALA dose level. We conclude that compared to each patient's own baseline, PALA at 250 mg/m² failed to appreciably inhibit ACTase activity at 24 hours in most patients. More consistent inhibition of ACTase activity was seen with PALA at or above 1266 mg/m², but toxicity was prohibitive with 2848 mg/m² PALA. Even with the highest PALA doses, ACTase activity was back to baseline by 96 hours in most patients. PALA at 1266 mg/m² given 24 hours prior to the start of 72 hour infusional 5-FU plus high-dose leucovorin was associated with acceptable toxicity and did not appear to compromise 5-FU dose-intensity. Finally, because of interpatient variability in the degree of ACTase inhibition following PALA, biochemical monitoring of target enzyme activity may permit more rational adjustment of the PALA dose in individual patients.

REFERENCES

1. Collins, K.D., and Stark, G,R.: Aspartate transcarbamylase, interaction with the transition state analogue N-(phosphonacetyl)-L-aspartate. *J. Biol. Chem.*, 246:6599-6605, 1971.
2. Grem, J.L., King, S.A., O'Dwyer, P.J., and Leyland-Jones, B.: N-(Phosphon-acetyl)-L-Aspartate (PALA): a review of its biochemistry and clinical activity. *Cancer Res.*, 48:4441 (1988).
3. Ardalan, B., Glazer, R.I., Kensler, T.W., Jayaram, H.N., Pham, T.V., MacDonald, J.S., and Cooney, D.A. Synergistic effect of 5-fluorouracil and N-

(phosphonacetyl)-L-aspartate on cell growth and ribonucleic acid synthesis in human mammary carcinoma. *Biochem. Pharmacol.*, 30:2045 (1981).

4. Liang C.M., Donehower, R.C., and Chabner, B.A. Biochemical interactions between N-(phosphonacetyl)-L-aspartate and 5-fluorouracil. *Mol. Pharmacol.*, 21:224 (1982).

5. Major, P.P., Egan, E.M., Sargent, L., and Kufe, D.W., Modulation of 5-FU metabolism in human MCF-7 breast carcinoma cells. *Cancer Chemother. Pharmacol.*, 8:87 (1982).

6. Martin, D.S., Stolfi, R.L., Sawyer, R.C., Spiegelman, S., Casper, E.S., and Young, C.W. Therapeutic utility of utilizing low doses of N-(phosphonacetyl)-L-aspartic acid in combination with 5-fluorouracil: a murine study with clinical relevance. *Cancer Res.*, 43:2317 (1983).

7. Ardalan, B., Singh, G. Silberman, H.A.: Randomized Phase I and Phase II study of short-term infusion of high-dose fluorouracil with or withour N-(phosphonacetyl)-L-aspartic acid in patients with advanced pancreatic and colorectal cancer. *J. Clin. Oncol.* 6:1053 (1988).

8. O'Dwyer, P.J., Paul, A.R., Walczak, J., Weiner, L.M., Litwin, S., and Comis, R.L.: Phase II study of biochemical modulation of fluorouracil by low-dose PALA in patients with colorectal cancer. *J. Clin. Oncol.* 8: 1497 (1990.

9. Grem, J.L., Hoth, D., Hamilton, M.J., et al: An overview of the current status and future directions of clinical trials of 5-fluorouracil and folinic acid. *Cancer Treat. Rep.* 71:1249 (1987).

10. The Advanced Colorectal Cancer Meta-Analysis Project. Modulation of fluorouracil by leucovorin in patients with advanced colorectal cancer: evidence in terms of response rate. *J. Clin. Oncol.* 10:896 (1992).

11. Calabro-Jones, P.M., Byfield, J.E., Ward, J.F., and Sharp, T.R.: Time-dose relationships for 5-fluorouracil cytotoxicity against human epithelial cancer cells in vitro. *Cancer Res.* 42:4413 (1982).

12. Moran, R.G., Scanlon, K.L.: Schedule-dependent enhancement of the cytotoxicity of fluoropyrimidines to human carcinoma cells in the presence of folinic acid. *Cancer Res.* 51:4618 (1991).

INCREASING THE EFFICACY OF 5-FLUOROURACIL WITH INTERFERONS: PRECLINICAL, CLINICAL, AND PHARMACOKINETIC STUDIES

Joseph A. Sparano and Scott Wadler

Albert Einstein Cancer Center
Montefiore Medical Center
Bronx, New York

INTRODUCTION

The interferons are a family of glycoproteins which possess potent antiviral, immunomodulatory, and antiproliferative effects in vivo[1]. The interferons also additively or synergistically enhance the efficacy of many cytotoxic agents against a number of cultured human adenocarcinoma, squamous cell carcinoma, and lymphoid tumor cell lines in vitro[1]. In particular, interferon-α synergistically augments the antineoplastic effect of 5-fluorouracil (5-FU) in cultured human colonic adenocarcinoma cell lines in vitro[2]. At the cellular level, the interferons act in a variety of ways to augment the antineoplastic effect of 5-FU by: (1) increasing the activity of thymidine phosphorylase[3], thereby augmenting the anabolism of 5-FU to its active metabolite, fluorodeoxyuridylate monophosphate, (2) enhancing inhibition of thymidylate synthase, the target enzyme of 5-FU, at the post-transcriptional level[4], (3) inhibiting thymidine salvage pathways[3], and (4) by enhancing 5-FU induced DNA damage[5].

In addition, the interferons induce a variety of effects on both host and tumor immunity,[6] providing another potential mechanism of interaction with 5-FU. In a murine model[7] of human colon carcinoma metastatic to the liver, the combination of 5-FU and murine interferon-γ resulted in a decrease in the liver metastases, whereas 5-FU and human interferon-γ had no effect; this occurred despite the fact that in vitro studies using the same cell line demonstrated synergy between 5-FU and both murine and human interferon-γ. Since murine interferon-γ is a potent stimulator of macrophage activity whereas human interferon-γ is devoid of any immunological effects in this murine model, these findings suggest that interferon-induced host immune activation was the basis for the enhanced in vivo activity of the combination.[7]

Interferon-α has a spectrum of toxicity which is non-overlapping with 5-FU.[8] Furthermore, animal models suggest that interferon-α may protect the host against lethal 5-FU-related toxicity.[9] These features, taken together with the preclinical data described, make interferon-α an attractive modulating agent to study in combination with 5-FU.

5-FU PLUS INTERFERON-α: CLINICAL STUDIES

Based on the aforementioned observations, a phase II trial of 5-FU plus interferon-α was performed at the Albert Einstein Cancer Center in patients with advanced colorectal cancer.[10] Patients received 5-FU, 750 mg/m^2 via continuous intravenous (IV) infusion daily for five days,

Novel Approaches to Selective Treatments of Human Solid Tumors: Laboratory and Clinical Correlation Edited by Y. M. Rustum, Plenum Press, New York, 1993

· 125

followed by 5-FU 750 mg/m^2 IV bolus weekly. In addition, interferon-α, 9 x 10^6 units was administered subcutaneously three times weekly. Twenty of thirty-two patients (63%, 95% confidence intervals 46%, 79%) achieved an objective partial response; with a median follow-up of 8 months, the median survival had not yet been reached.[10] Seven other single institution trials using an identical[11-13], nearly identical[14-16], or similar[17] regimen, and one multiinstitutional cooperative group trial using an identical regimen[18] have been reported (Table 1). The 95% confidence intervals for those trials[11-18] overlap or nearly overlap with the 95% confidence intervals of the initial trial performed at the Albert Einstein Cancer Center. The cumulative response rate for the aforementioned trials was 37% in evaluable patients.

Table 1. Clinical trials of intermediate-dose IV bolus 5-fluorouracil plus intermediate-dose interferon-α in patients with advanced colorectal carcinoma.

Reference	Group	Number/ Evaluable[1]	Response	95% Confidence Intervals
10	Einstein	32/32	20 (63%)	46%, 79%
11	Memorial	38/35	9 (26%)	11%, 41%
12	New England	42/33	13 (39%)	23%, 56%
13	Madrid	35/33	8 (24%)	11%, 42%
14	MD And	52/45	15 (35%)	22%, 50%
15	Hamburg	34/32	10 (31%)	15%, 47%
16	Nantes	22/16	5 (31%)	9%, 54%
17	Padova	21/21	9 (43%)	22%, 64%
18	ECOG	38/36	15 (42%)	27%, 58%
TOTAL				
All patients		314	104 (33%)	28%, 38%
Evaluable patients		283	104 (37%)	31%, 42%

[1] patients evaluable for response

Table 2. Toxicity of 5-FU/interferon-α therapy.

Ref.[1]	Eval.[2]	Grade 3-4 Toxicity[3] Leuk	Muc	Dia	Neuro	Death[4]
10	32	16%	9%	9%	6%	3 (9%)
11	38	8%	11%	13%	34%	0
12	40	43%	23%	20%	7%	0
13	35[5]	0	20%	20%	3%	2 (6%)
14	51	47%	37%	16%	4%	1 (2%)
15	32[5]	28%	9%	28%	0	2 (6%)
16	22	14%	27%	14%	27%	0
17	21[5]	14%	0	0	0	0
18	38	32%	5%	32%	5%	0

[1] reference
[2] number of patients evaluable for toxicity
[3] common toxicity criteria except where indicated; leuk - leukopenia; muc - mucositis; dia - diarrhea; neuro - neurologic
[4] treatment related death
[5] World Health Organization toxicity criteria

Neutropenia, stomatitis, and fatigue were the predominant toxic effects of 5-FU/interferon-α therapy in the initial study.[10] Reduction in the dose of 5-FU was required in 76% of patients, while reduction in the dose of interferon-α was required in 39% of patients in the ECOG trial.[18] Other groups have seen variable frequencies of severe neutropenia, diarrhea, and stomatitis (Table 2). The observed differences may be attributable to differing parameters for treatment modification and perhaps to differences in patient selection. In two trials[11,16], neurologic toxicity was common, particularly in patients greater than 60 years of age and in patients with extensive hepatic metastases.[11]

Treatment-related death occurred in eight patients (2.5%) treated in the nine studies described. Most treatment-related deaths were preceded by a syndrome characterized by watery diarrhea, sometimes accompanied by fever and/or severe neutropenia, comparable to the experience initially observed with 5-FU plus leucovorin.[19] In one of the first randomized trials comparing 5-FU plus leucovorin to 5-FU alone, treatment-related death occurred in 11 of 221 patients (5.0%) receiving the former compared with one of 107 patients (0.9%) receiving the latter[19]; after recognition by the principal investigators of that study that a similar watery diarrhea syndrome contributed to the majority of treatment-related deaths, the protocol was modified so that treatment was withheld for any degree of diarrhea or mucositis rather than grade 2 or greater toxicity. The impact of that change on the toxicity of the combination could not be evaluated, however, since it was implemented just prior to closure of the study. Likewise, since we have recognized a watery diarrhea syndrome in patients receiving 5-FU plus interferon-α, treatment-related mortality has been reduced by adopting the following policy: (1) for mild diarrhea (increase of 2-3 loose stools over pretreatment), withhold 5-FU, (2) for moderate diarrhea (increase of 4-6 loose stools over pretreatment) or severe diarrhea (increase of >6 stools per day or diarrhea associated with incontinence or abdominal cramping), withhold 5-FU, hospitalize, provide IV hydration, and initiate broad-spectrum parenteral antibiotics (particularly if occurring in association with neutropenia).

In reviewing the results of the nine clinical trials presented involving 5-FU/interferon-α for patients with advanced colorectal carcinoma, therefore, several conclusions can be made: (1) the response rates of the combination are higher than the expected response rate with 5-FU alone, (2) the response rates with the combination fall within or nearly within the confidence intervals of the initially reported 5-FU/interferon-α study, (3) the response rates with the combination are comparable to the response rates reported for treatment with 5-FU plus other modulating agents such as leucovorin[19] or N-(phosphonacetyl)-L-aspartate[20] (PALA), (4) toxicity was significant but manageable with appropriate modification of 5-FU and/or interferon-α, and (5) treatment-related deaths occurred, but may be preventable if treatment is withheld and appropriate supportive care measures are provided for patients experiencing moderate-severe diarrhea.

5-FU PLUS INTERFERON-α: PHARMACOKINETIC STUDIES

A number of studies have attempted to examine the effect of interferon-α on the pharmacokinetics of 5-FU, some of which are outlined in Table 3. Schuller et al[21] found that interferon-α (5×10^6 units) increased the half-life and the area under the curve (AUC), and decreased the clearance of 5-FU when administered as an IV bolus (750 mg/m^2); the effect was observed with a dose of interferon-α that was somewhat lower than that used in the phase II studies of 5-FU/interferon-α described (9×10^6 units)[10-18], but was not observed when even lower doses of interferon-α were used.[22] Grem et al[23] have also described a dose-dependent effect of interferon-α on the pharmacokinetics of IV bolus 5-FU when 5-FU (370-425 mg/m^2) was used in combination with leucovorin (500 mg/m^2); clearance was reduced in patients receiving 5×10^6 or 10×10^6 units/m^2 of interferon-α, but not in those receiving 3×10^6 units/m^2 of interferon-α. On the other hand, Danhauser et al[24] found that 5-FU clearance was reduced at all doses of interferon-α studied (0.1, 1, and 3×10^6 units/m^2); 5-FU was administered as a high dose five day continuous IV infusion (750 mg/m2/day) in that study. Both Grem et al[23] and Danhauser et al[24] found that diminished 5-FU clearance resulted in enhanced gastrointestinal toxicity. Lindley et al[25] also found that interferon-α (5×10^6 units/m^2) increased plasma 5-FU concentration when 5-FU was given as a low dose (300 mg/m^2/day) continuous infusion. On the other hand, our group[26] found no significant effect of interferon-α (5 x 10^6 units/m^2) on the pharmacokinetics of 5-FU when the data was analyzed using Cosinor analysis[27], a method which adjusts for the known diurnal variation which occurs in plasma 5-FU concentration when 5-FU is given as a continuous IV infusion.[28] Despite the absence of a pharmacokinetic effect of interferon-α in our study, the gastrointestinal toxicity of 5-FU was substantially enhanced, suggesting that under certain conditions enhanced 5-FU-related toxicity was not attributable to reduced 5-FU clearance.

Table 3. Clinical trials examining the effects of subcutaneous interferon-α on the pharmacokinetics of 5-fluorouracil ($\pm$ leucovorin).

Ref.	Schedule of 5-FU	Interferon-α	Effect of interferon-α on 5-FU Kinetics & Toxicity
21	Bolus 750 mg/m^2 $\pm$ leucovorin 200 mg/m^2	5 mu[1] TIW (α 2b[6])	1. AUC[2] increased 1.8 fold 2. Clearance decreased 0.5 fold 3. Leucovorin abrogated effect of IFN-α[3] on 5-FU kinetics
23	Bolus 370-425 mg/m^2 d2-6[4]	3, 5, or 10 mu/m^2 d1-7/14 (α 2a)	1. AUC increased 1.3,1.5 fold with 5,10 mu IFN-α, respectively. 2. IFN-α enhanced GI[5] and hematologic toxicity.
24	Infusion 750 mg/m^2 d1-5	0.5,1,or 3 mu/m^2/d d 1-5 (α 2b)	1. Clearance reduced in some patients at all dose levels of IFN-α.
25	Infusion 300 mg/m^2/d	5 x 10^6 u/m^2 (α 2a)	1. Plasma 5-FU concentration increased after IFN-α.
26	Infusion 300 mg/m^2/d	5 mu/m^2 TIW (α 2a)	1. No effect of IFN-α on 5-FU kinetics. 2. 5-FU-related toxicity increased with IFN-α.

[1] mu - million units; TIW - three times weekly
[2] AUC - area under the curve
[3] IFN-α - interferon-α
[4] d - day
[5] GI - gastrointestinal
[6] α2a - interferon-α2a; α2b - interferon-α2b

5-FU PLUS INTERFERON-α: MODULATION, INTENSIFICATION, OR BOTH ?

The aforementioned pharmacokinetic observations raise the question of whether the enhanced response observed with the 5-FU/interferon-α combination could be explained on the basis of interferon-α-induced "pharmacologic intensification" of 5-FU. Evidence supporting this hypothesis includes: (1) a dose response effect exists for 5-FU in the treatment of advanced colorectal carcinoma[29], (2) the response to 5-FU/interferon-α[10-18] is in the range observed with dose-intense bolus 5-FU regimens,[29] and (3) the dose of interferon-α used in the 5-FU/interferon-α studies is in the range reported to reduce the clearance and enhance the gastrointestinal toxicity of 5-FU.[21,23] On the other hand, our group found that while 5-FU-related gastrointestinal toxicity was enhanced by interferon-α, 5-FU clearance was unaffected when 5-FU was administered as a low-dose continuous infusion[26], suggesting that modulation of 5-FU was occurring at the cellular level. Supporting this observation, Findlay et al[30] found that interferon-α enhanced intratumoral 5-FU anabolite formation in hepatic metastatic tumors as measured by ^{19}F-magnetic resonance spectroscopy.

Therefore, it appears that interferon-α modulates the toxic and perhaps therapeutic effects of 5-FU via a number of potential mechanisms, including perturbation of the pharmacokinetics of 5-FU as well as biochemical modulation at the cellular level. Furthermore, the effect of interferon-α on the pharmacokinetics of 5-FU appears to be dependent not only on the dose of interferon-α but also upon the dose and schedule of 5-FU employed.

5-FU PLUS INTERFERON-α: FUTURE DIRECTIONS

Previous experience with 5-FU/leucovorin therapy in patients with advanced colorectal carcinoma suggests that the use of a modulating agent in combination with a standard cytotoxic agent represents a feasible approach.[19] Hence, based on reviewing the aforementioned clinical and laboratory investigations, there appears to be considerable promise for the use of interferon-α as a modulating agent to study in combination with 5-FU. Further investigation is required, however, regarding a number of issues, including identification of the optimal dose and schedule of interferon-α and 5-FU administration, as well as obtaining a more precise understanding of the biochemical basis of their interaction. It is possible that a lower dose of interferon-α may be equally effective in modulating the activity of 5-FU while being associated with less constitutional symptoms and hematologic toxicity. In fact, evidence suggests that higher doses of interferon-α[31] or lower doses of 5-FU[32] than those used in the Albert Einstein 5-FU/interferon-α regimen are associated with diminished likelihood of achieving response and, in the case of high-dose interferon-α, substantially more toxicity.[31] Concomitant use of 5-FU/interferon-α with other biological agents, such as granulocyte colony stimulating factor, may be capable of reducing the hematologic and mucosal toxicity of therapy as it has done with other drug regimens.[33] Other biological agents, such as β-interferon, may be more effective in enhancing the activity of 5-FU. Finally, preclinical evidence suggests that combination of 5-FU/interferon-α with other modulating agents, such as leucovorin[34] or PALA, may further enhance the cytotoxicity of the combination. The combination of two or more modulating agents with 5-FU, however, should proceed cautiously in carefully performed trials evaluating the clinical and pharmacokinetic consequences of such an approach. For example, Schuller et al[21] found that leucovorin abrogates the effect of interferon-α on the pharmacokinetics of 5-FU. Moreover, clinical trials evaluating the combination of 5-FU/interferon-α and leucovorin have not resulted in superior results thus far.[35-37] While these promising approaches are being investigated, prospective clinical trials comparing 5-FU/interferon-α to 5-FU alone or 5-FU plus other modulating agents are being performed in order to determine the potential benefit, if any, of the combination.

REFERENCES

1. S. Wadler and E.L. Schwartz, Antineoplastic activity of the combination of interferon and cytotoxic agents against experimental and human malignancies: a review, *Cancer Res.* 50:3673 (1990).

2. S. Wadler, R. Wersto, V. Weinberg, D. Thompson, D., and E.L. Schwartz, Interaction f fluorouracil and interferon in human colon cancer cell lines: cytotoxic and cytokinetic effects, *Cancer Res.* 50:5735 (1990).

3. E.L. Schwartz, M. Hoffman, C.J. O'Connor, and S. Wadler, Stimulation of 5-fluorouracil metabolic activation by interferon-α in human colon carcinoma cells,. *Biochemical and Biophysical Research Communications.* 182:1232 (1992).

4. E. Chu, S. inn, D. Boarman, and C.J. Allegra, Interaction of interferon γ and 5-fluorouracil in the H630 human colon carcinoma cell line, *Cancer Res.* 50:5834, (1990).

5. S. Wadler, X. Mao, and E.L. Schwartz, Recombinant alfa-2a-interferon augments 5-fluorouracil effects on nucleotide (dNTP) pools and DNA double strand breaks in human colon cancer cell lines, *Proc Am Assoc Cancer Res.* 33:2539 (1992).

6. D. Goldstein and J. Laslo, Interferon therapy in cancer: from imaginon to interferon, Cancer Res. 46:4315 (1986).

7. K. Morika, D. Fan, Y.M. Denkins, et al, Mechanisms of combined effects of γ-interferon and 5-fluorouracil on human colon cancers implanted into nude mice, *Cancer Res.* 49:799 (1989).

8. J.M. Kirkwood and M.S. Ernstoff, Interferons in the treatment of human cancer, *J Clin Oncol.* 2:336 (1984).

9. R.L. Stolfi, D.S. Martin, and R.C. Sawyer, Modulation of 5-fluorouracil-induced toxicity in mice with interferon or the interferon induce, polyinosinic-polycytidylic acid, *Cancer Res.* 43:561 (1983).

10. S. Wadler and P.H. Wiernik, Clinical update on the role of fluorouracil and recombinant interferon alfa-2a in the treatment of colorectal carcinoma, *Semin Oncol.* 17(suppl 1):16 (1990).

11. N. Kemeny, A. Younes, K. Seiter, et al, Interferon alpha-2a and 5-fluorouracil for advanced colorectal carcinoma: assessment of activity and toxicity, *Cancer.* 66:2470 (1990).

12. M. Huberman, E. McClay, M. Atkins, et al, Phase II trial of 5-fluorouracil and recombinant alpha interferon in advanced colorectal cancer, *Proc Am Soc Clin Oncol.* 10:153 (1991).

13. E. Diaz Rubio, J. Jimeno, C. Camps, et al, Treatment of advanced colorectal cancer with recombinant interferon alpha and fluorouracil: activity in liver metastasis, *Cancer Investigation.* 10:259, (1992).

14. R. Pazdur, J.A. Ajani, Y.Z. Patt, et al, Phase II study of fluorouracil and recombinant interferon alfa-2a in previously untreated advanced colorectal carcinoma, *J Clin Oncol.* 8:2027 (1990).

15. H. Weh, D. Platz, D. Braumann, et al, Treatment of metastatic colorectal carcinoma with a combination of fluorouracil and recombinant interferon alfa-2b: preliminary data of a phase II study, *Semin Oncol.* 19:180 (1992).

16. J.Y. Douillard, J. Leborgne J, J.Y. Danielou, et al, Phase II trial of 5-fluorouracile (5-FU) and recombinant alpha interferon (rαIFN) (Intron A) in metastatic, previously untreated colorectal cancer, *Proc Am Soc Clin Oncol.* 10:139 (1991).

17. A. Fornasiero, O. Daniele, C. Ghiotto, S.M.L Aversa, P. Morandi, and V. Florentino, Alpha-2 interferon and5-fluorouracil in advanced colorectal cancer, 1837X *Tumor.* 76: 385 (1990).

18. S. Wadler, B. Lembersky, M. Atkins, J. Kirkwoood, and N. Petrelli, Phase II trial of fluorouracil and recombinant interferon alfa-2a in patients with advanced colorectal carcinoma: an Eastern Cooperative Oncology Group study, *J Clin Oncol.* 9:1806 (1991).

19. N. Petrelli, H.O. Douglass, Jr., L. Herrera, et al, The modulation of fluorouracil with leucovorin in metastatic colorectal carcinoma: a prospective randomized phase III trial, *J Clin Oncol.* 7:1419, 1989.

20. D.S. Martin, and N.E. Kemeny, Overview of N-(Phosphonacetyl)-L-Aspartate + fluorouracil in clinical trials, *Semin Oncol.* 19:228 (1992).

21. J. Schuller, M. Czejka, G. Schernthaner, U. Fogl, W. Jager, and M. Micksche, Influence of interferon α 2b with or without folinic acid on pharmacokinetics of fluorouracil, *Semin Oncol.* 19:93 (1992).

22. Schuller, J, Personal Communication.

23. J.L. Grem, N. McAtee, R.F. Murphy, et al, A pilot study of interferon alfa-2a in combination with fluorouracil plus high-dose leucovorin in metastatic gastrointestinal carcinoma, *J Clin Oncol.* 9:1811 (1991).

24. L. Danhauser, T. Gilchrist, J. Friemann, A. Markowitz, A. Yeomans, C. Hunter, and J. Gutterman, Effect of recombinant interferon-α2b on the plasma pharmacokinetics of fluorouracil in patients with advanced cancer, *Proc Am Assoc Cancer Res.* 32:1052 (1991).

25. C. Lindley, S. Bernard, M. Gavigan, et al, Interferon-alpha increases 5-fluorouracil (5-FU) plasma levels 16-fold within one hour: results of a phase I study, *J Interferon Res.* 10:5 (1990).

26. J.A. Sparano, S. Wadler, R. Diasio, R. Spears, E.L. Schwartz, A. Einzig, and P.H. Wiernik, Phase I trial of prolonged infusion 5-fluorouracil and interferon alpha, *Proc Am Assoc Cancer Res.* 33:3185 (1992).

27. F. Halberg, E.A. Johnson, W. Nelson, W. Runge, R. Sothern, Autorhythmometry procedures for physiologic self-measurements and their analysis, *Physiol Teacher.* 1:1 (1972).

28. B.E. Harris BE, R. Song R, S. Soong S, R.B. Diasio, Relationship between dihydropyrimidine dehydrogenase activity and plasma 5-fluorouracil levels with evidence for circadian variation of enzyme activity and plasma drug levels in cancer patients receiving 5-fluorouracil by protracted continuous infusion, *Cancer Res.* 50: 197 (1990).

29. W.M. Hryniuk, W.M, A. Figueredo, and M. Goodyear, M, Applications of dose intensity to problems in chemotherapy of breast and colorectal cancer. *Semin Oncol* 14(suppl 4):3 (1987).

30. M. Findlay, M. Leach, J. Glaholm, et al, Monitoring interferon (Intron A) modulation of 5-fluorouracil in patients with colorectal cancer using ^{19}F magnetic resonance spectroscopy: correlation with clinical effects and implications for further clinical trials, *Proc Am Soc Clin Oncol.* 11:495 (1992).

31. S. Wadler, M. Goldman, A. Lyver, P.H. Wiernik, Phase I trial of 5-fluorouracil and recombinant α2b-interferon in patients with advanced cancer, *Cancer Res.* 50:2056 (1990).

32. P.I. Clark, M.L. Slevin, R.H. Reznik, et al, Two randomized phase II trials of intermittent intravenous versus subcutaneous alpha-2 interferon alone (Trial 1) and in combination with 5-fluorouracil (Trial 2) in advanced colorectal cancer, *Int J Colorect Dis.* 2:26 (1987).

33. J.L. Gabrilove, A. Jakubowski, H. Scher, et al, Effect of granulocyte colony-stimulating factor on neutropenia and associated morbidity due the chemotherapy for transitional-cell carcinoma of the urothelium, *N Eng J Med.* 318:1414 (1988).

34. J.A. Houghton, D.A. Adkins, A. Rahman, P.J. Houghton, Interaction between 5-fluorouracil, [6RS] leucovorin, and recombinant human interferon-α2a in cultured colon adenocarcinoma cells, *Cancer Communications.* 3:225 (1991).

35. J. Press, Fluorouracil plus interferon + folinic acid in regional and systemic therapy in colorectal cancer, *Semin Oncol.* 19:220 (1992).

36. J.A. Put, P.H.M, de Mulder, J.Th.M. Burghouts, and D.J.Th. Wagener, Fluorouracil continuous infusion plus alfa interferon plus oral folinic acid in advanced colorectal cancer, *Semin Oncol.* 19:208 (1992).

37. H.J. Schmoll, C.H. Kohne-Wompner, W. Hiddemann, et al, Interferon alpha-2b, 5-fluorouracil, and folinic acid combination therapy in advanced colorectal cancer: preliminary results of a phase I/II trial, *Semin Oncol.* 19:191 (1992).

ENHANCED CYTOTOXICITY OF 5-FLUOROURACIL COMBINED WITH [6RS]LEUCOVORIN AND RECOMBINANT HUMAN INTERFERON-α2a IN COLON CARCINOMA CELLS

Janet A. Houghton, David A. Adkins, and Peter J. Houghton

Department of Biochemical and Clinical Pharmacology
St. Jude Children's Research Hospital
Memphis, TN 38101

INTRODUCTION

We had proposed previously that one mechanism of intrinsic resistance to 5-fluorouracil (FUra) in colon adenocarcinomas was suboptimal concentrations of intracellular 5,10-methylenetetrahydrofolate (CH_2-$H_4PteGlu_n$).[1] Whereas the concentration of this reduced folate may not be rate limiting for thymidylate synthesis *de novo*, it may be suboptimal to allow maximal interaction between the FUra metabolite, 5-fluorodeoxyuridylate (FdUMP), and thymidylate synthase.[1-5] Supplementation with a reduced folate, therefore, elevates intracellular levels of CH_2-$H_4PteGlu_n$ and enhances the rate of formation or stabilization of the ternary complex. In human colon tumor xenografts, pools of CH_2-$H_4PteGlu_n$ and $H_4PteGlu_n$ expanded by 2- to 5-fold in response to 24 hr infusions of [6RS]leucovorin ([6RS]LV), elevating species containing from 2 to 5 glutamate residues.[6,7]

This concept appears to have translated into clinical utility. In Phase III randomized clinical trials in adults presenting with colorectal caricnoma, response rates to FUra-[6RS]LV in comparison to FUra administered alone are 33-48% vs 7-15%, respectively,[8-11] with significant increases in time to disease progression[8,9,11] and increased patient survival[9,11] reported. Although the use of FUra with [6RS]LV has improved response rates, there is a need to build upon this combination to develop more efficacious therapy for colorectal carcinoma.

Recently, there has been an interest in the clinical utility of FUra in combination with interferons (IFN's), specifically rIFN-α2a. Single institutional trials utilizing 9 x 10^6 IU of rIFN-α2a three times weekly and FUra (750 mg/m²/day x 5) given by infusion i.v. in previously untreated patients report response rates as high as 76%,[12] or lower, in the range of 26-35%.[13,14] These trials had been initiated from reports of studies conducted in cultured colon adenocarcinoma cells that had shown potentiation of the growth inhibitory or cytotoxic activity of FUra by IFN's.[15-18]

These studies suggested that IFN effects are dependent on initial inhibition of

Novel Approaches to Selective Treatments of Human Solid Tumors: Laboratory and Clinical Correlation Edited by Y. M. Rustum, Plenum Press, New York, 1993

133

thymidylate synthase by the fluoropyrimidine. The study of Chu et al.[16] suggested that rIFN-γ abrogates the FUra-induced increase in total thymidylate synthase that may be responsible for reducing cellular sensitivity to FUra. As [6RS]LV enhances the inhibition of thymidylate synthase by FdUMP, it appeared to us that the combination of FUra, [6RS]LV, and rIFN-α2a may be more effective that FUra combined with each modulator independently. We subsequently extended our studies to examine the interaction of rIFN-α2a as a direct modulator of the cytotoxic activity of FUra combined with [6RS]LV. The studies we describe below demonstrate the potentiation of FUra cytotoxicity by [6RS]LV or rIFN-α2a and substantially greater potentiation by rIFN-α2a when FUra and [6RS]LV were combined. Our results also suggest 1) that the mechanism of potentiation of FUra by rIFN-α2a was independent of any inhibition of dThd salvage in either cell line and 2) that the interaction appeared independent of thymine-less stress *per se* but required the presence of a 5-fluoropyrimidine.

MATERIALS AND METHODS

Materials

5-methyltetrahydrofolate ([6RS]5-CH₃-H₄PteGlu) and [6RS]LV wcrc purchased from Sigma Chemical Co., St. Louis, MO: FUra (50 mg/mL) was from SoloPak Laboratories, Franklin Park, IL, and rIFN-α2a (6×10^6IU/mL) was from Hoffmann La-Roche Inc., Nutley, NJ; both were the pharmaceutical preparations. CB3717 was a gift from Dr. Ken Harrap, Institute of Cancer Research, Sutton, Surrey, England. Falcon culture plates were obtained from Becton Dickinson Labware, Lincoln Park, NJ. Folate-free RPMI-1640 medium was formated by GIBCO Laboratories, Grand Island, NY, and dFBS was purchased from Hyclone Laboratories, Inc., Logan, UT. All other chemicals were obtained from Sigma or were of reagent grade.

Cell Lines

The human colon adenocarcinoma cell line, GC₃/M, was described previously[19,20] and was subsequently cloned; one clone (GC₃/cl) was utilized further.[21] GC₃/cl has a doubling time of 24 hr. Cells were grown in folate-free RPMI-1640 medium containing 10% dFBS and 712 μM Ca^{++} and were adapted to growth in physiological concentrations of 5-CH₃-H₄PteGlu; (80 nM; [6RS] form), equivalent to physiologic concentrations of reduced folate levels found *in vivo*.

Clonogenic Assays

Cells were plated at densities of 6,000 cells/well in 6-well plates. After allowing cells to attach for 16 to 24 hr, triplicate wells were treated with varied concentrations of FUra, rIFN-α2a, 10-propargyl-5,8-dideazafolate (CB3717), or [6RS]LV (1 μM) alone or in combination for 72 hr. After a further 4 days plates were rinsed once in 0.9% saline and dried and stained with 0.1% crystal violet. Colonies were subsequently enumerated using an Artek model 880 counter. Sixty cells represented the minimum number of cells accepted as a colony. IC₅₀ is defined as the concentration of FUra required to inhibit colony formation by 50%. [6RS]LV (1 μM) previously was determined to be the minimal concentration required to maximally potentiate FUra cytotoxicity. Data were analyzed statistically using a two-way analysis of variance and subsequently using the Newman Keuls' range test for differences between means.[22]

RESULTS

GC$_3$/cl cells were exposed to various concentrations of FUra alone or in combination with [6RS]LV (1 μM), rIFN-α2a (5,000 IU/mL) or both modulators either in the absence or in the presence of dThd (20 μM) for 72 hr. A representative experiment is shown in Figure 1.

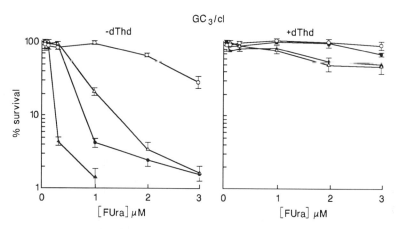

Figure 1. Effects of rIFN-α2a (5,000 IU/mL) or [6RS]LV (1 μM) used as single modulators or combined with various concentrations of FUra in GC$_3$/cl cells. Cells were treated in the absence of dThd with (O) FUra alone, or FUra combined with (●) [6RS]LV, (▲) [6RS]LV + rIFN-α2a, or in the presence of dThd (20 μM) with (O) FUra alone, or FUra combined with (●) [6RS]LV, (▲) rIFN-α2a, or (▲) [6RS]LV + rIFN-α2a. Each point is the mean ± SD of triplicate wells per group. The number of colonies per control well was 340 ± 9. Data show a representative experiment from three separate experiments.

At 5,000 IU/mL, rIFN-α2a was not cytotoxic. The IC$_{50}$ for FUra was 2.46 μM and was decreased by 3.7-fold in combination with [6RS]LV, by 3.4-fold with rIFN-α2a, and by 13-fold in the presence of both [6RS]LV and rIFN-α2a. The activity of FUra-[6RS]LV or FUra-rIFN-α2a was potentiated a further 3.5- to 3.8-fold by the addition of the second modulator. Potentiation observed in these groups was significant (P<0.001). Only small differences were observed between FUra-[6RS]LV and FUra-rIFN-α2a groups that were significant at 1 μM FUra (P<0.0001). The IC$_{50}$ values for data combined from independent experiments are shown in Table 1. When cells were exposed in the presence of dThd (20 μM), FUra ± [6RS]LV cytotoxicity was completely reversed, although cytotoxicity obtained in the presence of rIFN-α2a ± [6RS]LV was only partially reversed.

When the concentration of rIFN-α2a was reduced to 500 IU/mL (Table 1), the IC$_{50}$ for FUra alone (2.07 μM) was reduced by 3.2-fold when combined with either rIFN-α2a or [6RS]LV. When all three agents were combined, however, the IC$_{50}$ for FUra was reduced to 0.19 μM (10.9-fold potentiation). Modulation of the response to FUra-[6RS]LV or FUra-rIFN-α2a by the second modulator was 3.4-fold. Modulation of FUra cytotoxicity was highly significant for all groups exmained (P<0.0001). Although slightly lower, there was still substantial potentiation of FUra cytotoxicity at this concentration of rIFN-α2a.

When rIFN-α2a was reduced to a concentration of 50 IU/mL in GC$_3$/cl, the degree of potentiation of FUra cytotoxicity alone (1.4-fold), or in combination with [6RS]LV (4.6-fold) was less than observed with the two higher concentrations of rIFN-α2a (Table 1). Differences between groups, however, achieved a level of significance of P<0.001.

We subsequently examined the effect of varied concentrations of rIFN-α2a (50-5,000 IU/mL) on the activity of a non-cytotoxic concentration of FUra (0.3 μM) administered alone or in combination with [6RS]LV (1 μM; Figure 2). The lack of cytotoxicity of rIFN-α2a administered alone is shown also. The increasing cytotoxic

Table 1. Comparison of IC$_{50}$[a] values for combinations of FUra, [6RS]LV, and rIFN-α2a in GC$_3$/cl cells exposed for 72 hr.

Treatment	GC$_3$/cl	
	IC$_{50}$(μM) ± SD(N)[b]	Fold
FUra	2.07 ± 0.40 (5)	--
FUra + [6RS]LV	0.68 ± 0.03 (5)	3.2
FUra + rIFN-α2a (5,000 IU/mL)	0.61 ± 0.12 (2)	3.4
(500 IU/mL)	0.64 ± 0.11 (2)	3.2
(50 IU/mL)	1.52 (1)	1.4
FUra + [6RS]LV+rIFN-α2a (5,000 IU/mL)	0.15 ± 0.05 (2)	13.8
(500 IU/mL)	0.19 ± 0.08 (2)	10.9
(50 IU/mL)	0.45 (1)	4.6

[a]IC$_{50}$ = concentration of FUra required to inhibit colony formation by 50%. [b]N = number of separate experiments using triplicate wells for each drug concentration. Where N = 2, SD = average deviation. [c]ND = not determined.

activity of the three-agent combination was evident as the concentration of rIFN-α2a was increased. In the presence of a fixed concentration of FUra and [6RS]LV, 10% cell kill was achieved at 50 IU/mL rIFN-α2a, increasing to 40% and 73% at 500 and 5,000 IU/mL, respectively, (P<0.02 at 300 IU/mL rIFN-α2a, and P<0.0001 at rIFN-α2a concentrations of >500 IU/mL).

To determine whether thymidylate synthase inhibition *per se* was a requirement for initiation of a cellular response or rIFN-α2a, the activity of various concentrations of the quinazoline-based thymidylate synthase inhibitor CB3717 was examined either alone or combined with rIFN-α2a (500 IU/mL, Figure 3). The IC$_{50}$ value for CB3717 was 0.34 μM and was similar when CB3717 was combined with rIFN-α2a (0.32 μM).

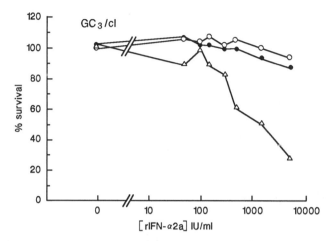

Figure 2. Clonogenic survival of GC₃/cl cells exposed for 72 hr to various concentrations of rIFN-α2a alone or in combination with FUra (0.3 μM) or FUra + [6RS]LV (1 μM). Data represent the mean ± SD of three cultures at each time point from single experiments. The number of colonies per control plate was 317 ± 17. Cells exposed to rIFN-α2a (O) alone or in combination with (●) FUra or (▵) FUra + [6RS]LV.

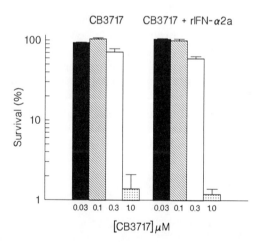

Figure 3. Clonogenic survival of GC₃/cl cells following a 72 hr exposure to CB3717 either (O) alone or (●) in combination with rIFN-α2a (500 IU/mL). Each point represents the mean ± SD of three wells per group. The number of colonies in control wells was 281 ± 1. Data were derived from single experiments.

DISCUSSION

IFN's were originally described as antiviral substances, but it is now apparent that they can have significant effects on cell structure and function.[23] Of note is that several studies[15-17] have demonstrated that rIFN's may potentiate the cytotoxicity of FUra, at concentrations of IFN that were not cytotoxic *per se*. Consequently, rIFN's may be regarded as modulators of FUra cytotoxicity. These studies suggested also that rIFN modulation occurred at the level of thymidylate synthase. Hence, increased inhibition of thymidylate synthase should enhance the activity of rIFN's. We[7] and others[24] have shown that [6RS]LV can expand the intracellular pools of CH_2-$H_4PteGlu_n$ and increase the inhibition of thymidylate synthase, probably by stabilizing the enzyme-FdUMP-folate ternary complex. Thus, equivalent cytotoxicity can be achieved at lower concentrations of FUra in the presence of [6RS]LV.[5,25,26] Consequently, the combination of FUra with [6RS]LV may prove additive with rIFN's. Since rIFN-α2a has been used in initial clinical trials combined with FUra, this particular subtype of IFN was evaluated in the present study.

In GC_3/cl colon adenocarcinoma cells, rIFN-α2a was not cytotoxic when administered alone at concentrations as high as 5,000 IU/mL and yet it was capable of increasing the cytotoxic activity of FUra. Of particular interest was the influence of rIFN-α2a on the cytotoxicity of FUra combined with [6RS]LV. rIFN-α2a and [6RS]LV administered as single modulators were approximately equivalent in their degree of potentiation of FUra cytotoxicity (3.2- to 3.4-fold). When combined, however, these agents further potentiatied FUra efficacy an additional 4-fold beyond that observed with either agent alone. These results suggest that the effect of [6RS]LV and rIFN-α2a in potentiating FUra cytotoxicity are at least additive and potentially act at independent loci. Studies by Wadler et al.[17] suggest that although non-cytotoxic concentrations of rIFN-α2a or rIFN-β can potentiate the cytotoxicity activity of FUra in two human colon cancer cell lines, it is necessary to expose cells to concentrations of FUra alone that cause some degree of cytotoxicity to mediate this effect. In GC_3/cl cells, however, rIFN-α2a decreased clonogenic survival at non-cytotoxic concentrations of FUra or FUra combined with [6RS]LV. Efficacy of the 3-agent combination may be regarded as synergistic, since two of the agents (rIFN-α2a, [6RS]LV) are non-cytotoxic. This also holds true for FUra-IFN combinations, as discussed by Wadler et al.[17] The dose-response relationship for FUra in combination with rIFN-α2a, [6RS]LV, or both agents simultaneously, was steep. For example, in Figure 1, when all three agents were combined, cell survival decreased from 87% to 4% between 0.1 and 0.3 μM FUra, respectively. Thus, small differences in the FUra concentration appeared to significantly influence the degree of cell kill achieved. It was evident that the potentiation of FUra or FUra-[6RS]LV cytotoxicity by rIFN-α2a was concentration dependent up to 5,000 IU/mL examined. Since concentrations of IFN-α up to 1,200 IU/mL[27,28] and $\geq$ 1.2 μM [6RS]LV[29-32] are clinically achievable in human serum, the three-agent combination has potential for activity *in vivo*. It is not clear at this point what exact duration of exposure or sequence is required in these lines or others to achieve maximal potentiation of FUra or FUra-[6RS]LV cytotoxicity, although Wadler et al.[17] reported that a 2 hr exposure was insufficient, while exposure for 24 hr to FUra-rIFN-α2a elicited a response.

With regard to the mechanism of interaction between FUra, rIFN-α2a, and [6RS]LV, there have been reports suggesting that IFN's may influence dThd salvage by inhibition of the uptake of dThd[33] or may act at the level of thymidine kinase.[34] In the experiments presented, however, studies were conducted in dialyzed serum lacking dThd, where dThd salvage would be minimal. The cytotoxicity of FUra and potentiation of FUra or FUra-[6RS]LV cytotoxicity by rIFN-α2a and reversibility of the effects by dThd does suggest, however, that modulation by rIFN-α2a occurs only after some level of inhibition of thymidylate synthase. Only partial reversal of the cytotoxic action of FUra-rIFN-α2a±[6RS]LV by dThd in GC$_3$/cl suggests that part of the modulating action of rIFN-α2a may be due to a dThd-independent or even thymidylate synthase-independent mechanism. Lack of potentiation by rIFN-α2a of the cytotoxic action of CB3717, a specific quinazoline-based inhibitor of thymidylate synthase,[35,36] suggests that thymine-less stress *per se* does not increase cell sensitivity to rIFN-α2a. Data thus suggest that a fluoropyrimidine rather than purely thymidylate synthase inhibition is required in the interaction mechanism but that potentiation of enzyme inhibition increases the extent of the interaction. Interaction either at the level of the enzyme or DNA following the action of the fluoropyrimidine is thus indicated in colon adenocarcinoma cells.

Of importance in this study is the identification and characterization of further potentiation by rIFN-α2a of FUra cytotoxicity in the presence of [6RS]LV, which has not been described previously. Chu et al.[16] found no enhancement of FUra cytotoxicity in the presence of 1 or 20 μM [6RS]LV in the H630 colon adenocarcinoma cell line. However, the high concentrations of folic acid (2.3 μM) present in complete RPMI-1640 medium may be sufficient to already allow maximal interaction between FdUMP and thymidylate synthase in this line. It is evident that with clinical management of patients with colorectal caricnoma, significant increases in response rates to FUra-[6RS]LV combinations have been achieved in comparison to the administration of FUra alone.[8-11] While results from one single institutional trial of FUra in combination with rIFN-α2a have been encouraging (76% response rates), data from randomized trials are needed to determine the comparative efficacies of FUra combined with [6RS]LV and/or rIFN-α2a. Thus, rather than evaluating IFN-α with FUra alone clinically, it may be of greater therapeutic benefit to combine all three agents to further increase response rates and patient survival.

ACKNOWLEDGEMENTS: This research was supported by United States Public Health Service, National Institutes of Health, National Cancer Institute, grants CA-32613, CA-23099, and CA-21765, and by the American Lebanese Syrian Associated Charities (ALSAC).

REFERENCES

1. J.A. Houghton, S.J. Maroda, J.O. Phillips, and P.J. Houghton, Biochemical determinants of responsiveness to 5-fluorouracil and its derivatives in human colorectal adenocarcinoma xenografts, *Cancer Res.* 41:144 (1981).
2. J.A. Houghton, L.G. Williams, S. Radparvar, and P.J. Houghton, Characterization of the pools of 5,10-methylenetetrahydrofolates and tetrahydrofolates in xenografts of human colon adenocarcinoma, *Cancer Res.* 48:3062 (1988).
3. A. Lockshin and P.V. Danenberg, Biochemical factors affecting the tightness of 5-fluorodeoxyuridylate binding to human thymidylate synthase, *Biochem. Pharmacol.* 30:247 (1981).
4. S. Radparvar, P.J. Houghton, and J.A. Houghton, Effect of polyglutamylation of 5,10-methylenetetrahydrofolate on the binding of 5-fluoro-2'-deoxyuridylate to thymidylate synthase purified from a human colon adenocarcinoma xenograft, *Biochem. Pharmacol.* 38:335 (1989).

5. B. Ullman, M. Lee, D.W. Martin, and D.V. Santi, Cytotoxicity of 5-fluoro-2'-deoxyuridine: requirement for reduced folate cofactors and antagonism by methotrexate, *Proc. Natl. Acad. Sci. USA* 75:980 (1978).

6. J.A. Houghton, L.G. Williams, S.S.N. de Graaf, P.J. Cheshire, J.H. Rodman, D.C. Maneval, I.W. Wainer, P. Jadaud, and P.J. Houghton, Relationship between dose rate of [6RS]leucovorin administration, plasma concentrations of reduced folates, and pools of 5,10-methylenetetrahydrofolates and tetrahydrofolates in human colon adenocarcinoma xenografts, *Cancer Res.* 50:3493 (1990).

7. J.A. Houghton, L.G. Williams, P.J. Cheshire, I.W. Wainer, P. Jadaud, and P.J. Houghton, Influence of dose of [6RS]leucovorin on reduced folate pools and 5-fluorouracil-mediated thymidylate synthase inhibition in human colon adenocarcinoma xenografts, *Cancer Res.* 50:3940 (1990).

8. J.H. Doroshow, P. Multhauf, L. Leong, K. Margolin, T. Litchfield, S. Akman, B. Carr, M. Bertrand, D. Goldberg, D. Blayney, O. Odujinrin, R. Dehop, J. Shuster, E. Newman, Prospective randomized comparison of fluorouracil versus fluorouracil and high-dose continuous infusion leucovorin calcium for the treatment of advanced measurable colorectal cancer in patients previously unexposed to chemotherapy, *J. Clin. Oncol.* 8:491 (1990).

9. C. Erlichman, S. Fine, A. Wong, and T. Elhakim, A randomized trial of fluorouracil and folinic acid in patients with metastatic colorectal carcinoma, *J. Clin. Oncol.* 6:469 (1988).

10. N. Petrelli, L. Herrera, Y. Rustum, P. Burke, P. Creaven, J. Stulc, L.J. Emrich, A. Mittelman, A prospective randomized trial of 5-fluorouracil versus 5-fluorouracil and high-dose leucovorin versus 5-fluorouracil and methotrexate in previously untreated patients with advanced colorectal carcinoma, *J. Clin. Oncol.* 5:1559 (1987).

11. M.A. Poon, M.J. O'Connell, C.G. Moertel, H.S. Wieand, S.A. Cullinan, L.K. Everson, J.E. Krook, J.A. Mailliard, J.A. Laurie, L.K. Tschetter, and M. Weisenfeld, Biochemical modulation of fluorouracil: evidence of significant improvement of survival and quality of life in patients with advanced colorectal caricnoma, *J. Clin. Oncol.* 7:1407 (1989).

12. S. Wadler, E.L. Schwartz, M. Goldman, A. Lyver, M. Rader, M. Zimmerman, L. Itri, V. Weinberg, and P.H. Wiernik, 5-fluorouracil and recombinant α-2a-interferon: an active regimen against colorectal carcinoma, *J. Clin. Oncol.* 7:1769 (1989).

13. N. Kemeny, A. Younes, K. Seiter, D. Kelsen, P. Sammarco, L. Adams, S. Derby, P. Murray, and C. Houston. Interferon α-2a and 5-fluorouracil for advanced colorectal carcinoma, *Cancer* 66:2470 (1990).

14. R. Pazdur, J.A. Ajani, Y.Z. Patt, R. Winn, D. Jackson, B. Shepard, R. DuBrow, L. Campos, M. Quaraishi, J. Faintuch, J.L. Abbruzzese, J. Gutterman, and B. Levin, Phase II study of fluorouracil and recombinant interferon α-2a in previously untreated advanced colorectal carcinoma, *J. Clin. Oncol.* 8:2027 (1990).

15. L. Elias and J.A. Crissman, Interferon effects upon the adenocarcinoma 38 and HL-60 cell lines: antiproliferative responses and synergistic interactions with halogenated pyrimidine antimetabolites, *Cancer Res.* 48:4868 (1988).

16. E. Chu, S. Zinn, D. Boarman, and C.J. Allegra, Interaction of γ interferon and 5-fluorouracil in the H630 human colon carcinoma cell line, *Cancer Res.* 50:5834 (1990).

17. S. Wadler, R. Wersto, V. Weinberg, D. Thompson, and E.L. Schwartz, Interaction of fluorouracil and interferon in human colon cancer cell lines: cytotoxic and cytokinetic effects, *Cancer Res.* 50:5735 (1990).

18. S. Wadler and E.L. Schwartz, Antineoplastic activity of the combination of interferon and cytotoxic agents against experimental and human malignancies: a review, *Cancer Res.* 50:3473 (1990).

19. P.W. Woodman, D.L. Williams, and H.H. Edwards, Heterogeneity in cell populations established *in vitro* from a human colon adenocarcinoma xenograft. *In Vitro* 16:211 (1980).

20. P.J. Houghton, J.A. Houghton, G. Germain, and P.M. Torrance, Development and characterization of a human colon adenocarcinoma xenograft deficient in thymidine salvage, *Cancer Res.* 47:2117 (1987).

21. S. Radparvar, P.J. Houghton, G. Germain, J. Pennington, A. Rahman, and J.A. Houghton, Cellular pharmacology of 5-fluorouracil in a human colon adenocarcinoma cell line selected for thymidine kinase deficiency, *Biochem. Pharmacol.* 39:1759 (1990).

22. B.J. Winer, Stastitical principles in experimental design, 2nd ed., McGraw-Hill, New York (1971).

23. L.M. Pfeffer, Cellular effects of interferons, *in:* "Mechanisms of interferon action," L.M. Pfeffer, ed., CRC Press, Inc., Boca Raton, FL (1987).

24. K. Keyomarsi and R.G. Moran, Mechanism of the cytotoxic synergism of fluoropyrimidines and folinic acid in mouse leukemic cells, *J. Biol. Chem.* 263:14402 (1988).

25. R.M. Evans, J.D. Laskin, and M.T. Hakala, Effect of excess folates and deoxyinosine on the activity and site of action of 5-fluorouracil, *Cancer Res.* 41:3288 (1981).

26. K. Keyomarsi and R.G. Moran, Folinic acid augmentation of the effects of fluoropyrimidines on murine and human leukemic cells, *Cancer Res.* 46:5229 (1986).

27. C. Welander, Overview of preclinical and clinical studies of interferon α-2b in combination with cytotoxic drugs, *Invest. New Drugs* 5(Suppl):47 (1987).

28. J. Gutterman, S. Fine, J. Quesada, S.J. Horning, J.F. Levine, R. Alexanian, L. Bernhardt, M. Kramer, H. Spiegel, W. Colburn, P. Trown, T. Merrigan, and Z. Dziewanowski, Recombinant leukocyte A interferon: pharmacokinetics, single-dose tolerance, and biologic effects in cancer patients, *Ann. Intern. Med.* 96:549 (1982).

29. D. Machover, E. Goldschmidt, P. Chollet, C. Metzger, J. Zittoun, J. Marquet, J.-M. Vandenbulcke, J.-L. Misset, L. Schwarzenberg, J.B. Fourtillan, H. Gaget, and G. Mathe, Treatment of advanced colorectal and gastric adenocarcinomas with 5-fluorouracil and high-dose folinic acid, *J. Clin. Oncol.* 4:685 (1986).

30. E. Newman, J. Doroshow, M. Bertrand, P. Burgeson, D. Villacorte, D. Blayney, D. Goldberg, B. Carr, L. Leong, K. Margolin, G. Cecchi, and R. Staples, Pharmacokinetics of high-dose folinic acid (DL-CF) administered by continuous intravenous (i.v.) infusion, *Proc. Am. Assoc. Cancer Res.* 26:158 (1985).

31. J.A. Straw, E.M. Newman, and J.H. Doroshow, Pharmacokinetics of leucovorin (D,L-5-formyltetrahydrofolate) after intravenous injection and constant intravenous infusion, *NCI Monogr.* 5:41 (1987).

32. N.J. Petrelli, Y.M. Rustum, H. Bruckner, and D. Stablein, The Roswell Park Memorial Institute and Gastrointestinal Tumor Study Group phase III experience with the modulation of 5-fluorouracil by leucovorin in metastatic colorectal adenocarcinoma, *Adv. Exp. Med. Biol.* 244:143 (1988).

33. D. Brouty-Boye and M.G. Tovey, Inhibition by interferon of thymidine uptake in chemostat cultures of L1210 cells, *Intervirology* 9:243 (1978).

34. M. Divizia and C. Baglioni, Lack of correlation between thymidine kinase activity and the antiviral or antiproliferative response to interferon, *Virology* 133:216 (1984).

35. R.C. Jackson, A.L. Jackman, and A.H. Calvert, Biochemical effects of a quinazoline inhibitor of thymidylate synthetase, (N-(4-(N-((2-amino-4-hydroxy-6-quinazolinyl)methyl)prop-2-ynyla benzoyl)-L-gluatmic acid (CB3717), on human lymphoblastoid cells, *Biochem. Pharmacol.* 32:3783 (1983).

36. A.L. Jackman, G.A. Taylor, A.H. Calvert, and R.K. Harrap, Modulation of anti-metabolite effects. Effects of thymidine on the efficacy of the quinazoline-based thymidylate synthetase inhibitor, CB3717, *Biochem. Pharmacol.* 33:3269 (1984).

REGULATION OF THYMIDYLATE SYNTHASE IN HUMAN COLON CANCER
CELLS TREATED WITH 5-FLUOROURACIL AND INTERFERON-GAMMA

Edward Chu and Carmen J. Allegra

NCI-Navy Medical Oncology Branch
National Cancer Institute, NIH
NMOB 8/5101 - Naval Hospital
Bethesda, Maryland 20889

INTRODUCTION

5-Fluorouracil (5-FU) remains, at present, the single most active agent for the treatment of human colorectal cancer. When used as a single agent against advanced disease, it is associated with an overall response rate of only 15-20%, and therapy with 5-FU is unable to prolong the survival of treated patients [1-3]. Since few other agents have been identified for the treatment of human colorectal cancer, considerable attention has focused on elucidating the basic mechanisms of 5-FU action. The cytotoxic effects of 5-FU have been traditionally ascribed either to inhibition of the critical target enzyme thymidylate synthase (TS) by the 5-FU metabolite 5-fluoro-2'-deoxyuridine-5'-monophosphate (FdUMP) with subsequent inhibition of thymidylate and DNA biosynthesis, to incorporation of the 5-FU metabolite 5-fluorouridine-5'-triphosphate (FUTP) into RNA with resultant inhibition of RNA synthesis and function, or to incorporation of the 5-FU metabolite 5-fluoro-2'-deoxyuridine-5'-triphosphate (FdUTP) into DNA with resultant inhibition of DNA synthesis and function [1-11]. The relative contribution of each of these metabolic processes remains unclear at this time.

One of the principal obstacles to the clinical efficacy of 5-FU is the rapid emergence of cellular resistance. Various mechanisms of resistance have been well characterized in a number of in vitro and in vivo model systems. They include increased levels of target enzyme TS, alterations in binding affinity of TS for the 5-FU metabolite FdUMP, decreased intracellular pools of the reduced folate substrate 5,10-methylenetetrahydrofolate, increased activity of catabolic enzymes such as acid and alkaline phosphatase leading to decreased accumulation of the active 5-FU metabolites, and decreased levels of anabolic enzymes with consequent decreased formation of active metabolites [1,3,5,12-22]. Various investigators have recently described acute increases in TS enzyme activity in in vitro, in vivo and clinical systems following short-term exposure to the fluoropyrimidines [23-28]. Although the underlying mechanism(s) for this process has not been identified, it has been proposed that this acute induction of TS enzyme may represent a mechanism by which malignant cells develop cellular resistance to 5-FU [27,28].

*Novel Approaches to Selective Treatments of Human Solid Tumors: Laboratory
and Clinical Correlation* Edited by Y. M. Rustum, Plenum Press, New York, 1993

With the emerging use of the biological response modifiers, there has been considerable interest in combining these agents with antineoplastic compounds such as 5-FU in an attempt to enhance their cytotoxicity and therapeutic selectivity as well as prevent and/or overcome the development of drug resistance. A number of pre-clinical studies have demonstrated synergistic antiproliferative interactions between 5-FU and each of the interferons (IFN), alpha, beta and gamma, in various murine and human tumor cell lines, including HeLa, myeloma (KMM-1), myeloid leukemia, and colon adenocarcinoma (HT-29, MCA-38, and H630) cells [29-36]. Elias and Crissman [37] described synergistic cytotoxic effects of 5-FU and IFN-gamma against murine colon cancer cells and HL-60 human promyelocytic leukemic cells. They postulated that the mechanism of synergy involved enhanced inhibition of TS given the ability of thymidine to completely protect against the cytotoxic effects of the combination. Their studies further demonstrated that treatment of HL-60 cells with IFN-gamma led to a 10-fold increase in intracellular FdUMP levels with consequent enhanced inhibition of TS enzyme [38]. A similar increase in the levels of FdUMP in HT-29 human colon cancer cells following treatment with IFN-alpha was observed by Schwartz et al [39]. The increased 5-FU anabolism was associated with a significant increase in the activity of pyrimidine nucleoside phosphorylase (PyNP), suggesting that the effect of IFN-alpha on PyNP gene expression may be an important biochemical process that modulates 5-FU cytotoxicity. Recent investigations by Houghton et al [40] demonstrated marked potentiation of 5-FU cytotoxicity when combined with both recombinant human IFN-alpha and leucovorin. Their results suggested that the site of interaction of this three-drug combination was either at the level of TS or at some other DNA-associated locus.

In the present study, the underlying mechanisms of interaction between 5-FU and IFN-gamma in a human colon cancer H630 cell line were examined. IFN-gamma at non-growth inhibitory concentrations significantly enhanced 5-FU-associated cytotoxicity. Exposure to 5-FU was associated with an increase in both TS enzyme activity and TS protein expression. IFN-gamma treatment repressed the 5-FU-mediated increase in TS enzyme expression. Further studies revealed that the increase in TS following 5-FU exposure and the inhibitory effects of IFN-gamma on TS protein expression are both regulated at a post-transcriptional level. These studies suggest that induction of TS may represent a biologically relevant mechanism of resistance to 5-FU and that this process may be effectively circumvented with the use of IFN-gamma.

MATERIALS AND METHODS

Cell Culture

The characteristics of the human colon cancer H630 cell line have been previously well described [41]. Monolayer cultures of H630 cells were grown in 75-cm^2 plastic tissue culture flasks (Falcon Labware, Oxnard, CA) in growth medium consisting of RPMI-1640 with 10% dialyzed fetal bovine serum (Grand Island Biological Co., Grand Island, NY) and 2 mM glutamine and maintained in a humidified incubator at 5% CO_2 and 37°C. All other media components were obtained from Biofluids Co. (Rockville, MD).

In Vitro Cytotoxicity Studies

Plastic 25-cm^2 tissue culture flasks were seeded with 4.9 ml suspensions of 5 x 10^4 H630 cells in 10% dialyzed fetal bovine serum-containing medium and were incubated at 37°C. After 24-hr incubation, 0.1 ml of drug, at various concentrations, was added to each flask. Sterile water (0.1 ml) was added to controls. All experiments were performed in duplicate. Following a 72-hr incubation at 37°C, cells were trypsinized and counted using a Coulter counter (ZBI). The concentration of drug that resulted in 50%

inhibition of cell growth (IC_{50}) was determined from the plot of percent of control growth (cell number) versus the logarithm of drug concentration.

Incorporation of 5-FU Into Nucleotide Pools and Nucleic Acids

H630 cells were treated with [^{3}H]5-FU (1 µM, final specific activity 2.5 Ci/mmol) for 24 hours at 37°C. Cells were then washed three times with ice-cold PBS and fractionated for cold acid-soluble, RNA, and DNA fractions as previously outlined [41].

TS Binding Assay

H630 cells were washed three times with ice-cold PBS, harvested, and resuspended in 0.1 M KH_2PO_4, pH 7.2. Cell lysis was accomplished by sonication with three 2- to 3-sec bursts. Cell extracts were then centrifuged at 10,000 x g for 30 min, and the supernatants were immediately assayed for enzyme activity. Total (TS_T) and free (TS_F) levels were determined by the radioenzymatic FdUMP binding assay as previously described [41].

Isolation of Total RNA and RNA Blot Hybridization (Northern) Analysis

H630 cells were washed three times with ice-cold PBS and harvested from 150-cm^2 tissue culture flasks with a rubber policeman. Total RNA was extracted according to the method of Chomczynski and Sacchi [42]. For Northern blot analysis, 30 µg/sample of total cellular RNA was denatured, fractionated on a 1% formaldehyde-agarose gel, and transferred to a Nytran filter membrane as described previously [21]. The cDNA for human TS was a generous gift from Dr. T. Seno (Saitama Cancer Center Research Institute, Saitama-ken, Japan).

Measurement of TS Biosynthesis

H630 cells were treated with drug for 22 hours in medium containing 10% dialyzed fetal bovine serum. The medium was changed, cells were washed with methionine-free medium, and then incubated for an additional 2 hours in 3 ml of methionine-free medium and 10% dialyzed fetal bovine serum containing 100 µCi/ml methionine (Trans [^{35}S]-label; specific activity = 1013 Ci/mmol). Cells were then washed twice with ice-cold PBS and scraped into ice-cold lysis buffer according to the method of Harford [43]. TS-specific protein was immunoprecipitated with polyclonal TS antisera along with protein-A agarose (Bethesda Research Laboratories, Bethesda, MD). Samples were analyzed by autoradiography after electrophoresis in a 12.5% SDS-polyacrylamide gel using the buffer system of Laemmli [44].

Quantitation of TS mRNA and TS Protein from Autoradiographs

The levels of TS-specific and TS protein were determined by densitometric scanning of autoradiographs using a Hewlett-Packard ScanJet Plus scanner.

Protein Determination

Protein was quantitated using the method of Bradford [45].

RESULTS

Effect of IFN-gamma on 5-FU Cytotoxicity

H630 human colon cancer cells were treated continuously for 72 hours with various concentrations of 5-FU in the absence or presence of IFN-gamma. The concentration of IFN-gamma (30 Units/ml) used in these growth studies

TABLE 1. Effect of 5-FU and IFN-γ on Growth of H630 Human Colon Cancer Cells

Treatment	IC$_{50}$ (μM)
5-FU	5.5
5-FU/IFN-γ	0.3

was non-growth inhibitory to these cells. As seen in Table 1, the concentration of 5-FU required to inhibit growth of H630 cells by 50% was significantly decreased (18-fold) from 5.5 to 0.3 μM with the simultaneous addition of IFN-gamma. Both the growth-inhibitory effects of 5-FU alone and the combination of 5-FU/IFN-gamma were overcome by the addition of 20 μM thymidine. This finding suggested that the locus of interaction of the combination of 5-FU/IFN-gamma either was at the level of TS or involved some other DNA-mediated process.

Effect of IFN-gamma on 5-FU Nucleotide Pools and on Incorporation into Nucleic Acids

Since the level of the 5-FU metabolite FdUMP is a critical determinant of TS enzyme inhibition, the effects of IFN-gamma on formation of this metabolite were measured. There were no differences in the intracellular levels of FdUMP either in the absence or presence of IFN-gamma (Table 2). IFN-gamma treatment did not alter formation of FUTP, the 5-FU anabolite involved in RNA incorporation (Table 2). The effects of IFN-gamma on incorporation of radioactively labeled 5-FU into nucleic acids during a 24-hr incubation were next examined. The addition of IFN-gamma did not alter the level of incorporation of 5-FU into either RNA or DNA compared to cells treated with 5-FU alone (Table 2).

Effect of IFN-gamma on Inhibition of 5-FU-Mediated Induction of TS

The results from the previous experiments suggested that TS may be an important site of interaction between 5-FU and IFN-gamma. The effect of this combination on TS expression with regard to enzyme activity, protein expression and TS mRNA levels was subsequently investigated.

In our initial attempts to characterize the potential mechanisms of resistance to 5-FU in the H630 cell line, the total level of TS enzyme, as determined by the FdUMP binding assay, was increased by nearly 4-fold

TABLE 2. Effect of IFN-γ on 5-FU Nucleotide Pools and on Incorporation of 5-FU Into Nucleic Acids of H630 Cells

Treatment	FdUMP (pmol/mg protein)	FUTP	RNA (pmol/mg RNA)	DNA (pmol/mg DNA)
5-FU	2.4	3.6	125	5.8
5-FU/IFN-γ	2.7	3.7	132	4.8

H630 cells were incubated at 37°C for a 24-hr exposure to [6-^{3}H]5-FU (1 μM, 2.5 Ci/mmol). Cells were harvested and fractionated for cold acid-soluble, RNA, and DNA fractions.

TABLE 3. Effect of 24-Hour Exposure of 5-FU and IFN-γ on TS Protein, TS mRNA Levels, and TS Synthesis in H630 Cells

Treatment	Ratio of Treated vs Control Cells		
	TS-Total[1]	TS mRNA[2]	TS Synthesis[3]
5-FU (1 µM)	4	1.0	3.5
IFN-γ (30 units/ml)	1.3	1.0	1.3
5-FU/IFN-γ	1.6	1.0	1.5

[1] This value represents the ratio of TS-Total in drug-treated cells relative to control cells as determined by the radio-enzymatic FdUMP binding assay.

[2] This value represents the ratio of TS mRNA in drug-treated cells relative to control cells as determined by densito-metric analysis of RNA hybridization blots.

[3] This value represents the ratio of newly synthesized TS in drug-treated cells relative to control cells as determined by densitometric analysis of autoradiograms.

following exposure to 1 µM 5-FU over a 24-hour time period (Table 3). This increase peaked at 24 hours (3-fold) and remained elevated for up to 36 hours (2.5-fold). Western immunoblot analysis revealed that these changes in TS enzyme activity in response to 5-FU exposure were associated with similar changes in TS protein levels. To determine the molecular basis by which TS protein expression was controlled, TS mRNA levels following 5-FU treatment were next measured by means of Northern blot analysis. The level of TS mRNA remained unchanged in 5-FU-treated cells when compared to control, untreated cells.

The effect of IFN-gamma on the 5-FU-mediated increase in TS enzyme expression was subsequently determined. IFN-gamma alone, at a concentration of 30 Units/ml, did not alter TS enzyme activity or TS protein expression when compared to control cells. Treatment with 1 µM 5-FU resulted in a 4-fold increase in TS expression. With the addition of IFN-gamma to cells treated with 1 µM 5-FU, the 5-FU-associated induction of TS expression was ablated, maintaining TS enzyme and TS protein at nearly control levels. When TS mRNA levels were measured in cells treated under the same conditions, there were no differences noted in cells treated with either, 5-FU, IFN-gamma, or 5-FU/IFN-gamma (Table 3). Radioactive [S^{35}]methionine labeling studies were performed to determine the amount of TS biosynthesis in response to 5-FU treatment. There was a 3.5-fold increase in newly synthesized TS following 5-FU exposure. In contrast, treatment either with IFN-gamma alone or with the combination of 5-FU/IFN-gamma resulted in net levels of newly synthesized TS not significantly different from that seen in control, untreated cells. Preliminary studies demonstrated that the stability of TS protein, i.e., TS enzyme half-life, was approximately the same in cells treated with no drug, 5-FU, IFN-gamma, or 5-FU/IFN-gamma. These findings suggest that the effects of 5-FU and IFN-gamma on TS protein expression are both regulated at a translational level.

DISCUSSION

A number of studies have recently described acute overexpression of the target enzyme TS following short-term exposure to the fluoropyrimidines [23-28]. With regard to the clinical setting, Swain et al [28] reported a 3-fold increase in total levels of TS in metastatic skin biopsy specimens taken from patients with breast cancer 24 hours following 5-FU treatment. The results of the present study demonstrate that a similar process of TS induction occurs in the H630 human colon cancer cell line. The level of both TS enzyme activity and TS protein expression are increased in response to 5-FU treatment. Moreover, IFN-gamma, at concentrations that are non-growth inhibitory and that do not affect TS enzyme expression, effectively inhibits the 5-FU-associated induction of TS. Consequently, H630 cells, which are inherently resistant to 5-FU, become 18-fold more sensitive to the cytotoxic effects of 5-FU in the presence of IFN-gamma. The biological relevance of this observation is that the concentration of 5-FU over time (area under the concentration-time curve) normally required to inhibit H630 cells is not clinically achievable. However, with simultaneous IFN-gamma treatment, the concentration of 5-FU required to inhibit growth by 50% is well within the clinically achievable range.

Several investigators have suggested that induction of TS enzyme levels following 5-FU exposure may represent a mechanism by which cellular resistance to 5-FU can develop. Our results demonstrate that exposure to 5-FU results in increased levels of both TS enzyme activity and TS protein expression with no corresponding changes in TS mRNA levels. Further studies show that TS expression in response to 5-FU is controlled at a translational level. We have recently demonstrated in a rabbit reticulocyte in vitro translation system that TS mRNA translation is controlled in a negative autoregulatory manner by its own protein end product TS [46]. Of particular interest was the observation that incubation of human recombinant TS protein with either of the normal substrate ligands dUMP or 5,10-methylenetetra-hydrofolate or with the 5-FU metabolite FdUMP completely repressed the inhibitory effect of TS protein on TS mRNA translation. This finding suggested that either the native conformational state of TS protein or active site occupancy of TS by these ligands may be critical determinants of TS mRNA translational efficiency. Treatment of cells with the fluoropyrimidines would result in the intracellular accumulation of the pyrimidine nucleotides dUMP and FdUMP, both of which can interact with TS protein to decrease the level of free TS. Their interaction with TS would repress formation of the TS protein/mRNA complex, resulting in enhanced translational efficiency and an increased intracellular level of TS protein. Thus, the present study lends further support to the model of TS translational autoregulation and suggests that this process is biologically relevant. Moreover, the ability to translationally regulate TS expression appears to provide an efficient mechanism for malignant cells to protect themselves against a cytotoxic stress such as 5-FU.

In summary, these studies suggest that the acute induction of TS represents a biologically important mechanism by which H630 cells develop resistance to 5-FU. Further, these studies identify a novel mechanism of interaction between 5-FU and IFN-gamma. IFN-gamma negatively regulates the 5-FU-mediated induction of TS expression at a translational level and, in so doing, enhances inhibition of this important target enzyme by 5-FU. Further characterization of the molecular basis for the interaction between 5-FU and IFN-gamma should provide important insights into the regulation of thymi-dylate synthase and should offer new therapeutic approaches to circumvent the development of cellular resistance to the fluoropyrimidines.

Acknowledgement

The authors would like to thank Kathy Moore for her editorial assistance in the preparation of the manuscript.

REFERENCES

1. H.M. Pinedo and G.F.J. Peters, Fluorouracil: biochemistry and pharmacology, J. Clin. Oncol. 6:1653-1664 (1988).
2. C. Heidelberger, Fluorinated pyrimidines and their nucleosides, in: "Antineoplastic and Immunosuppressive Agents," A. Sartorelli and D. Johns, eds, Springer-Verlag, New York, pp 193-231 (1975).
3. C. Heidelberger, P.V. Danenberg and R.G. Moran, Fluorinated pyrimidines and their nucleosides, Adv. Enzymol. Related Areas Mol. Biol. 54: 57-119 (1989).
4. D.V. Santi, C.S. McHenry and H. Sommer, Mechanism of interaction of thymidine synthetase with 5-fluorodeoxyuridylate, Biochemistry 13: 471-481 (1974).
5. B. Ardalan, D. Cooney, H. Jayaram, C. Carrico, R. Glazar, J. Macdonald and P.S. Schein, Mechanisms of sensitivity and resistance of murine tumors to 5-fluorouracil, Cancer Res. 40:1431-1437 (1980).
6. S. Spiegelman, R. Sawyer, R. Nayak, E. Ritzi, R. Stolfi and D. Martin, Improving the antitumor activity of 5-fluorouracil by increasing its incorporation into RNA via metabolic modulation, Proc. Natl. Acad. Sci. USA 77:4966-4970 (1980).
7. D.S. Wilkinson and J. Crumley, The mechanism of 5-fluorouridine toxicity in Novikoff hepatoma cells, Cancer Res. 36:4032-4038 (1976).
8. R.I. Glazar and A.L. Peale, The effect of 5-fluorouracil on the synthesis of nuclear RNA in L1210 cells in vitro, Mol. Pharmacol. 16: 270-277 (1979).
9. D.W. Kufe, P.P. Major, E.M. Egan and E. Loh, 5-Fluoro-2'-deoxyuridine incorporation in L1210 DNA, J. Biol. Chem. 256:8885-8888 (1981).
10. P.P. Major, E. Egan, D. Herrick and D.W. Kufe, 5-Fluorouracil incorporation in DNA of human breast carcinoma cells, Cancer Res. 42: 3005-3009 (1982).
11. Y-C. Cheng and K. Nakayama, Effects of 5-fluoro-2'-deoxyuridine on DNA metabolism in HeLa cells, Mol. Pharmacol. 23:171-174 (1983).
12. D. Kessel, T.C. Hall and I. Wodinsky, Nucleotide formation as a determinant of 5-fluorouracil response in mouse leukemia, Science 154: 911-913 (1966).
13. J.A. Houghton, S.J. Maroda, J.O. Phillips and P.J. Houghton, Biochemical determinants of responsiveness to 5-fluorouracil and its derivatives in xenografts of human colorectal adenocarcinomas in mice, Cancer Res. 41:144-149 (1981).
14. M.A. Mulkins and C. Heidelberger, Biochemical characterization of fluoropyrimidine-resistant murine leukemic cell lines, Cancer Res. 42:965-973 (1982).
15. M.B. Yin, S.F. Zakrzewski and M.T. Hakala, Relationship of cellular folate cofactor pools to the activity of 5-fluorouracil, Mol. Pharmacol. 23:190-197 (1983).
16. D.J. Fernandes and S.K. Crawford, Resistance of CCRF-CEM cloned sublines to 5-fluorodeoxyuridine associated with enhanced phosphatase activities, Biochem. Pharmacol. 34:125-132 (1985).
17. S.H. Berger, C-H. Jenh, L.F. Johnson and F. Berger, Thymidylate synthase overproduction and gene amplification in fluorodeoxyuridine-resistant human cells, Mol. Pharmacol. 28:461-467 (1985).

18. J.L. Clark, S.H. Berger, A. Mittelman and F. Berger, Thymidylate synthase gene amplification in a colon tumor resistant to fluoropyrimidine chemotherapy, Cancer Treat. Rep. 71:261-265 (1987).
19. S.H. Berger, K.W. Barbour and F. Berger, A naturally occurring variation in thymidylate synthase structure is associated with a reduced response to 5-fluoro-2'-deoxyuridine in a human colon tumor cell line, Mol. Pharmacol. 34:480-484 (1988).
20. E. Chu, G-M. Lai, S. Zinn and C.J. Allegra, Resistance of a human ovarian cancer line to 5-fluorouracil associated with decreased levels of 5-fluorouracil in DNA, Mol. Pharmacol. 38:410-417 (1990).
21. E. Chu, J.C. Drake, D.M. Koeller, S. Zinn, C.A. Jamis-Dow, G.C. Yeh and C.J. Allegra, Induction of thymidylate synthase associated with multidrug resistance in human breast and colon cancer cell lines, Mol. Pharmacol. 39:136-143 (1990).
22. C. Aschele, A. Sobrero, M.A. Faderan and J.R. Bertino, Novel mechanism(s) of resistance to two different clinically relevant dose schedules, Cancer Res. 52:1855-1864 (1992).
23. C.P. Spears, A.H. Shahinian, R.G. Moran, C. Heidelberger and T.H. Corbett, In vivo kinetics of thymidylate synthase inhibition in 5-fluorouracil-sensitive and -resistant murine colon adenocarcinomas, Cancer Res. 42:450-456 (1982).
24. W.L. Washtien, Increased levels of thymidylate synthetase in cells exposed to 5-fluorouracil, Mol. Pharmacol. 25:171-177 (1984).
25. M.H.O. Berne, B.G. Gustavsson, O. Almersjo, P.C. Spears and R. Frosing, Sequential methotrexate/5-FU: FdUMP formation and TS inhibition in a transplantable rodent colon adenocarcinoma, Cancer Chemother. Pharmacol. 16:237-242 (1986).
26. M. Berne, B. Gustavsson, O. Almersjo, C.P. Spears and J. Waldenstrom, Concurrent allopurinol and 5-fluorouracil: 5-fluoro-2'-deoxyuridylate formation and thymidylate synthase inhibition in rat colon carcinoma and in regenerating rat liver, Cancer Chemother. Pharmacol. 20:193-197 (1987).
27. K. Keyomarsi and R.G. Moran, Mechanism of the cytotoxic synergism of fluoropyrimidines and folinic acid in mouse leukemic cells, J. Biol. Chem. 263:14402-14409 (1988).
28. S.M. Swain, M.E. Lippman, E.F. Egan, J.C. Drake, S.M. Steinberg and C.J. Allegra, Fluorouracil and high-dose leucovorin in previously treated patients with metastatic breast cancer, J. Clin. Oncol. 7:890-899 (1989).
29. M. Namba, T. Miyoshi, T. Kanamori, M. Nobuhara, T. Kimoto and S. Ogawa, Combined effects of 5-fluorouracil and interferon on proliferation of human neoplastic cells in culture, Gann 73:819-824 (1982).
30. T. Miyoshi, S. Ogawa, T. Kanamori, M. Nobuhara and M. Namba, Interferon potentiates cytotoxic effects of 5-fluorouracil on cell proliferation of established human cell lines originating from neoplastic tissues, Cancer Lett. 17:239-241 (1983).
31. M. Inoue and Y.H. Tan, Enhancement of actinomycin-D and cis-diamminedichloroplatinum(II)-induced killing of human fibroblasts by human beta interferon, Cancer Res. 43:5484-5488 (1983).
32. D. Le, Y.K. Yip and J. Vilcek, CYtolytic activity of interferon-gamma and its synergism with 5-fluorouracil, Int. J. Cancer 34:495-500 (1984).
33. S. Yamamoto, H. Tanaka, T. Kanamori, M. Nobuhara and M. Namba, In vitro studies of cytotoxic effects of anticancer drugs by interferon on a human neoplastic cell line (HeLa), Cancer Lett. 20:131-138 (1983).
34. Y. Kimoto, Antitumor effect of interferons with chemotherapeutic agents, Gan. To Kayaku Ryoho 13:293-301 (1986).
35. K. Gohji, S. Macda, T. Sugiyama, J. Ishigumi and S. Kamidona, Enhanced inhibition of anticancer drugs by human recombinant gamma-interferon for human renal cell carcinoma in vitro, J. Urol. 137:539-543 (1987).

36. M.S. Mitchell, Combining chemotherapy with biological response modi-
    fiers in treatment of cancer, J. Natl. Cancer Inst. 80:1445-1450
    (1988).
37. L. Elias and H.A. Crissman, Interferon effects on the adenocarcinoma 38
    and HL-60 cell lines: antiproliferative responses and synergistic
    interactions with halogenated pyrimidine antimetabolites, Cancer
    Res. 48:4868-4873 (1988).
38. L. Elias and J.M. Sandoval, Interferon effects upon fluorouracil metab-
    olism by HL-60 cells, Biochem. Biophys. Res. Commun. 130:379-388
    (1989).
39. E.L. Schwartz, M. Hoffman, C.J. O'Connor and S. Wadler, Stimulation of
    5-fluorouracil metabolic activation by interferon-alpha in human
    colon carcinoma cells, Biochem. Biophys. Res. Commun. 182:1232-
    1239 (1992).
40. J.A. Houghton, D.A. Adkins, A. Rahman and P.J. Houghton, Interaction
    between 5-fluorouracil, [6RS]leucovorin, and recombinant human
    interferon-alpha-2a in cultured colon adenocarcinoma cells, Cancer
    Commun. 3:225-231 (1991).
41. E. Chu, S. Zinn, D. Boarman and C.J. Allegra, Interaction of gamma
    interferon and 5-fluorouracil in the H630 human colon carcinoma
    cell line, Cancer Res. 50:5834-4840 (1990).
42. P. Chomczynski and N. Sacchi, Single-step method of RNA isolation by
    acid guanidinium thiocyanate-phenol-chloroform extraction, Anal.
    Biochem. 162:156-159 (1987).
43. J. Harford, An artifact explains the apparent association of the trans-
    ferrin receptor with a ras gene product, Nature 311:493-495 (1984).
44. U.K. Laemmli, Cleavage of structural proteins during the assembly of
    the head of bacteriophage T$_4$, Nature 227:680-685 (1986).
45. M. Bradford, A rapid and sensitive method for the quantitation of
    microgram quantities of protein utilizing the principle of protein-
    dye binding, Anal. Biochem. 72:248-254 (1976).
46. E. Chu, D.M. Koeller, J.L. Casey, J.C. Drake, B.A. Chabner, P.G. Elwood,
    S. Zinn and C.J. Allegra, Autoregulation of human thymidylate syn-
    thase messenger RNA translation by thymidylate synthase, Proc.
    Natl. Acad. Sci. USA 88:8977-8981 (1991).

BIOCHEMICAL MODULATION OF 5-FLUOROURACIL BY PALA:
MECHANISM OF ACTION

Daniel S. Martin

From Developmental Chemotherapy, Memorial Sloan Kettering Cancer Center, Cornell University Medical College, New York, NY; and Catholic Medical Center of Brooklyn & Queens, Inc., New York, NY

Address reprint requests to Daniel S. Martin, Cancer Research, 89-15 Woodhaven Blvd., Woodhaven, NY 11421

CELLULAR HETEROGENEITY AND BIOCHEMICAL MODULATION

Selectivity is, of course, the key to all chemotherapy. However, selectivity is very difficult to achieve against cancer cells in vivo because the biochemical differences between cancer and normal cells are quantitative rather than qualitative. Consequently, anticancer agents have a narrow therapeutic index and, therefore, chemotherapy is frequently toxic to the patient as well as to the tumor.

There is, in addition to this difficulty, a large therapeutic problem brought about by tumor cell "qualitative" biochemical heterogeneity within the neoplastic cell population[1-2]; namely, the presence of subsets of cancer cells within an individual tumor that differ in a qualitative biochemical sense (i.e., a subset differs in not being at all sensitive to an agent with therapeutic activity against another subset).

In addition, there is the further difficulty that biochemical heterogeneity usually extends "quantitatively" within each subset of malignant cells. "Quantitative" biochemical heterogeneity means that a subset of cancer cells that is sensitive to an individual anticancer agent possesses a gradient of responsiveness to that agent. The cancer cells within a particular subset differ in that, while all cells of the subset are sensitive to a single effector agent, some cells are more vulnerable than others to a particular dose. Due to this gradient of sensitivity, and the low chemotherapeutic indices of anticancer agents, eradication of even slightly resistant cells of the drug-sensitive subset is impossible at the agent's low in vivo-tolerated dose. When this occurs this component of the malignant population is untreated and can then grow to dominance as an apparently drug-resistant tumor. These cells initially are actually only pseudoresistant, but under the described in vivo chemotherapeutic treatment conditions, will appear unresponsive to chemotherapy and grow into a large tumor recurrence[3].

To avoid the latter lethal eventuality, the use of biochemical modulation can be employed to create new intracellular biochemical conditions in the quasi-drug-resistant (but actually drug-sensitive) cells that then will permit their destruction by in vivo tolerated doses of the effector agent. Thus, one approach to improving the selectivity of anticancer

Novel Approaches to Selective Treatments of Human Solid Tumors: Laboratory and Clinical Correlation Edited by Y. M. Rustum, Plenum Press, New York, 1993

153

agents (as well as to circumvent the development of drug resistance) is to utilize selective biochemical modulation to increase the therapeutic activity of an individual effector agent, such as FUra.[3-4]

MECHANISM(S) OF CYTOTOXICITY OF FUra

Pharmacodynamics (knowledge of the intracellular biochemical effects of a drug and its mechanism(s) of action) is of key importance to biochemical modulation.[5-7] Thus, improving an effector agent's selectivity through biochemical modulation requires an understanding of the drug's probable mechanism of action. In particular, and as exemplified by the N-(phosphonacetyl)-L-aspartate (PALA)-5-FU clinical paradigm[3-9] pharmacodynamic information of an anticancer agent is of basic utility to the medical oncologist.

FUra exerts its cytotoxic effects by at least two major mechanism's of action[3-4]: 1) inhibition of thymidylate synthase (TS) by the FUra metabolite, 5-fluoro-2'-deoxyuridine-5'-mono-phosphate (FdUMP), an effect that kills cells by limiting the only de novo source of thymidylate for DNA synthesis; and 2) incorporation of FUra into RNA at the level of 5-fluorouridine triphosphate (FUTP) (Fig. 1), the resulting fraudulent (FU)RNA causing anticancer activity due to erroneous processing of RNA with consequent adverse effects on one or more enzymes[10-21] The incorporation of FUra in RNA proceeds via FUTP in a reaction catalysed by RNA polymerase, and is a time- and concentration-dependent process. In intact cells FUTP constitutes the major fraction of acid-soluble FUra derivatives.[22]

Whether the DNA-directed effect (i.e., inhibition of TS), or the RNA-directed effect (i.e., (FU)RNA), is more important in producing tumor cytotoxicity is controversial. Certainly, the early prevalent view was that the anti-TS mechanism was the main antitumor mechanism of fluoropyrimidines. By 1984, enough (FU)RNA data had been reported for a review article to note, "it is surprising that the notion of 5-FU cytotoxicity has been so widely accepted when many conflicting reports have appeared in the literature."[23] In recent years, despite the absence of simultaneous analysis of both the DNA- and RNA-directed effects in most studies of the combination of leucovorin (LV) and FUra, the spate of positive clinical reports claiming enhancement of antitumor efficacy by the LV/FUra combination, has led some to state that "the RNA incorporation of 5-FU plays only a minor role in tumor cytotoxicity."[24] In contrast, a very recent review of the metabolism and mechanism of action of FUra stated: "Because FUra is toxic to cells in the presence of thymidine and in some cells there is a good correlation between the incorporation of FUra into RNA and cytotoxicity, it is widely accepted that the incorporation of FUra into RNA is an important element of FUra cytotoxicity . . . and . . . (importantly) . . . usually occurs at higher concentrations than are required for DNA-directed toxicity."[25] For example, where both of FUra's major biochemical effects, the degree of TS inhibition, and the amount of (FU)RNA, have been concurrently evaluated in tumor cells, "low" FUra doses have produced inhibition of TS that has caused cytotoxicity only in some cell lines, whereas "high" FUra doses could be correlated with (FU)RNA and cytotoxicity in all the cell lines.[26] It is also revealing of the significance of high FUra dosage to mechanism of action and therapeutic efficacy, that in in vivo murine tumor studies comparing "high" (MTD) FUra and low-dose FUra at equal weekly-dose intensities, high (MTD) FUra was therapeutically superior, inhibited TS activity essentially equally and maximally, and produced increased incorporation of FUra into RNA. Moreover, at still greater doses of FUra than the MTD (with the animals protected from FUra toxicity by uridine "rescue"), TS inhibition could not be further enhanced (even with the addition of LV), but both (FU)RNA and therapeutic efficacy were further increased; thus, since TS could not be further inhibited at doses above MTD, the increased chemotherapeutic efficacy correlated with increased (FU)RNA.[43] The latter studies were preclinical, and the issue of which of the two mechanisms is the more important has not been clarified at the clinical level, largely because safe methodology for sensitive analysis of (FU)RNA in patients is not yet available.

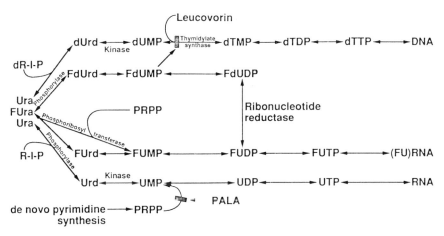

Fig. 1. Outline of biochemical pathways taken by 5-fluorouracil (FUra) to its principal loci of action, the blocking of thymidylate synthase and incorporation into RNA to form (FU)RNA. Note that FUra tracks the pathways of normal uracil (Ura) metabolism and, therefore, must compete with Ura-containing metabolites for enzymatic attention at every anabolic step. Greater intracellular levels of FUra favor the competition of FUra over Ura. Modulation with PALA, which in low dosage can inhibit de novo pyrimidine synthesis selectively in the tumor, releases thereby the PRPP pools normally employed for this synthesis, and by making available greater amounts of this necessary substrate thereby facilitate greater anabolic conversion of FUra to FUMP by the enyzme, phosphoribosyl transferase. Moreover, this inhibition of pyrimidine biosynthesis lowers the intracellular levels of Ura nucleotides, which futher favors FUra-nucleotides to outcompete Ura-containing nucleotides, such as FUTP over UTP for incorporation into RNA, or as FdUMP over dUMP to block thymidylate synthase.

However, it is generally agreed that high FUra dose intensity per se is therapeutically important. And, as well be explained below, biochemical modulation of FUra with PALA can substantially increase, in effect, the intracellular level of FUra metabolites and markedly increase the incorporation of FUra into RNA with consequent and selective augmentation of FUra's antitumor efficacy.

BIOCHEMICAL MODULATION OF FUra WITH PALA

To understand the PALA-FUra interaction, it must be understood that FUra is a "prodrug" that gains anti-tumor activity only after conversion to the nucleotide level, and that, regardless of whether FUra acts through a DNA- or RNA-mechanism, FUra must compete with uridine nucleotides at every metabolic step of its way toward its DNA- and/or RNA-target site(s) (Fig. 1). Therefore, an agent that lowers uracil nucleotide pools (particularly in tumor tissue) will favor greater metabolic targeting of FUra-containing nucleotides and thereby enhance FUra's anti-tumor efficacy. PALA, an inhibitor of de novo pyrimidine sythesis, is such an agent.

PALA irreversibly inhibits aspartate transcarbamylase, the second enzyme in the de novo pathway for the biosynthesis of pyrimidine, by competing with its natural substrate, carbamyl phosphate[27]. Inhibition of de novo synthesis results in a lowering of uridine triphosphate (UTP) pools. When PALA is administered well before FUra, the resulting decrease in pyrimidine pools favors greater utilization of FUra at its metabolic targets, resulting, for example, in increased incorporation of FUra into tumor RNA and enhanced anti-tumor activity in a number of animal tumor models.[5,10-11,18-20,28-32]

Thus, the basis for the synergism appears to be the change in the FUTP/UTP ratio, resulting in increased incorporation of FUTP into RNA. In effect, then, PALA administered well before FUra to allow lowering of the intracellular pyrimidine pools in tumor tissue at the time of FUra administration, results in a substantial increase in the level of FUra incorporation into the RNA of tumor cells. The optimal treatment interval is approximately 24 hours.[5,38] In addition, PALA results in increased intracellular phosphoribosyl-pyrophosphate (PRPP) (Fig. 1), through the reduced utilization of PRPP due to PALA inhibition of de novo pyrimidine synthesis; in turn, the increased availability of PRPP favors the formation of FUra nucleotides.[33-35] See Fig. 1.

Since PALA's target enzyme, aspartate transcarbamylase, is apparently in low concentration in tumor tissue,[36] a low, but biochemically active, dose of PALA may selectively deplete pyrimidine pools in cancers and safely modulate the anticancer activity of a high dose of FUra in cancer patients, as it does in tumor-bearing animals. It is possible to inhibit more selectively an enzyme present in cancer tissue in small amounts, while producing much less inactivation of the same enzyme in normal tissues containing larger amounts.[37]

SIGNIFICANCE OF THE APPROPRIATE DOSAGE RATIO BETWEEN AGENTS

Dosage ratio between agents can be a crucial detail in the design of clinical protocols, and the PALA/FUra combination is a paradigm of these relationships.

In tumor-bearing animals, moderate to high doses of PALA alone display anticancer activity (as measured by inhibition of tumor growth), and any ratio of such therapeutic doses of PALA and FUra in combination (e.g., high PALA to low FUra, or moderate PALA to high FUra) is able to display enhanced antitumor activity. However, in the clinical trials (where anticancer activity is measured by tumor regression), even high doses of PALA alone are devoid of demonstrable therapeutic activity[39]. Unfortunately, originally only a high PALA dosage in combination with FUra was investigated in the clinical trials of this combination[40]. The toxicity of this high PALA dosage permitted tolerable drug combination only with low FUra dosage, and the resulting antitumor activity of this combination in the clinic was found no better than the clinical maximal tolerated dose (MTD) of FUra alone in historical controls. The use of a dose of a modulating agent high enough to require a significant reduction of the dose of the effector agent (when the latter has a steep dose-response curve and is at its MTD in the historical controls) is likely to be self-defeating in comparison with the historical controls employing high-dose therapeutic activity of the effector agent (i.e., FUra) as a single agent.

Logically, then, a low-PALA "modulating" dose (i.e., a biochemically active dose, even if low) might permit a clinically tolerable combination with a high FUra dose at or close to its MTD and thereby might effect useful synergistic anti-tumor activity over that of the MTD of FUra alone. Since PALA's target enzyme, aspartate transcarbamylase, is in low concentration in tumor cells, selectivity should be attained in the presence of a low biochemically active dose of PALA.[36] Moore et al[36] noted that PALA does have biochemical effect on human tumors and that "a 50-70% decrease in UTP might well be sufficient to alter the effect of . . . (FUra) . . . in susceptible tumors."

NEW FINDINGS THAT WERE REQUIRED FOR APPROPRIATE TRANSFER OF THE PALA-5-FU COMBINATION TO THE CLINIC

On the basis of the preceding facts and reasoning, appropriate application of the above logic would require: 1) demonstration of a low dose of PALA in laboratory tumors in vivo that emulates PALA's clinical findings in being non-therapeutic but has biochemical activity; 2) determining whether such a low PALA dose can usefully enhance the in vivo anti-tumor activity of a high dose of FUra; 3) if the laboratory answers are encouraging, identifying a similar, low, "modulating" dose of PALA in patients; and 4) clinically testing this low dose in combination with the highest tolerated dose of FUra, which, it would be hoped, would be the clinical MTD of FUra.

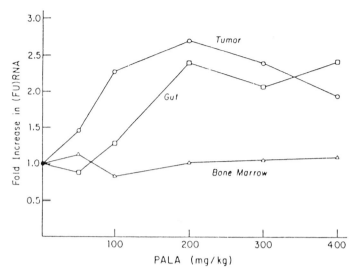

Fig. 2. Effect of PALA on dose on the level of (FU)RNA in murine (CD8F1) breast cancer intestinal epithelium, and bone marrow. Only low dose PALA (100 mg/kg) was selective in causing more FU incorporation into the RNA of the tumor than in the gut. PALA has no effect on (FU)RNA in the bone marrow, and doses higher than 100 mg/kg resulted in little difference between (FU)RNA levels in tumor and gut.

ATTAINMENT OF THE REQUIRED PRECLINICAL DATA

A study of the PALA-FUra combination in the laboratory demonstrated that a low and non-therapeutic dose of PALA (100 mg/kg) could lower UTP tumor pools by 40% in vivo, and thereby selectively potentiate the anti-tumor effects of the MTD of FUra without undue toxicity.[5]

Since the incorporation of FUra into RNA has been causally associated with cytotoxicity in our preclinical tumor system[10-11,21,32] the effect of various doses of PALA administered 24 hours before FUra on the incorporation of FUra into RNA in the murine breast tumor, intestinal epithelium, and bone marrow was examined. Results (Fig. 2) indicated that in bone marrow, PALA did not affect the level of (FU)RNA regardless of the PALA dosage administered. This negative result is consistent with the lack of PALA hematologic toxicity in mice reported by Harrison et al[41]. In contrast, the latter investigators reported a PALA-induced gastrointestinal toxicity. In accord with this finding, Fig. 2 records that PALA augmented gut levels of (FU)RNA. It is pertinent that substantial elevations of (FU)RNA in intestine were seen only with PALA dosages of 200 mg/kg or higher, whereas PALA at 100 mg/kg caused only a slight elevation in the gut (FU)RNA[5]. In contrast, the latter low dose of PALA produced substantial elevation of (FU)RNA in the tumor -- in keeping with the desired selectivity -- and resulted in safe therapeutic synergism in combination with a full (MTD) dose of FUra.[5]

ATTAINMENT OF THE REQUIRED CLINICAL DATA

On the basis of these encouraging preclinical findings, a subsequent clinical biochemical pharmacology and phase I study by Casper et al[6] determined that a low dose of PALA could effectively inhibit pyrimidine synthesis in patients; indeed, essentially equivalent inhibition was produced by PALA at 250 or 500, or 1000, or 2000 mg/m^2. The impact of PALA on the inhibition of pyrimidine synthesis was evident in 24 hours and lasted at least 5 days. Doses of PALA higher than 250 mg/m^2 could only be administered in combination with FUra at doses of FUra that were

157

below its MTD; however the low, "modulating" dose of PALA (250 mg/m^2) could be administered weekly in sequenced combination with the weekly "historical" MTD of FUra (600 mg/m^2) without causing undue toxicity. This low PALA/high FUra dosage ratio has undergone clinical trial to evaluate its potential for therapeutic benefit.

A phase I-II trial by Ardalan et al[8] utilized the above recommended weekly low bolus PALA dose (250 mgm^{2}IV), followed in 24 hours by a 24-hour continuous infusion of FUra at its weekly MTD alone (2,600 mg/m^2), and reported promising anti-tumor activity.

O'Dwyer et al[9] subsequently reported a confirmatory phase II study in patients with advanced colorectal cancers employing Ardalan's weekly schedule of low-dose bolus PALA/high dose 24-hour continuous infusion FUra, and reported that the regimen was well-tolerated and produced a gratifying 43% response rate.

Kemeny et al[42] used the same schedule of low dose PALA (250 mg/mg^2) followed 24 hours later by bolus FUra. There was an overall response rate of 38% with a 50% response rate in patients receiving high dose FUra (800 mg/m^2 weekly) after PALA.

THE APPLICATION OF BIOCHEMICAL MODULATION TO CLINICAL TRIAL --LESSONS OF THE PALA/5-FU EXPERIENCE

The possibilities for improvement in combination chemotherapy may well depend on a clearer understanding of how an agent affects intracellular biochemistry, and on how deliberate further biochemical manipulation by other agents may facilitate therapeutic gain. The potential for clinical benefit may only be realized by measuring in patients the intracellular biochemical change produced by a particular dose of an agent and the time interval it takes to produce this
effect.

Appropriate ratios of agents, and the sequence and time interval between administration of agents, are critical determinants of success in preclinical studies of biochemical modulation. These parameters need to be scientifically (not arbitrarily) incorporated into the design of Phase I clinical protocols as the appropriate endpoints (rather than the maximum tolerated dose or MTD) for the determination of dose and interval in any Phase I study evaluating biochemical modulation. It is necessary to determine in patients, by direct biochemical measurements at the tissue level, the dose and temporal relationship between agents that reproduces the pertinent biochemical changes in human tumors that produced the therapeutic success of that particular drug combination in the preclinical model, if the Phase II study is to be accepted as an appropriate clinical test of the preclinical findings.

FURTHER MODULATION OF THE PALA/FUra COMBINATION

Modulation at multiple sites of FUra action can further enhance FUra's antitumor activity.[44] The conversion of FUra to FUMP is dependent on supplies of PRPP (Fig. 1). PRPP is an obligatory substrate in de novo pyrimidine and purine synthesis, and inhibition of either (e.g., PALA) or both of these pathways can make more PRPP available for FUra anabolism. 6-methylmercaptopurine riboside (MMPR), an inhibitor of de novo purine synthesis at the early step of phosphoribosyl amidotransferase, increases PRPP levels, and, when appropriately administered prior to FUra, increases the conversion of FUra to its nucleotides (e.g., FUTP), and results in enhanced incorporation of FUra into RNA, and augmentation of FUra's antitumor activity.[37,18,19,29,32,45] In addition to its antipurine action, MMPR, in high dosage, has been reported to decrease pyrimidine concentrations.[46,47] For the above reasons, it is reasonable that the addition of MMPR to PALA could provide further modulation of FUra activity.

The purine antagonist, MMPR, also has been shown to deplete levels of adenosine triphosphate (ATP), the key energy source in biosynthesis, active transport and DNA

Table 1

Therapeutic Comparison of PALA + MMPR + 6-AN Chemotherapy with and without the Addition of 5-Fluorouracil (FU) in Mice Bearing Spontaneous, Autochthonous CD8F1 Breast Tumors[a].

Treatment[b]	Percent Body Weight Change	Dead/Total	Partial Regressions
1. $PALA_{100}-17hr->MMPR_{150}+6AN_{10}$	-10	3/67 (4%)	24 (38%)
2. $PALA_{100}-17hr->MMPR_{150}+6AN_{10}-2\frac{1}{2}hr->FU_{75}$	-10	5/66 (7%)	41 (67%)

[a] Pooled data: Experiments R536; R537; R538; R539; R540; R541. Spontaneous, autochthonous CD8F1 breast tumors averaging 260mgs at the time of initiation of treatment.

[b] The indicated treatment was administered at 10-11 day intervals. Subscripts refer to doses in mg/kg.

Observations were recorded 6 weeks after initiation of treatment (i.e. approximately 9 days after the fourth course of treatment).

159

repair. Disruption in NAD^+ synthesis and metabolism could have adverse effects on the generation of ATP from ADP in oxidative phosphorylation. Limitation of adenine or NAD^+, or both, is the key to ATP depletion. Therefore, the nicotinamide antagonist, 6-aminonicotinamide (6-AN), was added to MMPR and PALA, and the triple combination (PALA/MMPR/6-AN) was found to markedly lower intracellular ATP levels and to reduce all four ribonucleoside pools[3]; the latter reduction generally correlates with a reduction in the corresponding deoxyribonucleoside triphosphate pools.[48] Thus, because the DNA damage produced by FUra is subject to repair, the ability of the PALA-MMPR-6-AN modulatory drug combination to deplete both the "building blocks" (i.e., the deoxyribonucleosides) and the energy source (i.e., ATP) required for DNA repair, could be expected to increase the anticancer activity of FUra.

Also, the underlying molecular mechanism of fluoro-pyrimidine-induced cell death has been shown to be due to apoptosis or programmed cell death,[49,50] a unique biochemical feature of which is NAD^+ and ATP depletion.[51-54] Therefore, it was thought that prior administration of the modulating combination, PALA + MMPR + 6-AN, to the apoptosis-inducing anticancer agent, FUra, might result in complementary therapeutic activity.

Table 1 records an impressive increase in tumor regression rates when FUra is administered in conjunction with PALA, MMPR and 6-AN in the therapy of advanced, spontaneous, autochthonous murine breast tumors. These are striking results -- a 67% PR rate in a spontaneous tumor that has demonstrated a remarkable chemotherapeutic correlation with human breast cancer![55] Although many biochemical findings associated with this therapy have been documented[56], the precise mechanism of action most responsible for the striking therapeutic results are not clear.

PALA, however, as a biochemical modulator employed successfully in both preclinical[5,7] and clinical studies,[8,9] has lead the way for greater investigation of the strategy of biochemical modulation for the enhancement of anticancer chemotherapy. The lasting lesson from the PALA experience is that biochemical treatment strategies can only be optimized when based on cellular pharmacodynamics.

ACKNOWLEDGEMENT

Supported in part by Public Health Service Grant CA25842 from the National Cancer Institute and in part by the Chemotherapy Foundation, New York, NY.

REFERENCES

1. L.E. Schnipper, Clinical implications of tumor cell heterogeneity, New Engl J Med 314:1423-1431 (1986).
2. G.H. Heppner, and B.E. Miller, Therapeutic implications of tumor heterogeneity, Semin Oncol 16:91-105 (1989).
3. D.S. Martin, Purine and pyrimidine biochemistry, and some relevant clinical and preclinical cancer chemotherapy research, in Powis G, Prough RA (eds): Metabolism and Action of Anti-Cancer Drugs, London, Taylor and Francis, (1987), pp. 91-140.
4. D.S. Martin, Biochemical modulation: Perspectives and objectives, in Harrap K, Connors T (eds): New Avenues in Developmental Chemotherapy, London, Academic Press, (1987), pp 113-162.
5. D.S. Martin, R.L. Stolfi, R.C. Saywer, et al, Therapeutic utility of utilizing low doses of N-(phosphonacetyl)-L-aspartic acid in combination with 5-fluorouracil: A murine study with clinical relevance, Cancer Res 43:2317-2321 (1983).
6. E.S. Casper, K. Vale, L. J. Williams, et al, Phase I and clinical pharmacological evaluation of biochemical modulation of 5-fluorouracil with N-(phosphonacetyl)-L-aspartic acid, Cancer Res 43:2324-2329, (1983).
7. D.S. Martin, R.L. Stolfi, R. C. Sawyer, et al, The application of biochemical

modulation with a therapeutically inactive modulating agent in clinical trials of cancer chemotherapy, Cancer Treat Rep 69:421-423 (1985).

8.   B. Ardalan, G. Singh, and H. Silberman, A randomized phase I and II study of short-term infusion of high-dose fluorouracil with or without N-(phosphonacetyl)-L-asparatic acid in patients with advanced pancreatic and colorectal cancers, J. Clin Oncol 6:1053-1058 (1988).

9.   P. J. O'Dwyer, A. R. Paul, J. Walczak, et al, Phase II study of biochemical modulation of fluorouracil by low-dose PALA in patients with colorectal cancer, J. Clin. Oncol 8:1497-1503 (1990).

10.   S. Speigelman, R. Sawyer, R. Nayak, et al, Improving the anti-tumor activity of 5-fluorouracil by increasing its incorporation into RNA via metabolic modulation, Proc. Natl. Acad Sci USA 77:4966 (1980).

11.   R.C. Sawyer, R.L. Stolfi, R. Nayak, et al, Mechanism of cytotoxicity in 5-fluorouracil chemotherapy of two murine solid tumors, in Tattersall MHN, Fox RM (eds): Nucleosides and Cancer Treatment, New York, NY, Academic Press, (1981), pp 308-338.

12.   R. Heimer, and A.C. Sartorelli, RNA polymerase II transcripts as targets for 5-fluorouridine cytotoxicity: Antagonism of 5-fluorouridine actions by a-amanitin, Cancer Chemother Pharmacol 24:80-86 (1989).

13.   D.A. Greenhalgh, and J. H. Parish, Effect of 5-fluorouracil combination therapy on RNA processing in human colonic carcinoma cells, Br J Cancer 61:415-419 (1990).

14.   D. S. Wilkinson, and H. C. Pitot, Inhibition of ribosomal ribonucleic acid maturation in Novikoff hepatoma cells by 5-fluorouracil and 5-fluorouridine. J Biol Chem 248:63-68 (1973).

15.   B. J. Dolnick, and J. J. Pink, Effects of 5-fluorouracil on dihydrofolate reductase dihydrofolate reductase mRNA from methotrexate-resistant KB cells, J Biol Chem 260:3006-3014 (1985).

16.   S-L. Doong, and B.J. Dolnick, 5-Fluorouracil substition alters pre-mRNA splicing in vitro, J Biol Chem 263:4467-4473 (1988).

17.   L. D. Nord, and D. S. Martin, Loss of murine tumor thymidine kinase activity in vivo following 5-fluorouracil (FUra) treatment by incorporation of FUra into RNA, Biochem Pharmacol 42:2369-2375 (1991).

18.   D. W. Kufe, and E. M. Egan, Enhancement of 5-fluorouracil incorporation into human lymphoblast ribonucleic acid, Biochem Pharmacol 30:129-133 (1981).

19.   D. W. Kufe, and P. P. Major, 5-Fluorouracil incorporation into human breast carcinoma RNA correlates with cytoxicity, J Biol Chem 256:9803-9805 (1981).

20.   B. Ardalan, R. I. Glazer, T. W. Kensler, et al, Synergistic effect of 5-fluorouracil and N-(phosphonacetyl)-L-aspartate on cell growth and ribonucleic acid synthesis in a human mammary carcinoma, Biochem. Pharmacol 30:2045-2049 (1981).

21.   D. S. Martin, R. L. Stolfi, and S. Spiegelman, Striking augmentation of the in vivo anticancer activity of 5-fluorouracil (5-FU) by combination with pyrimidine nucleosides: An RNA effect, Proc. Am Assoc Cancer Res 19:221 (1978).

22.   G. Weckbecker, and D. S. Keppler, Substrate properties of 5-fluorouridine diphospho sugars detected in hepatoma cells, Biochem Pharmacol 33:2291-2298 (1984).

23.   F. Valeriote, and G. Santelli, 5-Fluorouracil (FUra), Pharmac Ther 24:107-132 (1984).

24.   R. J. Epstein, Drug-induced DNA damage and tumor chemothersensitivity, J Clin Oncol 8:2062-2084 (1990).

25.   W. B. Parker, and Y-C. Cheng, Metabolism and mechanism of action of 5-fluorouracil, Pharmac Ther 48:381-395 (1990).

26.   R. M. Evans, J. D. Laskin, and M. T. Hakala, Assessment of growth-limiting events caused by 5-fluorouracil in mouse cells and in human cells, Cancer Res 40:4113-4122 (1980).

27.   K. D. Collins, and G. R. Stark, Aspartate transcarbamylase interaction with the transition state analogue N-(phosphonacetyl)-L-aspartate, J. Biol. Chem 246:6599-6605 (1971).

28. D. S. Martin, R. Nayak, R. Sawyer, et al, Enhancement of 5-fluorouracil chemotherapy with emphasis on the use of excess thymidine, Cancer Bull 30:219-222 (1978).

29. D. S. Martin, R.L. Stolfi, R. C. Sawyer, et al, An overview of thymidine, Cancer 45:1117-1128 (1980).

30. R. K. Johnson, J. J. Clement, and W. S. Howard, Treatment of murine tumors with 5-fluorouracil in combination with de novo pyrimidine synthesis inhibitors PALA or pyrazofurin, Proc Am Assoc Cancer Res 21:292 (1980).

31. B. Ardalan, R. Glazer, T. Kensler, et al, Biochemical mechanism for the synergism of 5-fluorouracil (5-FU) and phosphonacetyl-L-aspartate (PALA) in human mammary carcinoma cells, Proc Am Assoc Cancer Res 21:8 (1980).

32. D. S. Martin, R. L. Stolfi, R. C. Sawyer, et al, Biochemical modulation of 5-fluorouracil and cytosine arabinoside with emphasis on thymidine, PALA, and 6-methylmercaptopurine riboside, in Tattersall MHN, Fox RM (eds): Nucleosides and Cancer Treatment. Sydney, Academic Press, (1981), pp. 339-382.

33. G. J. Peters, E. Laurensse, A. Leyva, et al, The concentration of 5-phosphoribosyl 1-pyrophosphate in monolayer tumor cells and the effect of various pyrimidine antimetabolites, Int J Biochem 17:95-99 (1985).

34. P. P. Major, E. M. Egan, L. Sargent, et al, Modulation of 5-FU metabolism in human MCF-7 breast carcinoma cells, Cancer Chemother. Pharmacol 8:87-91 (1982).

35. A. A. Miller, E. C. Moore, R. B. Hurlbert, et al, Pharmacological and biochemical interactions of N-(phosphonacetyl)-L-aspartate and 5-fluorouracil in beagles, Cancer Res 43:2565-2570 (1983).

36. C. E. Moore, J. Friedman, M. Valdivieso, et al, Aspartate carbamoyltransferase activity, drug concentrations and pyrimidine nucleotides in tissue from patients treated with N-(phosphonacetyl)-L-aspartate, Biochem Pharmacol 31:3317-3321 (1982).

37. W. W. Ackerman, and V. R. Potter, Enzyme inhibition in relation to chemotherapy, Proc Soc Biol Med 72:1-9 (1949).

38. C. M. Liang, R. C. Donehower, and B. A. Chabner, Biochemical interactions between N-(phosphonacetyl)-L-aspartate and 5-fluorouracil, Mol Pharmacol 21:224-230 (1982).

39. J. L. Grem, S. A. King, P. J. O'Dwyer, et al, Biochemistry and clinical activity of N-(phosphonacetyl)-L-aspartate: A review, Cancer Res 48:4441-4454 (1988).

40. D. S. Martin, and N.E. Kemeny, Overview of PALA + 5-fluorouracil in clinical trials, Semin Oncol 18:228-233, (1991) (suppl 8).

41. S. H. Harrison, H. D. Giles, and E. P. Denine, Hematologic and histopatholic evaluation of N-(phosphonacetyl)-L-aspartate (PALA) in mice, Cancer Chemother Pharmacol 2:183-187 (1979).

42. N. E. Kemeny, and P. Costa, Phase II trial of PALA and FU in metastatic colorectal carcinoma, Proc Am Soc Clin Oncol 10: (1991).

43. L. D. Nord, R. L. Stolfi, and D. S. Martin, Biochemical modulation of 5-fluorouracil with leucovorin or delayed uridine rescue. Correlation of antitumor activity with dosage and FUra incorporation into RNA, Biochem. Pharmacol 43:2543-2549 (1992).

44. D. S. Martin, R. L. Stolfi and R. C. Sawyer, Improved therapeutic index with sequential N-phosphonacetyl-L-aspartate plus high-dose methotrexate plus high-dose 5-fluorouracil and appropriate rescue, Cancer Res 43:4653-4661 (1983).

45. P. J. O'Dwyer, G. Hudes, J. Colofiore, et al, Phase I trial of Fluorouracil modulation by N-phosphonacetyl-L-aspartate and 6-methylmercaptopurine riboside dose and schedule through biochemical analysis of sequential tumor biopsy specimens, J Natl Cancer Inst 83:1235-1240 (1991).

46. R. A. Woods, R. M. Henderson, and J. F. Henderson, Consequences of inhibition of purine biosynthesis de novo by 6-methylmercaptopurine ribonucleoside in cultured lymphoma L5178 cells, Eur J Cancer 14:765-770 (1978).

47. G. B. Grindey, J. K. Lowe, A. Y. Direker et al, Potentiation by guanine nucleosides of the growth-inhibitory effects of adenosine analogues on L1210 and Sarcoma 180 cells in culture, Cancer Res 36:379-383 (1976).

48. D. Hunting, J. Hordern, and J. F. Henderson, Effects of altered ribonucleotide concentrations on ribonucleotide reduction in intact Chinese hamster ovary cells, Can J Biochem 59:821-829 (1981).

49. N. Kyprianou, and J. T. Isaacs, Thymineless death in androgen-independent prostatic cancer cells, Biochem Biophys Res Commun 165:73-81 (1989).

50. M. A. Barry, C. A. Behnke, and A. Eastman, Activation of programmed cell death (apoptosis) by cisplatin, other anticancer drugs, toxins, and hyperthermia, Biochem Pharmacol 40:2353-2362 (1990).

51. I. U. Schraufstatter, D. B. Hinshaw, P. A. Hyslop, et al, Oxidant injury of cells: DNA strand-breaks activate polyadenosine diphosphate polymerase and lead to depletion of nicotinamide adenine dinucleotide, J Clin Invest 77:1312-1320 (1986).

52. P.A. Hyslop, D.B. Hinslaw, W.A. Halsey, Jr., et al, Mechanisms of oxidant-mediated injury. The glycolytic and mitochondrial pathways of ADP phosphorylation are major intracellular targets inactivated by hydrogen peroxide, J. Biol. Chem., 263:1665-1675 (1988).

53. A.R. Boobis, D.J. Fawthrop, and D.S. Davies, Mechanism of cell death, Trends Pharmacol. Sci., 10:275-280 (1989).

54. N.A. Berger, S.J. Berger, and S.L. Gerson, DNA repair, ADP ribosylation and pyridine nucleotide metabolism as targets for cancer chemotherapy, Anti-Cancer Drug Design 2:203-210 (1987).

55. R.L. Stolfi, L.M. Stolfi, R.C. Sawyer, and D.S. Martin, Chemotherapeutic evaluation using clinical criteria in spontaneous, autochthonous murine breast tumors, J. Natl. Cancer Inst., 80:52-55 (1988).

56. R.L. Stolfi, J.R. Colofiore, L.D. Nord, J.A. Koutcher, and D.S. Martin, Biochemical modulation of tumor cell energy: regression of advanced spontaneous murine breast tumors with a 5-fluorouracil-containing drug combination, Cancer Res. 52:4074-4081 (1992).

DISCUSSION OF DR. WADLER'S/DR./HOUGHTON'S/DR. LOEFFLER'S
DR. CHU'S AND DR. MARTIN'S PRESENTATION

Audience: I wonder if you could comment, since I'm uncertain you've done the experiments varying the amount of thymidylate synthase in these assays but binding to the RNA. I wonder if you could comment on the relationship between how much thymidylate synthase in concentration terms you require to get this effect and how that relates to the concentration of thymidylate synthase that you calculate in dividing cells?

Dr. Chu: That's a very good question. In fact if one does some rough calculations and the problem is unfortunately one doesn't really know the level the true level of TS mRNA within a cell, but if one does some rough calculations, and we've done it actually in one of our human colon cancer cell lines where we know the level of TS protein. The molar excess of TS protein to mRNA is actually somewhere within that cell line in the order of 10-15 fold and in most of the experiments, in all the experiments that we've done either with the in vitro translation or even the competition were at similar level of about 10-15 fold excess so it appears that at the concentrations that we're dealing with that they're biolgically relevant. Does that answer your question?

Dr. Rustum: Dr. Houghton, this question is for you on DNA damage induced by 5-FU together with leucovorin and interferon. Was the damage single- or double-strand breaks?

Dr. Houghton: What we actually measured at that point in time the total of DNA strand breaks is measured by alkaline elution. We since note that these combinations can induce double-strand breaks. But I don't know at this point in time is whether all the strand breaks can be accounted for as double-strand breaks. We're currently doing those calculations.

Dr. Rustum: How about DNA repair? Have you looked at repair?

Dr. Houghton: No. That is an area we need to look at.

Dr. Diaz-Rubio: I have some comments about the presentation for Dr.Wadler in relation to 5-fluorouracil/interferon experience. As you know, we have done a study before with the same dose that you used. In 54 patients, the overall response rate was 24%. Of interest, responses were seen in liver metastases but not in other organs. In the future do you feel it is necessary to reduce the dose of interferon?

Dr. Wadler: Yes, I'm very familiar with your study and it was a very interesting study. There's been no breakdown overall of patients with or without liver metastasis who have responded to therapy although it's perfectly logical that this may be the case. In terms of the toxicities, we went back for instance and looked at the Memorial study where there was a 24% response rate too and very high neurotoxicity much higher than any other studies. The age of the patients were relatively comparable to those of the ECOG study, however, the CEA levels in the Memorial study were about 3 times as high as the median CEA levels than the ECOG trial suggesting that these were patients with much larger tumor burdens and much sicker patients. I mean it's reasonable because at the time they were doing the phase II trial they had a phase III ongoing as well so there may have been sometimes biased in terms patients going into one study or the other. It's certainly unintentional but it can happen. So, that's suggested that patients who had higher tumor burdens and maybe sicker may have greater toxicity again not a terribly surprising finding. When we went back and looked, of course in our original study, the thing that impressed us most was we had a large number of patients with massive tumor burdens and some patients with poor performance status were entered onto this trial who responded and some gave us dramatic responses which kind of contradict what I just said. Of course, many of our patients with massive tumor burdens had massive tumor burdens in the liver and those are the patients who, I showed you those responses which were very dramatic and that would go along with what you're saying. So the issues you're raising are very valid and interesting question and and I think need to be sorted out in a more systematic fashion, but I think your observations are interesting.

Dr. Mihich: I have a question for Dr. Houghton but Dr. Chu is also involved. Maybe I missed your reporting it but under the condition when you saw a increase in DNA damage did you see differences in thymidylate syntetase levels? The question is related to the fact that is it possible that you are dealing with two different sites of interaction by interferon or is DNA damage a consequence of the reversal of the increase in thymidylate synthetase that would be otherwise seen?

Dr. Houghton: We have clearly shown from our studies that thymidylate synthase is not involved as a target site. We have 3 pieces of evidence that demonstrate that. The studies conducted with thymidylate synthase deficient cells, studies conducted in the well-type GC3 parent line which clearly showed that CB3717 is not potentiated such obvious facts are not potentiated by interferon and also from the direct measurements of thymidylate synthase that we conducted at 24 hrs. All of those 3 pieces of evidence confirm that thymidylate synthase is not the primary interaction site of these cells.

Dr. Mihich: Do you suggest that there are differences in sites and different cell types because these were different cell types or is there any evidence by anyone that would answer the question whether there would be two sides or sequence? Maybe there are different sites and different cell types but in some cell types both might be co-existent. Does anyone have any evidence in this regard?

Dr. Houghton: Until somebody does that we won't know.

Audience: Does interferon modulate the response as well as the duration of response? Does it effect long-term development of resistance? If you gave the chemotherapeutic agent with interferon over a period of time under selection pressure would you prolong the consequences of resistance?

Dr. Houghton: I don't know at this point.

Dr. Mihich: It's obviously a complex question one that can't be answered here but I think that there's 3 things going on. One question, I can guess at the answer, this is an observation, it's really a seminal observation in this area by Dr. Martin and colleagues. This really is one of the most interesting things ever done where Dr. Martin showed that interferon had a protective effect in mice and that in mice given lethal doses of 5-FU could then be treated with interferon and they would survive. So, there's a suggestion of protection of normal host tissues there. The second thing that's going on is that there does seem to be some enhancement of the direct cytotoxic effects. Maybe through some of the mechanisms suggested by Dr. Houghton, effects on DNA. The third piece of evidence is one from Dr. Chu that it maybe the altering host resistance to 5-FU in other words the ability to inhibit cells from making more TS would be one mechanism of overcoming endogenous resistance. So I think that there's 3 things that going on simultaneously both enhanced cytotoxicity, overcoming resistance and possibly host resistance that are interacting. Now where do all these things fit in? I think it's hard to tell. Certainly I think we have to wait before we can say that the addition of interferon or interferon + leucovorin augments duration of response or survival. We really have to wait for the results of the phase III trial, the ECOG trial that's ongoing now. I think that will probably answer that question.

IMPLICATIONS OF CHRONOBIOLOGY FOR 5-FLUOROURACIL (5-FU) EFFICACY

F. Lévi, S.Brienza, G. Metzer, P. Deprés-Brummer,
F. Bertheault-Cvitkovic, R. Zidani, R. Adam, J.L. Misset

Laboratoire "Rythmes biologiques et Chronothérapeutique" and Centre
de Chronothérapie, Service des Maladies Sanguines, Immunitaires et
Tumorales, and Service de Chirurgie, Hôpital Paul Brousse, Villlejuif, France

INTRODUCTION

The drug 5-fluorouracil (5-FU) has remained the main active drug against gastrointestinal malignancies. Both its tolerability and/or its efficacy have been increased through combination with folinic acid (FA) (1-4) or its administration by continuous venous infusion (5, 6). Both such regimens usually resulted in a threefold to fourfold improvement of tumor response rate in patients with metastatic colorectal cancer, as compared with standard 5-FU treatment. These figures, however, still were low (30 %) and affected survival modestly (1-6). In addition, a correlation between 5-FU dose intensity (D.I.) and response rate was reported in patients with metastatic colorectal cancer (7). Thus any method which allows a significant increase in the D.I. of 5-FU may result in improved anticancer efficacy.

Both the toxicity and the antitumor efficacy of cancer chemotherapeutic drugs predictably vary by more than 50 % according to dosing time in mice or rats (8-14). Such changes in drug pharmacodynamics result from the organization in time of biological functions. Biological rhythms usually persist in a constant environment, since they have a genetic basis (15). Twenty-four hour circadian rhythms are governed or coordinated by central biological clocks, the suprachiasmatic nucleus being the most important one (16, 17). As a result, biological rhythms characterize absorption, transport, distribution and elimination processes, as well as the susceptibility of cells to drug effects (16, 17). The relevance of an adequate selection of dosing time for optimizing therapy in patients was shown for numerous agents including corticosteroids, NSAID's, anticoagulants, bronchodilators, cancer chemotherapy and ... light (18, 19). Few randomized trials have yet tested the relevance of circadian drug timing for improving quality of life or survival (20).

Chronotherapy - drug administration according to biological rhythms - has undergone initial testing in clinical oncology ten years ago. Two early randomized trials revealed that significantly less toxicity and/or higher dose intensity resulted from early morning dosing of doxorubicin or theprubicin and late afternoon or early evening infusion of cisplatin. Despite the relatively small sample size of these trials (≈ 30 patients each), similar results were achieved (21, 22).

The recent development of programmable-in-time pumps was a key step, making the evaluation of chronotherapy principles a realistic target. Preclinical studies, clinical Phase I, II, and III trials of cancer chronotherapy could now be planned with reliable devices avoiding additional hospitalization for night infusions. Using these devices,

*Novel Approaches to Selective Treatments of Human Solid Tumors: Laboratory
and Clinical Correlation* Edited by Y. M. Rustum, Plenum Press, New York, 1993

169

phase I trials have shown that circadian-modified delivery was less toxic than flat infusion for floxuridine, doxorubicin, oxaliplatin and alpha-interferon (23-26). The short half-life of 5-FU, its well-known metabolism and its rather specific intracellular targets make it potentially amenable to optimization through chronotherapy. We initiated such clinical investigations of chronotherapy with this drug in 1986.

I - PRECLINICAL STUDIES OF CHRONOPHARMACOLOGY

Dosing-time dependent toxicity

Three different groups have tested the relevance of 5-FU dosing time with regard to drug lethal toxicity in mice. Survival rate was 2 to 8 times higher if a single high dose of 5-FU was injected near the middle of the rest pan of mice, irrespective of strain or sex (figure 1) (27-29). The hematological toxicity of 5-FU was also significantly lower in the early rest span, as compared to early activity span (30), with a subsequent rebound of leukocyte count following drug dosing at the most toxic time, both in mice or in rats (30, 31). Nonetheless, toxicity to the intestinal mucosa of rats, as gauged by both the incidence of diarrhea and the impairment of water absorption may be reduced following 5-FU injection at night (32). These data may well indicate that 5-FU is less toxic to the bone marrow when it is dosed near the middle of the rest span of mice or rats, but it may be more toxic to the jejunal mucosa at this same time.

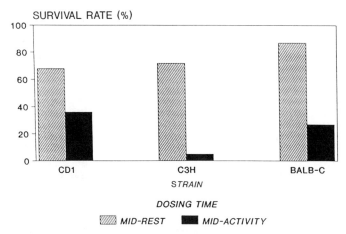

Figure 1. Circadian rhythm in 5-FU toxicity. Survival rate of mice according to 5-FU dosing time. Results from 3 independent studies are referred to the 24-hr-rest/activity cycle. After Popovic et al. (27), Burns et al. (28) and Gonzalez et al. (29).

Antitumor efficacy

In a two-stage circadian study, subgroups of mice bearing the murine colon carcinomas colon 38 or colon 26 were treated with 5-FU once a week in the early rest span (at 2.30 HALO - Hours After Light Onset) or in the early activity span (12.30 HALO), respectively (30). The antitumor effect of treatment at 2.30 HALO was significantly the best one against both tumors. Toxic effects (leukopenia) were observed only in the 12.30 HALO treatment group. Thus, a good correlation was observed between time of optimal effectiveness and that of least hematologic toxicity. In another study, dosing 5-FU in the early rest or early activity span resulted in minimal differences in growth inhibition of a human squamous cell carcinoma xenograft in nude mice (33), despite the fact that this strain has retained a circadian system (34). These latter apparently negative data may however result from a limited comparison of two time points, which respectively corresponded to a high and to a low point in the proportion of tumor S-phase cells. They emphasize, however, that this parameter may not be a critical one to take into account for optimizing 5-FU cytotoxicity through circadian timing.

Metabolism and cellular proliferation in target host tissues.

Circadian changes characterize 5-FU metabolism in mice or rats. Thus, the activity of liver dehydropyrimidinedehydrogenase, the rate-limiting enzyme in 5-FU catabolism displays maximal activity during the rest phase of mice or rats (35, 36). This time indeed corresponded to an increase in 5-FU catabolism in isolated perfused rat liver (37). However, liver thymidine phosphorylase (dThd-Pase), which can convert 5-FU into FUdR, was not rhythmic (36).
Other enzymes involved into fluoropyrimidine anabolism or catabolism were recently shown to exhibit large circadian changes (38-41). Taken as a whole, these data indeed suggest that 5-FU is oriented towards anabolism (FdUMP and FUMP) near mid-activity and towards catabolism (FUH_2,...) near mid-rest in normal tissues .

Twenty-four hour changes in liver and intestinal blood flow also alter cellular exposure to 5-FU and influence its metabolism and its cytotoxicity. The distribution of labeled microspheres to these organs following intracarotid injection was investigated in rats at four different times. The estimated blood flow was 50 % larger near the middle of the activity span of rats in both organs (42).

Target organs such as the bone marrow or the intestinal mucosa exhibit circadian changes in metabolic and mitotic activity. An extensive review of these topics is beyond the scope of this article. Let us, however, recall that most studies have reported that DNA synthetic activity in murine jejunal or colon mucosa was higher at the end of the nocturnal (activity) span or at the beginning of the diurnal (rest) span in mice or rats (43-47). Large, yet predictable, changes in the proportion of myeloid progenitors of murine bone marrow (CFUs, CFU_{GM}, F-CFU) were found along the 24 hr-time scale, with the highest values usually occuring in the second half of the activity span, or at the beginning of the rest span of mice (48-50). Such rhythm in CFU_{GM} was shown as one of the mechanism of the circadian rhythm in both the lethal and the hematologic toxicities of theprubicin, a new anthracycline analog (50). Figure 2 briefly summarizes these data.

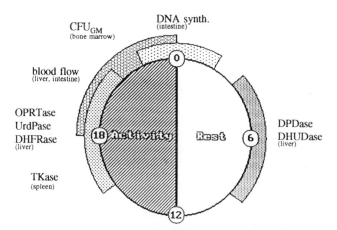

Figure 2. Distribution of peak times of several biological functions relevant for 5-FU metabolism or cytotoxicity in mice or rats. Time, on the internal circle is expressed in hours after light onset - HALO (0, 6, 12 or 18 HALO). Mice or rats rest during the 12 h-light span and are active during the dark span. After data from Harris et al. (35), Daher et al. (36), Diasio et al. (38), Kouni et al. (39), Zhang et al. (40), Malmary-Nebot et al. (41), Labrecque et al. (42), Scheving et al. (43), Haus et al. (44), Waldrop et al. (46), Levi et al. (50).

II - CLINICAL PHARMACOKINETICS

In a joint study with the Centre Antoine Lacassagne (Nice, France) we demonstrated that despite 5-FU was infused at a constant rate to 7 patients with bladder carcinoma, its plasma level varied rhythmically along the 24 hr-scale (51). Mean plasma concentration was lowest at 13.00 h and doubled at 1.00 h at night. This circadian rhythm was similar on day 1, 3, and 5 of infusion. Similar results have been reported in three other studies (52-54). All four investigations involved 4 or 5 day flat infusion of 5-FU (450 to 1000 mg/m²/d). In one of them, 5-FU was infused alone (52) ; in our first study, 5-FU infusion was initiated 15 h after the end of a 30 min-cisplatin infusion (51) ; in another study, cisplatin was concurrently infused at a constant rate to 10 patients with advanced lung cancer (53). Finally, in our second study, 5-FU was associated to concurrent 5-day flat infusion of both D-L FA (300 mg/m²/d) and oxaliplatin (20 mg/m²/d) in 4 patients with metastatic colorectal cancer (54). Figure 3 gives an example of such rhythm. In another study by Harris et al., 5-FU (300 mg/m²/d) was continuously infused for 14 d in 7 patients with gastrointestinal cancer (55). A significant circadian rhythm was also documented, yet the highest mean plasma level was found near 12.00 h and the lowest one near midnight. These results emphasize the stability of the circadian mechanisms involved into 5-FU disposition and metabolism.

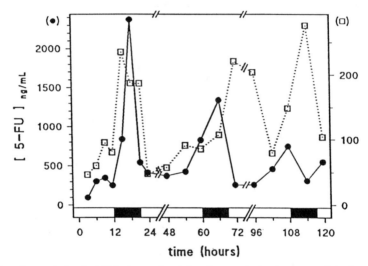

Figure 3. Circadian variation in 5-FU plasma level despite constant rate venous infusion of 5-FU (600 mg/m²/d) for 5 days. FA (300 mg/m²/d) and oxaliplatin (20 mg/m²) were also concurrently infused at a constant rate. Both patients had metastatic colorectal cancer (liver involvement). Cosinor analysis yielded the following parameters : subject 1 p = 0.003 ; 24 hr mean (± SEM) : 132 ± 12 ng/ml ; amplitude (± SD) : 77 ± 51 ng/ml ; acrophase (time of maximum, ± SD) = 3.55 hrs ± 160 min. ; subject 2 : p = 0.03 ; 24 h-mean = 610 ± 61 ng/ml ; amplitude = 479 ± 441 ng/ml ; acrophase = 2.20 hrs ± 260 min. Also note five-fold difference in 24 hr mean levels.

We were struck, however, by the 12 h-phase difference between the circadian rhythm in 5-FU following a flat infusion for 4 to 5 days vs 14 days. A major effect of platinum complexes can be eliminated, since
1) no Pt complex was administered in one study (52),
2) cisplatin was given 15 hrs after the onset of 5 day-continuous infusion of 5-FU in our first study, and the circadian rhythm in plasma 5-FU concentration remained similar on day 1, 3 or 5 of infusion (51),
3) Pt complexes may interact with 5-FU pharmacokinetics or metabolism, but such interaction is limited to a few hours following Pt complex exposure (56, 57).

The daily dose level administered is most likely to be relevant. Thus, all 4- or 5-day schedules involved the administration of daily doses which were 1.5 to 3 times higher than the 14 day schedule. As a result, the mean 24 hr plasma levels ranged from 340 to 470 ng/ml in the 4- or 5-day schedules (51, 54) and it was 16 ng/ml in the 14-day schedule (Table 1) (55).

Table 1. Circadian rhythm in plasma 5-FU concentration during continuous venous infusion at a constant rate in cancer patients . Tentative comparison between results from 5-day vs 14-day infusion (After Petit et al. (51) and Harris et al. (55).

Duration (days)	Median dose $(mg/m^2/d)$	24 h-mean (ng/ml)	peak time (h)	ref.
5	700	340	1.00 (night)	51
14	300	16	11.25 (day)	55

Such hypothesis is supported by results from 1) a chronopharmacokinetics study of bolus 5-FU and 2) investigations of circadian rhythmicity of dehydropyrimidine dehydrogenase (DPD, the rate limiting enzyme of 5-FU catabolism) (60).

Thus, 5-FU (15 mg/kg - eg. $\approx$ 600 mg/m^2) was injected intravenously (bolus) at 1.00, 7.00, 13.00 or 19.00 h to 28 patients with metastatic gastrointestinal cancer in a randomized sequence, each injection being separated by 96 hr from the next one. Both plasma pharmacokinetics and hematologic toxicity were assessed. 5-FU dosing at 1.00 h resulted in the longest half-life, the largest VdSS and AUC and in the lowest clearance (CL$_B$), as well as in the least depression of leukocyte count. All these differences were statistically validated (56).

The activity of DPD was measured every 4 hr for 24 hr in human mononuclear cells. Similar results were found both in 5 healthy subjects (59) and in 7 patients receiving continuous venous infusion of 5-FU at a constant rate (55). In both studies DPD varied two to six-fold, with the highest activity occuring near 1.00 h. at night. Quite interestingly, peak 5-FU concentration and peak DPD activity occurred 12 hr apart, in those patients receiving low dose 5-FU for 14 days (55). This indeed suggests a prominent role for DPD rhythm as a mechanism in 5-FU rhythm. Nonetheless, DPD activity is saturable (36), and other mechanisms may influence 5-FU disposition. Among these factors, liver blood flow, as estimated by indocyanine green plasma clearance, exhibited a 50 % increase in the second half of the night and in the early morning in 10 healthy supine subjects. Lowest values were found at 13.00 h (61). Quite strikingly, 5-FU clearance reportedly had a similar value as liver blood flow (58). This suggests that the main mechanism of the circadian rhythm in 5-FU plasma levels is the rhythm in DPD activity when low doses of 5-FU are infused, whereas the rhythm in liver blood flow may be a more relevant mechanism when high daily doses of 5-FU are delivered. These data are summarized in figure 4.

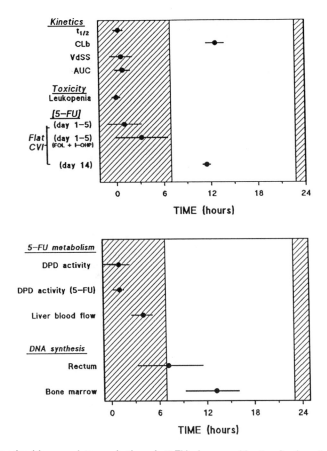

Figure 4. Summarized human data on rhythms in 5-FU pharmacokinetics (top) and some metabolic or mitotic activities in target tissues (bottom). Night is represented as a hatched area. Each dark point represents the estimated peak time (acrophase) for the considered variable, with its 95 % confidence interval,. After Nowakowska-Dulowa (58), Petit et al. (51), Metzger et al. (54), Harris et al. (55), Tuchman et al. (59), Lemmer et al. (61), Smaaland et al. (66), Buchi et al. (67).

Other clinical requisites

The primary target organs of 5-FU toxicity also display large amplitude rhythms in healthy human subjects. Thus, an increased incidence of mitoses occurred at 1.00 hr in the skin (62), whereas a trough in DNA synthetic activity, as gauged by ex-vivo ^{3}H-TdR incorporation or flow cytometric studies was found between 4.00 h and 9.00 h in this tissue (63).

Mitotic activity in human bone marrow was higher at midnight. Peak DNA synthetic activity, as gauged by ex-vivo ^{3}H-TdR synthesis or by the cytometry-assessed proportion of S-phase cells occurred between 12.00 h and 18.00 h (64-66).

DNA synthetic activity (ex-vivo ^{3}H-TdR incorporation) was the highest near 8.00 h in the normal rectal mucosa of 16 normally fed or fasting healthy subjects (67). Several enzymatic activities of the brush border of human jejunum also displayed prominent circadian rhythmicity (68). This was also the case for several enzymatic activities in the superficial cells of the human oral mucosa (69).

III - CIRCADIAN SCHEDULING REDUCES 5-FU TOXICITY

Since mice or rats tolerated 5-FU best when it was dosed near the middle of the rest span (day-time), and biological rhythms are most easily modelled by a sinewave function, we devised a quasi sinusoidal schedule for 5-FU continuous delivery over 5 days (figure 4). A programmable-in-time pump prototype was made available to us (Chronopump, Autosyringe - Baxter Travenol, Hookset, NH, USA). Peak flow rate was programmed at 4.00 h and KVO infusion rate was scheduled from 18.00 h to 22.00 h. The 5-FU containing 60-ml syringe was changed daily at 18.00 h. Our goal was to investigate whether such circadian scheduling of 5-FU, as extrapolated from murine toxicity data, would allow to increase the usual recommended dose intensity. Thus, on a 5-day continuous venous flat infusion, 5-FU is usually given at doses ranging from 800 to 1200 mg/m^2/d x 5 d every 28 d. (1000 to 1500 mg/m^2/wk) (Figure 5).

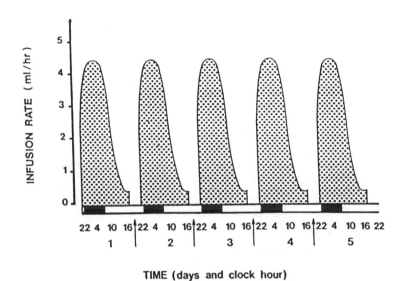

TIME (days and clock hour)

Arrows indicate daily syringe changes.

Figure 5. Schedule of 5-FU delivery. Peak delivery was scheduled to occur at 4.00 hrs, daily for 5 consecutive days.

An intrapatient dose escalation scheme was planned. At first course of therapy, patients received 1000 mg/m^2/d x 5 d. Courses were scheduled every 21 days (at 16 days' interval). Subsequently, the dose level was increased by 200 mg/m^2/d if toxicity was less than grade 2. If grade 2 toxicity was achieved the tolerated dose was considered as being reached for this patient. If toxicity was grade 3 or higher, the patient was allowed to recover up to a total of 5 wks, then he was treated at the dose level preceeding that responsible for the toxicity. Thirty-five patients with metastatic colorectal cancer entered this trial from October 1986 to July 1988. 41 % of the patients had received prior treatment and 63 % had a W.H.O. performance status of 2 or greater ; 54 % patients had 2 or more metastatic sites. Three hundred and fifty one courses were given to outpatients (3 to 25 per patient). All patients were evaluated for toxicity and response. Disease progressed in five patients before reaching a toxic dose, thus 30 patients were assessable for dose escalation. Figure 6 indicates that 80 % patients received 1400

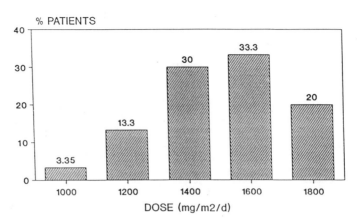

Figure 6. Distribution of highest daily dose of 5-FU chronotherapy given to patients with metastatic colorectal cancer. Thirty patients were assessable for this endpoint.

$mg/m^2/d \times 5$ d, and 55 % received higher doses. An objective response was achieved in 30 % of the 35 patients and median survival was 16 months.

In a pilot study in 16 patients with pancreatic cancer, we further validated that such circadian scheduling also allowed to safely deliver 1400 $mg/m^2/d \times 5$ d every 3 wks. A 23 % response rate was achieved, with an 11-months median survival and a rather good quality of life (71). Such recommended dose and schedule corresponds to a D.I. of 2333 mg/m^2 of 5-FU, i.e. 55 % to 200 % higher than the recommended D.I. for flat 5-FU delivery. Thus, this circadian scheduling of 5-FU served as a basis for further optimization through combination with other drugs.

IV - CIRCADIAN SCHEDULING OF 5-FU WITH FOLINIC ACID

Both biochemical and chronopharmacologic treatment methods were combined to optimize treatment efficacy further. The drug FA is known to stabilize the complexing of 5-fluorodeoxyuridine monophosphate, the intracellular cytotoxic form of 5-FU, with thymidylate synthetase, a key enzyme in DNA metabolism (72, 73). Cisplatin was shown to block methionine entry into tumor cells <u>in vitro</u> and increase both endogenous methionine synthesis and thymidylate synthetase activity. As a result, tumor cells became more susceptible to injury by 5-FU (74). The severe clinical toxicity and/or the apparent lack of increased antitumor efficacy of chemotherapeutic regimens associating cisplatin and 5-FU with or without FA (3, 75, 76) led most oncologists to avoid such combination chemotherapy in patients with gastrointestinal malignancies, despite initial encouraging results (77).

Because oxaliplatin (1,2-diammino-cyclohexane (trans-1)oxalatoplatin(II) ; l-OHP), a new third generation platinum complex, is not associated with renal and has minimal hematologic toxicity (78, 79), this drug was considered to be a good candidate for further platinum modulation of 5-FU and FA cytotoxicity. The association of all three drugs was synergistic against murine L1210 leukemia (79). We hypothesized that (1) high doses of all three drugs and (2) proper scheduling of drug delivery were needed to achieve clinical synergy.

The drugs 5-FU (700 mg/m^2/d) and FA (300 mg/m^2/d) combined with l-OHP (25 mg/m^2/d) were infused continuously for 5 days every 3 wks at 16-day intervals (Figure 7) (80). Such schedule and dose level had been selected following a) a randomized pilot study of flat vs chronomodulated schedule of all three drugs in 8 patients and b) a dose-finding study in 10 previously-treated patients. In the present Phase II trial, l-OHP was infused for 12 hrs from 10.15 h to 21.45 h., with a sinusoidally varying delivery rate and peak delivery at 4.00 h. Subsequently, 5-FU and FA were infused concurrently from 22.15 h to 9.45 h, with peak delivery at 4.00 h. A 6-ml flush with 5 % glucose was programmed between the infusion of l-OHP and that of 5-FU and FA to minimize the risk of precipitate formation. Such a complex chronomodulated delivery schedule of three drugs was administered to outpatients with a programmable-in-time multichannel ambulatory pump (IntelliJect^R, Aguettant, Lyon, France). This pump is equipped with four 30-ml disposable syringes connected to the same central venous line by a manifold.

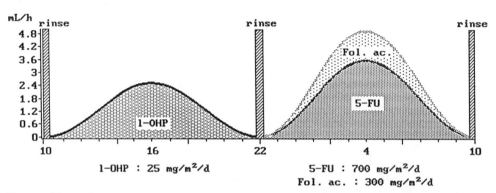

Figure 7. Drug delivery schedule as automatically administered for 5 consecutive days to outpatients who were ambulatory with the use of a multichannel programmable-in-time pump. A 20-minute rinse with 5 % glucose was programmed between l-OHP and 5-FU - FA infusion.

From April 1988 to May 1990, 93 consecutive eligible patients were entered into the study ; 49 % had received prior therapy, 43 % had performance status of 2 or greater and 43 % had 2 or more organs involved. A total of 839 courses were delivered to outpatients. No hematologic or skin toxicity was encountered. Dose limiting toxicities (grade 3-4) were vomiting (8 % courses - no anti-HT$_3$ serotonin receptor drug was given), diarrhea (5 %) or stomatitis (2 %). Peripheral sensitive neuropathy was cumulative. It started to be observed after the 7th course and eventually led to l-OHP withdrawal in 14 patients, with complete recovery within 3 months.

Of 93 patients, 54 had an objective response to therapy (58 % ; 95 % confidence limits, 48 % to 68 %). Of those, six had CR (6.4 %). The sites of objective response included liver, lungs and/or abdominopelvic localizations. There was SD in 31 patients and PD in 6. The objective response rate was similar in previously treated or untreated patients. Because of the effectiveness of this therapy, 18 patients (6 with CR and 12 with PR > 50 %) had successful removal or residual potential tumor masses, previously regarded as unresectable. A histologic CR was documented in four patients (4 %). The same protocol was continued subsequently for six courses after radical surgical excision of residual tumor as an attempt to prevent recurrence. The median estimated progression-free survival was 10 months for all assessable patients (n = 87). The median duration of response was 10 months. The median survival was 15 months for all 93 patients included in this trial (80).

These results compare favourably with any systemic medical treatment thus far reported against metastatic colorectal cancer, both with regard to patient tolerance and treatment efficacy. Furthermore, they suggest such chronotherapy may increase survival as compared to standard chemotherapy. Thus median survival differed significantly according to performance status (PS), it was 21 months in those patients with PS = 0-I and 10 months in those patients with PS = II-IV (p from log-Rank test < 0.005). As a result, the median survival of patients with a good PS was ≈ 50 % longer than that reported in most trials of 5-FU - FA or continuous 5-FU (12-14 months). A performance status of 0 or I was usually an inclusion criteria for these trials (1-4, 6). A prolonged survival may also result in part from the fact that a total of 18 patients could undergo a complete resection of all residual liver and/or lung metastases (19 % ; 95 % confidence limits ; 11 to 27 %). In August 1992, i. e. after a median follow up of 3.2 years, these 18 patients were alive (2.3 to 4 yrs after protocol entry) and 9 of them were disease-free and treatment free.

Such effect of chronotherapy on survival is further suggested by the efficacy of such regimen against progressive metastatic disease despite ongoing standard chemotherapy. Nineteen of these 93 patients and 27 consecutive additional patients met these criteria. All these 46 patients had CT-scan and/or echography-proven disease progression while receiving 5-FU - FA or continuous venous 5-FU. 48% patients had failed two chemotherapy regimens. 25 patients (54 %) exhibited an objective response. Response rate was similar whether clinical resistance to 5-FU was primary or acquired. Median PFS was 10 months and median survival was 13 months (81). In August 1992, two of these patients were alive, disease free and treatment free.

V-PERSPECTIVES OF CHRONOTHERAPY WITH 5-FU CONTAINING REGIMENS

Such chronotherapy regimen with 5-FU, FA and l-OHP constitutes to date the most active regimen in patients whose disease progresses while on standard chemotherapy. It may also be best as first line treatment. In order to investigate some of the factors responsible for such apparent increased antitumor activity, we have undertaken several multiinstitutional trials. A Phase II study involved 5-day continuous venous infusion of l-OHP at a circadian-rhythm modulated rate to 30 heavily pretreated patients with metastatic colorectal cancer. We demonstrated an objective response in 3 patients (10 %) (25, 82). This is higher than previously reported for any Pt complex in this disease, and further warrants the association of l-OHP to 5-FU-FA chronotherapy.

The role of circadian scheduling with regard to both toxicity and efficacy is currently being investigated in an international multicenter randomized trial. This trial was initiated in May 1990 and had registered 240 patients in July 1992. Chronotherapy is compared to flat delivery of all 3 drugs. If the merits of such chronotherapy schedule are validated, it may become pertinent to investigate the role of circadian modulation of drug delivery vs setting peak and trough times at specific times of day or night.

Nonetheless, experiments in rats with continuous venous infusion of FUdR indicated that the circadian pattern and not the quasi-intermittency of circadian FUdR administration was primarily responsible for significant differences in both toxicity and antitumor efficacy (14).

Recently, chronotherapy with 5-FU was investigated using 14-day infusion of this drug with FA (83). This phase I trial of 14-day continuous venous infusion of 5-FU and FA was undertaken in 14 patients with various malignancies. Both drugs were delivered as an admixture, with highest flow rate at 4.00 h. Both 5-FU and FA doses could be safely escalated from 200 to 250 mg/m^2/d and from 5 to 20 mg/m^2/d respectively. These authors also suggest that peak delivery of this admixture at 21.00 h might even be better tolerated for 14 day - CVI (83). The main results of clinical trials with 5-FU are summarized in Table 2.

Table 2. Summarized main findings of reported trials of chronomodulated 5-FU continuous venous infusion.

Schedule duration (d)	peak time	other drugs (dose, mg/m²/d)	device	cancer type	N. pts (prev. tt)	recommended 5-FU dose (mg/m²)	resp. rate (%)	surv. (mo.)
5d q 21d	4.00	none	AS 20 C	colon	35 (15)	1400	30	16
id.	id.	FA (300)	IntelliJect	colon	93 (48)	700	58	15
id.	id.	& I-OHP (25)	id.	id. (all resistant)	46	id.	54	13
5d q 21d	4.00	none	AS 20 C	pancreas	16 (5)	1400	23	11
14d q 28d	4.00	FA (20)	NR	various	14 (NR)	250	NR	NR

NR : not reported

After Lévi et al. (70, 80), Berthault-Cvitkovic et al. (71) and Bjarnason et al (83)

In conclusion, preclinical requisites, clinical pharmacokinetics and phase I trials indeed indicate that 5-FU disposition and pharmacodynamic effects are modulated by chronobiological rhythms. The availability of programmable-in-time pumps has made feasible to test the chronotherapy hypotheses - drug delivery according to biological rhythms. Phase II studies combining 5-FU, FA and oxaliplatin have yielded among the highest response rate achieved in patients with metastatic colorectal cancer. Indeed both primary and acquired resistance to 5-FU appear to be partly circumvented by chronotherapy. Consequences for survival are being explored in a randomized multicenter trial in metastatic colorectal cancer, whereas clinical trials of 5-FU chronotherapy are being developed in patients with other tumor types (breast, pancreas, biliary tract and non-small cell lung cancer.

ACKNOWLEDGEMENTS

This work was supported in part by the Association pour la Recherche sur le Temps Biologique et la Chronothérapie.

We are indebted to M. Levi for excellent editorial assistance.

REFERENCES

1. Machover D., Schwarzenberg L., Goldschmidt E., et al. Treatment of advanced colorectal and gastric adenocarcinomas with 5-FU combined with high dose folinic acid : a pilot study. *Cancer Treat. Rep.*, 1982, 66 : 1803-1807.
2. Erlichman C., Fine S., Wong A. et al. A randomized trial of fluorouracil and folinic acid in patients with metastatic colorectal carcinoma. *J. Clin. Oncol.*, 1988, 6 : 469-475.
3. Poon M., O'Connell M., Moertel G. et al. Biochemical modulation of fluorouracil : evidence of significant improvement of survival and quality of life in patients with advanced colorectal carcinoma. *J. Clin. Oncol.*, 1989, 7 : 1407-1417.
4. Petrelli N., Douglass H., Herrera L. et al. The modulation of fluorouracil with leucovorin in metastatic colorectal carcinoma : a prospective randomized phase III trial. *J. Clin. Oncol.*, 1989, 7 : 1419-1426.
5. Seiffert P., Baker L., Reed M. et al. Comparison of continuously infused 5-fluorouracil with bolus injection in treatment of patients with colorectal adenocarcinoma. *Cancer*, 1975, 36 : 123-128.

6. Lokich J., Ahlgren J., Gullo J. et al. Prospective randomized comparison of continuous infusion fluorouracil with a conventional bolus schedule in metastatic colorectal carcinoma : a mid-Atlantic Oncology Program study. *J. Clin. Oncol.*, 1989, 7 : 425-432.

7. Hryniuk W., Figueredo A., Goodyear M. Applications of dose-intensity to problems in chemotherapy of breast and colorectal cancer. *Semin. Oncol.*, 1987, 14 : 3-11.

8. Haus E., Halberg F., Scheving L.E. et al. Increased tolerance of leukemic mice to arabinosyl cytosine given on schedule adjusted to circadian system. *Science* (Washington DC), 1972, 177 : 80-81.

9. Lévi F., Hrushesky W., Blomquist J. et al. Reduction of cis-diamminedichloroplatinum nephrotoxicity in rats by optimal circadian drug timing. *Cancer Res.*, 1982, 42 : 950-955.

10. Hrushesky W., Lévi F., Halberg F; et al. Circadian stage dependence of cis-diamminedichloroplatinum lethal toxicity in rats. *Cancer Res.*, 1982, 42 : 945-949.

11. Mormont M.C., Boughattas N., Lévi F. Mechanisms of circadian rhythms in the toxicity and the efficacy of anticancer drugs : relevance for the development of new analogs. In : Lemmer B., ed. Chronopharmacology : cellular and biochemical interactions. New York : Marcel Dekker, 1989, 395-437.

12. Boughattas A.N., Lévi F., Fournier C. et al. Circadian rhythm in toxicities and tissue uptake of 1,2-diamminocyclohexane (trans-1)oxalatoplatinum(II) in mice. *Cancer Res.*, 1989, 49 : 3362-3368.

13. Boughattas A.N., Lévi F., Fournier C. et al. Stable circadian mechanisms of toxicity of two platinum analogs (cisplatin and carboplatin) despite repeated dosages in mice. *J. Pharmacol. Exp. Ther.*, 1990, 255 : 672-679.

14. Roemeling R.v., Hrushesky W. : Determination of the therapeutic index of floxuridine by its circadian infusion pattern. *J. Natl Cancer Inst.*, 1990, 82 : 386-393.

15. Dunlap J. Closely Watched clocks : molecular analysis of circadian rhythms in Neurospora and Drosophilia. *Trends in Genetics*, 1990, 65 : 135-168.

16. Klein D., Moore R.Y., Reppert S. eds *Suprachiasmatic nucleus. The mind's clock.* Oxford Univ. Pr. Inc., N.Y., USA; 1991, 467 pp.

17. Kornhauser J., Nelson D., Mayo K., et al. Regulation of jun-B messenger RNA and AP-1 activity by light and a circadian clock. *Science*, 1992, 255 : 1581-1585.

18. Touitou Y., Haus E., eds *Biological rhythms in clinical and laboratory medicine.* Springer Verlag, Berlin, Heidelberg, 1992, 730 pp.

19. Reinberg A., Smolensky M., Labrecque G. Eds. *Chronothérapeutique.* Flammarion, Paris, 1991.

20. Rivard G., Infante-Rivard C., Hoyoux C. et al. Maintenance chemotherapy for childhood acute lymphoblastic leukemia : better in the evening. *Lancet*, 1985, 2 : 1264-1266.

21. Hrushesky W. Circadian timing of cancer chemotherapy. *Science*, 1985, 228 : 73-75.

22. Lévi F., Benavides M., Chevelle C. et al. Chemotherapy of advanced ovarian cancer with 4'-0-tetrahydropyranyl adriamycin (THP) and cisplatin : a phase II trial with an evaluation of circadian timing and dose intensity. *J. Clin. Oncol.*, 1990, 8 : 705-714.

23. Bailleul F., Lévi F., Metzger G. et al. Chronotherapy of advanced breast cancer with continuous doxorubicin infusion via an implantable programmable device. 78th Ann. Meeting Amer. Assoc. Cancer Res., Atlanta (USA), May 20-23 1987. *Proc. Am. Ass. Cancer Res.*, 1987, 28: 771.

24. Roemeling R.v., Hrushesky W. Circadian patterning of continuous floxuridine infusion reduces toxicity and allows higher dose intensity in patients with widespread cancer. *J. Clin. Oncol.*, 1989, 7 : 1710-1719.

25. Caussanel J.P., Lévi F., Brienza S. et al. Phase I trial of 5-day continuous venous infusion of oxaliplatinum at circadian-modulated vs constant rate. *J. Natl. Cancer Inst.*, 1990, 82 : 1046-1050.

26. Després-Brummer P, Lévi F., Di Palma M. et al. A phase I trial of 21-day continuous venous infusion of a alpha-interferon at circadian rhythm modulated rate in cancer patients. *J. Immunother.*, 1991, 10 : 440-447.

27. Popovic P., Popovic V., Baughman J. Circadian rhythm and 5-fluorouracil toxicity in C$_3$H mice. In : *Biomed. Thermol.*, Alan Liss Inc., N.Y., USA, 1982, pp. 185-187.

28. Burns E., Beland S. Effects of biological time on the determination of the LD 50 of 5-fluorouracil in mice. *Pharmacology* (Basel), 1984, 28 : 296-300.
29. Gonzalez J., Sothern R., Thatcher G. et al. Substantial difference. in timing of murine susceptibility to 5-fluorouracil and FUdR. *Proc. Am. Ass. Ccancer Re*s., 1989, 30, 616 (abstract 2452).
30. Peters G., Van Dijk J., Nadal J., et al. Diurnal variation in the therapeutic efficacy of 5-fluorouracil against murine colon cancer. *In Vivo*, 1987, 1 : 113-118.
31. Minshull M., Gardner M. The effect of time of administration of 5-fluorouracil on leucopenia in the Rat. *Eur. J. Cancer Clin. Oncol.*, 1984, 20 : 857-858.
32. Gardner M., Plumb J. Diurnal variation in the intestinal toxicity of 5-fluorouracil in the rat. *Clin. Sci.*, 1981, 61 : 717-722.
33. Rydell R., Wenneberg J., Willen R. Circadian variation in cell cycle phase distribution in a squamous cell carcinoma xenograft ; effects of cisplatin and fluorouracil treatment. *In Vivo*, 1990, 4 : 385-390.
34. Beau J., Lévi F., Motta R. The influence of the athymic mutation nude on the components of the circadian rhythm of activity in mice. *Chronobiol. Intern.*, 1990, 7 : 371-376.
35. Harris B.E., Song R., He Y.J. et al. Circadian rhythm of rat liver dihydropyrimidine dehydrogenase. Possible relevance to fluoropyrimidine chemotherapy. *Biochem. Pharmacol.*, 1988, 37 : 4759-4762.
36. Daher G., Zhang R., Soon S.J., Diasio R. Circadian variation of fluoropyrimidine catabolic enzymes in rat liver : possible relevance to 5-fluorodeoxyuridine chemotherapy. *Drug Metab. Disp.*, 1991, 19 : 285-287.
37. Harris B.E., Song R., Soong S.J. et al. Circadian variation of 5-fluorouracil in isolated perfused rat liver. *Cancer Res.*, 1989, 49 : 6610.6614.
38. Diasio R., Zhang R., Lu Z. et al. Circadian variation of fluoropyrimidine metabolic enzymes : importance to fluorodeoxyuridine (FdURD) chemotherapy. *Proc 5th Intern. Conf. Chronopharmacol.*, Amelia Island, Fl., USA, July 12-16, 1992, IV-1 (abst.).
39. El Kouni M., Naquib F. Circadian rhythm of hepatic pyrimidine metabolizing enzymes and plasma uridine concentration in mice. *Proc 5th Intern. Conf. Chronopharmacol.*, Amelia Island, Fl., USA, July 12-16, 1992, IV-2 (abst.).
40. Zhang R., Lu E., Liu T. et al. Circadian rhythm of rat spleen cytoplasmic thymidine kinase : possible relevance to 5-fluorodeoxyuridine chemotherapy. *Proc 5th Intern. Conf. Chronopharmacol.*, Amelia Island, Fl., USA, July 12-16, 1992, IV-3 (abst.).
41. Malmary-Nebot M., Labat C., Casanovas A. et al. Aspect chronobiologique de l'action du méthrotréxate sur la dihydrofolate réductase. *Ann. Pharm. Fr.*, 1985, 43 : 337-343.
42. Labrecque G., Bélanger P., Doré F., Lalande M. Twenty-four variations in the distribution of labeled microspheres to the intestine, liver and kidneys. *Ann. Rev. Chronopharmacol.*, 1988, 5 : 445-448.
43. Scheving L.E., Burns E.R., Pauly J.E. et al. Circadian variations in cell division of the mouse alimentary tract, bone marrow and corneal epithelium. *Anat. Rec.*, 1978, 191 : 479-486.
44. Haus E., Lakatua D.J., Sackett-Lundeen L., et al. Circannual variation of intestinal cell proliferation in BDF1 male mice on three lighting regimens. *Chronobiol. Intern.*, 1984, 1 : 185-194.
45. Kennedy M., Tutton P., Barkla D. Comparison of the circadian variation in cell proliferation in normal and neoplastic colonic epithelial cells. *Cancer Lett.*, 1985, 28 : 169-175.
46. Waldrop R., Saydjari R., Rubin N. et al. DNA synthetic activity in tumor bearing mice. *Chronobiol. Intern.*, 1989, 6 : 237-243.
47. Rubin N., Shayestehmehr M., Chad-Wofford D. et al. Effect of colostomy on the circadian rhythm in DNA synthesis in the rat colon. *Chronobiol. Intern.*, 1992, 9 : 11-18.
48. Stoney P., Halberg F., Simpson H. Circadian variation of colony-forming ability of presumably intact murine bone marrow cells. *Chronobiologia*, 1975, 2 : 319-327.

49. Lévi F., Blazsek I., Ferlé-Vidovic A. Circadian and seasonal rhythms in murine bone marrow colony forming cells affect tolerance for anticancer agent 4'-tetrahydropyranyl Adriamycin (THP). *Exp. Hematol.*, 1988, 16 : 696-701.
50. Perpoint B., Le Bousse-Kerdiles C., Clay D. et al. In vitro pharmacology of recombinant mouse IL-3 recombinant mouse GM-CSF and recombinant human G-CSF on murine myeloïd progenitor cells. Submitted for publication.
51. Petit E., Milano G., Lévi F. et al. Circadian rhythm-varying plasma concentration of 5-fluorouracil during a five-day continuous venous infusion at a constant rate in cancer patients. *Cancer Res.*, 1988, 48 : 1676-1679.
52. Gudausras G., Goldie J. The pharmacokinetics of high dose continuous infusions. *Proc. Am. Assoc. Cancer Res.*, 1978, 19 : 364 (abstr.).
53. Thiberville L., Compagnon P., Moore N. et al. Accumulation plasmatique du 5-fluorouracile chez l'insuffisant respiratoire. *Rev. Mal. Resp.*, 1992, 111.
54. Metzger G., Comisso M., Massari C., Brienza S., Lévi F., Misset J.L. Differences in time course of plasma levels of 5-fluorouracil (5-FU) during constant or chronomodulated infusion in cancer patients *Proc. Am. Assoc. Cancer Res.*, 1992, 33 : 534 (abstr.).
55. Harris B., Song R., Soong S., Diasio R.B. Relationship between dihydropyrimidine dehydrogenase activity and plasma 5-fluorouracil levels : evidence for circadian variations of plasma drug levels in cancer patients receiving 5-fluorouracil by protracted continuous infusion. *Cancer Res.*, 1990, 50 : 197-201.
56. Bastian G., Demarq C., Leteure F. et al. Pharmacokinetics of 5-fluorouracil : effect of association with cisplatinum during long term infusion. *Proc. Am. Soc. Clin. Oncol.*, 1986, 5 : 55 (abstr.).
57. Milano G. Personal communication.
58. Nowakowska-Dulawa E. Circadian rhythm in 5-fluorouracil (FU) pharmacokinetics and tolerance. *Chronobiologia*, 1990, 17 : 27-35.
59. Tuchman M., Roemeling R. v., Lanning R. Source of variability of dehydropyrimidine dehydrogenase (DPD) activity in human blood mononuclear cells. In : Reinberg A., Smolensky M., Labrecque G., eds. *Annual Rev. Chronopharmacol.*, Oxford, Pergamon, 1988, 349-402.
60. Diasio R.B., Harris B.E. Clinical pharmacology of 5-fluorouracil. *Clin. Pharmacokinet.*, 1989, 16 : 215-237.
61. Lemmer B., Nold G. Circadian changes in estimated hepatic blood flow in healthy subjects. *Brit. J. Clin. Pharm.*, 1991, 32 : 627-629.
62. Scheving L.E. Mitotic activity in the human epidermis. *Anat. Rec.*, 1959, 135 : 7-19.
63. Brown W. A review and mathetical analysis of circadian rhythm in cell proliferation in mouse, rat and human epidermis. *J. Invest. Dermatol.*, 1991, 97 : 273-280.
64. Killman S.A., Cronkite Z.E.P., Fliedner T.M., Bond V.T. Mitotic indices of human bone marrow cells. 1. Number and cytologic distribution of mitoses. *Blood*, 1962, 19 : 743-750.
65. Mauer A.M. Diurnal variation of proliferative activity in the human bone marrow. *Blood*, 1965, 26 : 1-7.
66. Smaaland R., Laerum O., Lote K. et al. DNA synthesis in human bone marrow is circadian stage dependent. *Blood*, 1991, 77 : 2603-2611.
67. Buchi K., Moore J., Hrushesky W. et al. Circadian rhythm of cellular proliferation in the human rectal mucosa. *Gastroenteroly*, 1991, 101 : 410-415.
68. Markiewick A., Lelek A., Panz B., et al. Chronomorphology of jejunum in man. Proc. XVIII Intern. Conf. on Chronobiol., (Leiden, July 12-17th, 1987) *Chronobiologia*, 1987, 14 : 131 (abstr.).
69. Rietweld W., Boon M. Variation in size and glycogen content of exfoliating epithelial cells at different times of day. In : *Chronobiology*, 1982-1983, H. Kabat ed., S. Karger (Basel), 22-24.
70. Levi F., Brienza S., Misset J.L. et al. Circumvention of clinical resistance of metastatic colorectal cancer to 5-fluorouracil (5-FU) with circadian-rhythm modulated venous chemotherapy. *Proc. Am. Soc. Clin. Oncol.*, 1192, 11 : 171 (abstr.).

71. Berthault-Cvitkovic F., Soussan S., Brienza S. et al. Circadian-rhythm modulated chemotherapy with high-dose 5-fluorouracil : a pilot study in patients with pancreatic adenocarcinoma. 1992, submitted for publication.
72. Houghton J., Maroda S., Phillips J. et al. Biochemical determinants of responsiveness to 5-fluorouracil and its derivatives in xenografts of human colorectal adenocarcinoma in mice. *Cancer Res.*, 1989, 41 : 144-149.
73. Rustum Y., Trave F., Zakrewsky S.F. et al. Biochemical and pharmacologic basis for potentiation of 5-fluorouracil action by leucovorin. *NCI Monogr.*, 1987, 5 : 165-170.
74. Scanlon K., Newman E., Lu Y. et al. Biochemical basis for cisplatin and 5-fluorouracil synergism in human ovarian carcinoma cells. *Proc. Natl. Acad. Sci. USA*, 1986, 83 : 8923-8925.
75. Loehrer P., Turner S., Kubilis P. et al. A prospective randimized trial of fluorouracil versus fluorouracil plus cisplatin in the treatment of metastatic colorectal cancer : a Hoosier Oncology Group trial. *J. Clin. Oncol.*, 1988, 6 : 642-648.
76. Scheithauer W., Depisch D., Schiesscl R. ct al. Phase II evaluation of 5 fluorouracil, folinic acid and cisplatin in advanced-stage colorectal adenocarcinoma. *Oncology*, 1986, 46 : 217-221.
77. Cantrell J., Hart R., Taylor R. et al. Pilot trial of prolonged continuous infusion of 5-fluorouracil and weekly cisplatin in advanced colorectal cancer. *Cancer Treat. Rep.*, 1987, 71 : 615-618.
78. Mathé G., Kidani Y., Triana K. et al. A phase I trial of trans-l-diammino cyclohexane oxalato-platinum (l-OHP). *Biomed. Pharmacother.*, 1986, 40 : 372-376.
79. Mathé G., Kidani Y., Eriguchi M. et al. Oxalato-platinum or l-OHP, a third generation platinum complex : an experimental and clinical appraisal and preliminary comparison with cisplatinum and carboplatinum. *Biomed. Pharmacother.*, 1989, 43 : 237-250.
80. Lévi F., Misset J.L., Brienza S. A chronopharmacologic phase II clinical trial with 5-fluorouracil, folinic acid and oxaliplatinum using an ambulatory multichannel programmable pump : high antitumor effectiveness against metastatic colorectal cancer. *Cancer*, 1992, 69 (4) : 893-900.
81. Lévi F., Brienza S., Misset J.L. Circumvention of clinical resistance of metastatic colorectal cancer to 5-fluorouracil (5-FU) with circadian-rhythm modulated venous chemotherapy. *Proc. Am. Soc. Clin. Oncol.*, 1992, 11 : 171 (abstr.).
82. Levi F., Perpoint B., Garufi C. et al. Oxaliplatin activity against metastatic colorectal cancer. A phase II study of 5-day continuous venous infusion at circadian-rhythm modulated rate. 1992, submitted for publication.
83. Bjarnason G., Kerr I., Doyle N. et al. Phase I study of 5-fluorouracil and leucovorin by 14-day continuous infusion chronotherapy in patients with metastatic adenocarcinoma. *Proc. 5th Intern. Conf. Chronopharmacol.*, Amelia Island, Fl., USA, July 12-16 1992, IV-5 (abstr.).

GENERAL DISCUSSION

Dr. Mihich: This is a general question which has to do in part with Dr. Martin et al. and in part with Dr. Moran et al. In listening at the renaissance of the story of the RNA involvement as target for FU, I was reminded of the fact that some years back we tried thymidine and thymidine was very different from PALA in the sense that thymidine reduced catabolism of FU and increased blood levels there and also by competing the anabolism of thymidine, competing with the kinases on the one hand and feed-back inhibiting the reductase on the other hand were greatly reducing the thymidylate synthetase site and pushing much of the FU towards RNA. Whereas PALA seems to preserve thymidylate synthetase inhibition possibly while at the same time pushing FU into RNA. Dr. Moran this morning said it with a perhaps, perhaps the so called, he didn't say impure, but he called some pure inhibitors of thymidylate synthetase which by contrast means that the others are impure inhibitors of thymidylate synthetase. It might be better because perhaps there is a necessity of a co-existence in the proper proportions of thymidylate synthetase inhibition and of an action at the level of RNA. So that is the comment but which has an implicit question in it. Should we revisit thymidine if thymidine was mishandled like PALA was in a sense or do we know enough of the difference between thymidine and PALA that we are contented to leave it in a resting place?

Dr. Moran: I'm not going to touch it because in actual fact all I was doing this morning was trying to preface Dr. Martin with his studies on the decreasing TK mRNA which I find he didn't talk about. So I'm going to throw it back to Dr. Martin and give him a chance to talk about that now.

Dr. Martin: If you review the literature and not my data, you will find that for the last 20 or 30 years where people have simultaneously measured both TS and FU in RNA. The major effect has been due to FU in RNA as shown by thymidine and uridine reversal experiments. So, based upon that, and that's a lot of investigating, I would say that you will get more of an effect in terms of cytotoxicity out of a dose of FU which will accomplish both. So, there's a relatively small amount of TS in the cell and a fair amount of FdUMP can easily be made and that will swamp that TS. But there's a threshold level in RNA at which you begin to get the effect and the more FU you can give the more FU gets into RNA to reach that threshold effect and beyond. Now what Dr. Moran was talking about in terms of FU and RNA is that we recently published data showing that FU could knock out thymidine kinase. That means that you are simultaneously blocking salvage pathways through DNA when you have an Fura effect. So certainly at that level of DNA synthesis a high dose of FU will be preferable. When I say a high dose of FU, it doesn't mean that you have to give a lot of FU per se. There are modulators as we talked about all day that will in effect raise that level of FU intracellularly that will produce this effect. Now I haven't answered your thymidine question yet. I do think that thymidine should be explored further because I think it's effect on mononucleotide reductase is real and hasn't been well integrated with the effect in blocking catabolic pathways per se. So, as been said often in the last 6 months, the more we do the more we find out about all these things about FU which had been accepted for so long and I don't think that the answer is clear . For example, I think that certainly there's got to be some significance to FU and DNA in terms of everything I've just been talking about and this has not been simultaneously measured either in terms of what it might contribute. So I think that I can't answer your question other than to say that I do think there's a lot of work that still has to be done and can be done to unravel this thing.

Audience: I have a really short question for Dr. Allegra.

Dr. Allegra: Have you folks looked at other cytokines in addition to your gamma interferon?

Dr. Allegra: One of the difficulties with biologic response modifiers in the interferons in general at least preclinically and probably in the clinical setting is that and there has been some work from Dr. Fidler's group at M.D. Anderson which has suggested that in any given cell line or tumor, colon tumor, that they may only have about a third of the receptors the interferon receptors present either α, β or γ. So that may be one of the difficulties and why for instance in our hands α-interferon didn't seem to have any effects in the H 630 cell line alone.

Audience: I have a quick question for Dr. Levi and Dr. Hrushesky. Is there agreement as to when during the normal sleep cycle of a patient when the fluoropyrimidine levels will peak during continuous infusion? I was a little confused by the two talks it seems they were peaking at different times of the day.

Dr. Hrushesky: I think there is general concensus in the studies in which FU has been infused as a single agent. There are a couple of studies where other agents are given particularly the first one published within conjunction with a timed dose of platinum on day 1. That particular study seemed to have a different FU pattern for its peak but all, there have been now at least 4 or 5 studies demonstrating a similar circadian pattern during continuous constant infusion of FU as a single agent and perhaps Dr. Diasio can comment.

Dr. Diasio: That peak is at night around 2 in the morning for normal patients.

Dr. Houghton: I would like to address one point regarding interferons which may actually be confusing some people. Dr. Chu's was talking about the use of interferon-γ and basic studies I was talking about the use of interferon-α2A. These are very different compounds they are very different modulators and I think this needs to be clarified. Interferon-γ of course was originally isolated from cells of the immune system and the α-interferons originally came from leukocytes. The α,β-inteferons bind to the same receptor whereas interferon-γ binds to a completely different receptor. I think we to clarify here that we are talking about, although they are interferons, they are different classes of interferons.

FLUOROURACIL AND LEUCOVORIN IN ADVANCED BREAST CANCER[*]

James H. Doroshow, Kim Margolin, Lucille Leong, Steven Akman, Robert Morgan, Jr., James Raschko, George Somlo, Victor Hamasaki, Eleanor Womack, Edward Newman, and C. Ahn

Departments of Medical Oncology, Pediatrics, and Biostatistics
City of Hope Cancer Research Center
Duarte, CA 91010

INTRODUCTION

The prognosis for women with advanced breast cancer continues to be poor despite recent advances in several different treatment modalities. Patients whose disease has progressed on standard chemotherapeutic regimens have limited therapeutic options; response rates for second- or third-line therapies are in the range of 10-20%, and complete remissions are rare.[1] Therefore, the development of more effective treatment programs for patients with metastatic breast cancer remains an important area of investigation in clinical oncology.

Soon after the introduction of 5-fluorouracil (5-FU) into oncologic practice, it was found to possess significant therapeutic activity in patients with advanced breast cancer.[2] More recent data suggest that alterations in the schedule of administration of 5-FU (by continuous infusion for example[3]) may enhance the therapeutic efficacy of 5-FU in this disease. Because of the large body of preclinical evidence indicating that pharmacologic concentrations of reduced folates increase the duration and degree of thymidylate synthase inhibition after exposure to 5-FU *in vitro*, several recently completed phase II trials have addressed the efficacy of the combination of 5-FU and calcium leucovorin in patients with advanced breast cancer. Furthermore, current studies have also examined the use of the 5-FU and leucovorin combination as part of multiagent chemotherapeutic regimens for patients with advanced disease. In this report, the pertinent clinical investigations that have evaluated the use of this biochemical modulation strategy in the treatment of breast cancer as well as a recently-completed trial of 5-FU, leucovorin, and cis-platinum will be reviewed.

[*]This study was supported by Cancer Center Support Grant CA-33572. Requests for reprints should be addressed to James H. Doroshow, M.D., Department of Medical Oncology and Therapeutics Research, City of Hope National Medical Center, 1500 E. Duarte Road, Duarte, CA 91010. These results have been reported, in part, in *Proc. Amer. Soc. Clin. Oncol.*, 10:65 (1991).

Novel Approaches to Selective Treatments of Human Solid Tumors: Laboratory and Clinical Correlation Edited by Y. M. Rustum, Plenum Press, New York, 1993

187

TRIALS OF 5-FU AND LEUCOVORIN

The initial studies of the 5-FU/leucovorin combination were performed in patients who had been heavily-pretreated with chemotherapy. As shown in Table 1, several recently-reported clinical trials have demonstrated the utility of the combination of 5-FU and calcium leucovorin in women who have received one or more prior regimens for metastatic breast cancer. All of these studies[4-9] utilized a daily times five schedule of bolus 5-FU at a dose of 370-375 mg/m^2 with from 200 to 500 mg/m^2/day of leucovorin given as either a 15 to 30 min intravenous infusion completed immediately before the delivery of the 5-FU, or as a continuous, intravenous infusion for a total of 5.5 days beginning 24 hours prior to the first dose of the fluoropyrimidine. The objective response rates in these investigations ranged from 10-28%, with very few complete remissions. However, essentially all of the patients entered had progressed on a previous 5-FU-containing chemotherapeutic program; furthermore, the study by Swain *et al.* demonstrated that the addition of leucovorin did improve the inhibition

Table 1. Efficacy of 5-FU and leucovorin in breast cancer patients with extensive prior therapy.

RX Group	Regimen	Pt No./Results (CR+PR/%)	Reference
5FU/ CF >1 Rx	FU 370 mg/M2/dx5 CF 500 mg/M2/dx5 .5CI	60/ 10(17%)	JCO 7:439
		14/ 2(14%)	JCO 10:1278
		21/ 2(10%)	PASCO 10:59
	FU 375 mg/M2/dx5 1hr p CF CF 500 mg/M2/dx5 30min	50/ 12(24%)	JCO 7:890
		36/ 10(28%)	AJCO 14:30
		11/ 36 no chemo for mets	
	FU 370 mg/M2/dx5 CF 200 mg/M2/dx5 15min	36/ 16(44%) Prior + no prior Rx	Oncol 44:336
		Summary 145/ 26(18%)	

of thymidylate synthase by 5-FU in patients whose tumors were available to be sampled for multiple biochemical studies.[6] Thus, there was the strong suggestion from these intial trials that at least some patients could be salvaged with 5-FU by the provision of pharmacologic doses of reduced folates.

Based on these results, trials have been conducted at the Princess Margaret Hospital, the City of Hope Cancer Research Center, and by the Southwest Oncology Group in patients who had received no prior therapy for metastatic disease. Preliminary results are available from these studies examining the efficacy of 5-FU and leucovorin in patients with objectively measurable, advanced breast cancer. The data are summarized in Table 2 on the next page. In essence, these investigations[8-10] have demonstrated that the 5-FU and leucovorin combination has substantial clinical activity in patients who have not been heavily pretreated. The overall objective response rate from the three trials is 36% with a 95% confidence interval from 26-46%. Despite the absence of a randomized, phase III comparison, these results suggest that the modulation of 5-FU by reduced folates in patients with disseminated breast cancer may be associated with objective response rates similar to those of the most

Table 2. Utility of 5-FU and leucovorin in breast cancer patients previously untreated for metastatic disease.

RX Group	Regimen	Pt No./Results (CR+PR/%)	Reference
5FU/ CF No Rx	FU 370 mg/M2/dx5 CF 500 mg/M2/dx5.5CI	31/ 14(45%)	JCO 10:1278
	FU 370 mg/M2/dx5 CF 200 mg/M2/dx5	25/ 12(48%)	PASCO 7:41
	FU 370 mg/M2/dx5 CF 500 mg/M2/dx5CI	36/ 7(19%)	PASCO 10:59
		Summary No Prior Rx: 92/ 33(36%)	

active single agents in advanced disease (20-40% for doxorubicin and mitoxantrone, for example[11]). Furthermore, the toxicity profile for patients treated with the daily times five schedule of 5-FU used in these three trials was excellent, and supports the use of the 5-FU and leucovorin combination in patients with medical contraindications to treatment with an anthracycline.

Because of the frequency with which doxorubicin and/or mitoxantrone are utilized for patients with disseminated breast cancer, several recent studies have examined the feasibility of combining these drugs with 5-FU and leucovorin.[12-15] A summary of the trials of multiagent chemotherapy including 5-FU and leucovorin is provided in Table 3. The studies

Table 3. Combination chemotherapy studies with 5-FU, leucovorin, and an anthracycline or mitoxantrone.

RX Group	Regimen	Pt No./Results (CR+PR/%)	Reference
5FU/ CF/ Anth	FU 600 mg/M2/q14d 1hr CF 500 mg/M2/q14d 2hr DOX 20 mg/M2 q14d 12 wks later CTX daily po DOX 20 mg/M2/wk	25/ 8(32%) 18/ 25 Prog Non-DOX	Cancer 68:934
	FU 375 mg/M2/dx3 CF 200 mg/M2/dx3 EPI 75 mg/M2d1 CTX 600 mg/M2d1	20/ 12(60%) No Prior Rx	J Chemo 3:176
5FU/ CF/ MX	FU 1000 mg/M2/dx3CI CF 100 mg/M2/dx3 MITOX 10 mg/M2/d1	53/ 24(45%) 1 5 Prior Rx	JCO 9:1736
	FU 350 mg/M2/dx3 CF 300 mg/M2/dx3 1hr MITOX 12 mg/M2d1 Q21days	26/ 17(65%) Measurable 18/ 13(72%) Meas+NonMeas Prior Chemo Mets	JCO 9:1731

reported by Hainsworth and colleagues[14] and Jones *et al.*[15] are of substantial interest. In both reports, the 5-FU and leucovorin schedules were changed to accomodate the expected toxicities of the added mitoxantrone. The principal concern of both investigative teams was the possibility of increased mucositis; thus, the 5-FU/leucovorin combination was given for three, rather than five consecutive days. Both studies reported impressive therapeutic activity--45% objective responses in heavily-pretreated patients, 65% responders in untreated patients--with quite acceptable levels of toxicity. Thus, in patients with reduced performance status who are not resistant to doxorubicin, this combination is a reasonable alternative to standard programs such as FAC or CMF. There is less experience with 5-FU and leucovorin in combination with an anthracycline. While the trial reported by Palmeri and colleagues[13] supports the feasibility of combining cyclophosphamide and epirubicin with 5-FU and leucovorin, the 60% overall response rate in a small number of patients is not better than many previous reports in which leucovorin was not added to CAF or FAC, for example.[1] The novel schedule of 5-FU and leucovorin used with doxorubicin in the report from the Southwest Oncology group makes comparison with other doxorubicin-containing trials difficult.[12] It seems clear that additional trials will be required to determine whether leucovorin <u>can</u> or <u>should</u> be added to standard combination regimens for the treatment of advanced disease. Finally, it is appropriate to note that very preliminary phase I-II data exist for the combination of 5-FU and leucovorin with PALA[16], hydroxyurea[17], or methotrexate and cyclophosphamide[18] in the treatment of advanced breast cancer. Unfortunately, the small number of patients accrued with breast cancer in each of these trials prohibits an accurate evaluation of the efficacy of the combinations. Clearly, these are all interesting approaches to various biochemical modulation pathways that deserve further careful study.

5-FU, LEUCOVORIN, AND PLATINUM

A trial of the combination of 5-FU, leucovorin, and cisplatin has recently been completed at the City of Hope Cancer Research Center[19] that merits evaluation in the context of the results reviewed above. This trial, begun late in 1989, was based on pilot studies of this combination in advanced colorectal cancer and on evidence from the University of Indiana demonstrating the surprising efficacy of cisplatin as a single agent in patients with advanced, measurable breast cancer previously unexposed to chemotherapy.[20] Eligibility criteria, pretreatment evaluation and follow-up, and study design were modeled on our previous studies of 5-FU and leucovorin in advanced, measurable breast cancer.[5,9] Patients received the identical infusional leucovorin schedule, with bolus 5-FU at a dose of 370 mg/m^2/day for five days. Cisplatin was administered at a starting dose of 20 mg/m^2/day for five days as a 45 minute infusion; 30 minutes after the completion of the platinum, 5-FU was administered. Of the 58 patients entered, 55 were evaluable and 3 are too early in their course of treatment to be reported. No patients were found to be ineligible for the study. The median age was 55 years (range 25-67); the median performance status was 90%. The distribution of metastatic sites was typical with most patients having 3 or more sites of disease. 44 patients had received prior chemotherapy for metastatic disease; 38 had received doxorubicin and 7 had been treated with 5-FU and leucovorin.

As shown in Table 4, the objective response rate was 34% for the combination in heavily-pretreated women with advanced disease, approximately double that seen in our initial trial of 5-FU and leucovorin alone in a comparable group of patients. Furthermore, the response rate of 73% in untreated women compares favorably with essentially any anthracycline-containing combination program. The median response duration was 3 months with a range from 2-26+ months. Perhaps of most interest are the observations that only 1 of the seven patients refractory of 5-FU and leucovorin responded after the addition of the cisplatin, and that 10 of the 23 responders overall (and 10 of 15 responders who had been previously-treated) had been exposed to doxorubicin. Two of the seven complete responders had progressed on a doxorubicin-containing program. Responses were seen in all visceral sites; the median survival was 11 months. The toxicity profile demonstrated significant hematologic suppression with 25% of treatment courses associated with severe granulocytopenia in the absence of growth factor support. Mucositis, as previously noted with 5-FU and leucovorin, was significant. These results suggest that despite the added toxicity the addition of platinum to 5-FU and leucovorin may produce a regimen with significant activity in patients who are anthracycline-resistant. The recent trial from the National Cancer Institute demonstrating a 45% response rate for the combination of carboplatinum, 5-FU, and leucovorin in heavily-pretreated patients supports this suggestion.[21]

Table 4. 5-FU, leucovorin, and cisplatin in metastatic breast cancer.

No. of Patients Entered	58
No. of Patients Evaluable	55
Too Early	3
Complete Responses	7 (13%)
Partial Responses	16 (29%)
Overall Response Rate	42% (95% CI 29-55%)
Pts with Prior Chemotherapy	
3 CR's and 12 PR's	34% (95% CI 20-48%)
Pts with No Prior Chemotherapy	
4 CR's and 4 PR's	73% (95% CI 47-99%)
Response Duration	
Median	3 months
Range	2-26+ months

SUMMARY AND FUTURE TRENDS

It is clear from the studies summarized above that the combination of leucovorin and 5-FU can salvage 15-20% of heavily-pretreated patients with advanced breast cancer. In previously-untreated patients, the combination generates objective responses in over one third of women with a very modest and acceptable toxicity profile. It is also clear that the addition of mitoxantrone or cisplatin to 5-FU and leucovorin produces very effective regimens, that, at least in the case of the platinum combination, may be quite active in patients who have failed therapy with an anthracycline. All of these recently-completed trials, suggest that studies currently in progress aimed at improving the biochemical modulation of the fluoropyrimidines have real promise for enhancing the therapy of patients with advanced breast cancer further.

REFERENCES

1. Henderson IC, Hayes DF, Come S, et al: New agents and new medical treatments for advanced breast cancer. Semin Oncol 14:34-64, 1987

2. Ansfield FJ, Ramirez G, Mackman S, et al: A ten-year study of 5-fluorouracil in disseminated breast cancer with clinical results and survival times. Cancer Res 29:1062-1066, 1969

3. Huan S, Padzur R, Singhakowinta A, et al: Low-dose continuous infusion 5-fluorouracil: evaluation in advanced breast carcinoma. Cancer 63:419-422, 1989

4. Marini G, Simoncini E, Zaniboni A, et al: 5-Fluorouracil and high-dose folinic acid as salvage treatment of advanced breast cancer: an update. Oncology 44:336-340, 1987

5. Doroshow JH, Leong L, Margolin K, et al: Refractory metastatic breast cancer: salvage therapy with fluorouracil and high-dose continuous infusion leucovorin calcium. J Clin Oncol 7:439-444, 1989

6. Swain SM, Lippman ME, Egan EF, et al: Fluorouracil and high-dose leucovorin in previously treated patients with metastatic breast cancer. J Clin Oncol 7:890-899, 1989

7. Loprinzi CL, Ingle JN, Schaid DJ, et al: 5-Fluorouracil plus leucovorin in women with metastatic breast cancer. Am J Clin Oncol 14:30-32, 1991

8. Margolin K, Doroshow J, Green S, et al: Treatment of advanced breast cancer with 5-FU and high-dose folinic acid. Proc Amer Soc Clin Oncol 10:59, 1991(abstr)

9. Margolin KA, Doroshow JH, Akman SA, et al: Effective initial therapy of advanced breast cancer with fluorouracil and high-dose, continuous infusion calcium leucovorin. J Clin Oncol 10:1278-1283, 1992

10. Fine S, Erlichman C, Kaizer L, et al: Phase II trial of 5FU + folinic acid (FA) as first line treatment for metastatic breast cancer. Proc Amer Soc Clin Oncol 7:41, 1988(abstr)

11. Cowan JD, Neidhart J, McClure S, et al: Randomized trial of doxorubicin, bisantrene, and mitoxantrone in advanced breast cancer: a Southwest Oncology Group study. J Natl Cancer Inst 83:1077-1084, 1991

12. Ellis GK, Green S, Schulman S, et al: Alternating weekly doxorubicin and 5-fluorouracil/leucovorin followed by weekly doxorubicin and daily cyclophosphamide in stage IV breast cancer. A Southwest Oncology Group study. Cancer 68:934-939, 1991

13. Palmeri S, Gebbia V, Russo A, et al: Cyclophosphamide plus epidoxorubicin and 5-fluorouracil with folinic acid as a novel treatment in metastatic breast cancer: preliminary results of a phase II study. J Chemother 3:176-179, 1991

14. Hainsworth JD, Andrews MB, Johnson DH, et al: Mitoxantrone, fluorouracil, and high-dose leucovorin: an effective, well-tolerated regimen for metastatic breast cancer. J Clin Oncol 9:1731-1735, 1991

15. Jones SE, Mennel RG, Brooks B, et al: Phase II study of mitoxantrone, leucovorin, and infusional fluorouracil for treatment of metastatic breast cancer. J Clin Oncol 9:1736-1739, 1991

16. Ardalan B, Sridhar KS, Benedetto P, et al: A phase I, II study of high-dose 5-fluorouracil and high-dose leucovorin with low-dose phosphonacetyl-L-aspartic acid in patients with advanced malignancies. Cancer 68:1242-1246, 1991

17. Bhalla K, Birkhofer M, Bhalla M, et al: A phase I study of a combination of allopurinol, 5-fluorouracil and leucovorin followed by hydroxyurea in patients with advanced gastrointestinal and breast cancer. Am J Clin Oncol 14:509-513, 1991

18. Pronzato P, Amoroso D, Ardizzoni A, et al: Sequential administration of cyclophosphamide, methotrexate, 5-fluorouracil, and folinic acid as salvage treatment in metastatic breast cancer. Am J Clin Oncol 10:404-406, 1987

19. Leong L, Doroshow J, Akman S, et al: Phase II trial of 5-fluorouracil (5-FU), folinic acid (FA), and cis-platinum (CDDP) in metastatic breast cancer. Proc Amer Soc Clin Oncol 10:65, 1991(abstr)

20. Sledge GW,Jr., Loehrer PJ,Sr., Roth BJ, et al: Cisplatin as first-line therapy for metastatic breast cancer. J Clin Oncol 6:1811-1814, 1988

21. Allegra CJ, Mayer A, Reed E, et al: Therapy of patients with metastatic breast cancer (MBC) with 5-fluorouracil (FU), leucovorin (L), and carboplatin (CBDCA). Proc Amer Soc Clin Oncol 8:54, 1989(abstr)

DISCUSSION OF DR. DOROSHOW'S PRESENTATION

Audience: Would you comment on, Dr. Scanlon's results suggesting that platinum is a modulator of FUra action through increase in 5,10 methylenetetrahydrofolate pools resulting from inhibition of methionine uptake.

Dr. Doroshow: I think we're going to hear more about that in probably in less than an hour so I hate to say too much. Basically, one of the reasons that we started this trial and the reason for this particular schedule that is the sequencing of the platinum and the FUra is related to Dr. Scanlon's PNAS paper showing that enhancement of folate pools after platinum pretreatment. I think that as subsequent speakers will point out it's probable that platinum modulates the fluorouracil and it's also very possible that fluorouracil modulates the platinum activity. One thing to point out is that some patients who had extensive prior radiotherapy the dose of platinum had to be reduced to 10 mg/M^2 and some patients even 5 mg/M^2 platinum. Under these conditions objective responses were observed.

Audience: Anybody have any experience with PALA modulation in breast cancer? Dr. Ardalan did you have any experience you wanted to share with us in breast cancer?

Dr. Ardalan: As Dr. Doroshow treated very few patients, I think we've treated about 3 or 4 patients previously heavily pretreated and the problem there is of course their regimen of FUra was different than what they had before. They had a higher dose of FUra so nobody has looked at it carefully.

FLUOROURACIL MODULATION IN HEAD AND NECK CANCER

Everett E. Vokes

Department of Medicine and Radiation Oncology
University of Chicago Medical Center
5841 S. Maryland Avenue, MC2115
Chicago, IL 60637-1470

The majority of patients with head and neck cancer present with locoregionally advanced disease (1-3). For most of these patients, standard therapy consists of surgery followed by radiotherapy, unless the patient has unresectable disease due to the specific anatomic location (e.g. nasopharynx) or widespread involvement of neighboring structures, or is medically inoperable. In these cases, standard therapy consists of radiotherapy alone. However, less than 30% of patients are cured and locoregional disease persistence/ recurrence is the most common pattern of failure. Distant metastases, second malignancies, and medical problems related to smoking and alcohol consumption are significant additional causes of treatment failure and death (4,5). Chemotherapy has traditionally been investigated in patients with recurrent or metastatic disease (1-3). In that setting, response rates of 30% with a median response duration of 3 months are usually achieved. Commonly used regimens include single agent methotrexate or cisplatin, and the combination of cisplatin and a 4 to 5 day continuous infusion of fluorouracil. The latter combination, in particular, has been frequently investigated with response rates ranging from 20% to 74% (6).

The investigational use of chemotherapy in advanced head and neck cancer has focused on its use as induction (or neoadjuvant) chemotherapy (1-3, 6) prior to locoregional therapy and on concomitant chemoradiotherapy (7). The goals of these investigations are to increase survival rates and allow for less aggressive surgery (organ preservation). Randomized studies investigating induction chemotherapy have demonstrated a lower incidence of distant recurrence rates in patients receiving chemotherapy (8-11). In addition, larynx preservation (i.e. the substitution of surgery with chemotherapy) has been shown to be feasible (10). Locoregional recurrence rates however, have not been reduced (8-16) and, as a result, no randomized study has been able to demonstrate improved survival. Therefore, induction chemotherapy, including the combination of cisplatin and fluorouracil remains an investigational tool in advanced head and neck cancer and cannot be considered a part of standard therapy with the possible exception of larynx cancer, where it allows for organ preservation (although this goal might also be achieved with radiotherapy alone).

Novel Approaches to Selective Treatments of Human Solid Tumors: Laboratory
and Clinical Correlation Edited by Y. M. Rustum, Plenum Press, New York, 1993

Concomitant chemoradiotherapy, the simultaneous administration of chemotherapy and radiotherapy, is an alternative approach to multimodality therapy of head and neck cancer. It has resulted in statistically significant increases in disease free survival (7,17) and, in one study using bolus 5-FU, a small survival benefit was also demonstrated (18). These benefits have been small and have not led to a redefinition of standard therapy. Here, too, efforts at intensifying the chemotherapy component have been conducted and have involved modulation of 5-FU as reviewed below.

It has been shown repeatedly that patients achieving a complete response (CR) to initial therapy have a better prognosis than patients achieving partial response (PR) or no response (12-16). One goal of clinical studies can, therefore, be the identification of new regimens leading to higher CR-rates and, hopefully, improved overall survival rates. One possible strategy to achieve higher CR-rates has been the biochemical modulation of fluorouracil or of the cisplatin and fluorouracil combination. Modulation studies have been conducted in patients with recurrent and/or metastatic disease and in those with previously untreated locoregionally advanced disease. 5-FU modulation has included methotrexate, allopurinol, leucovorin, hydroxyurea, and interferon.

(a) Methotrexate and its analogues

Methotrexate and fluorouracil are two agents with activity in head and neck cancer. Browman et al have conducted studies in patients with recurrent disease investigating the sequential administration of methotrexate and 5-FU versus their simultaneous administration (19,20). In their first trial, 79 evaluable patients were randomized to receive methotrexate 200 mg/m^2 intravenously (IV) and 5-FU 600 mg/m^2 IV bolus either simultaneously or sequentially with methotrexate preceding 5-FU by one hour (19). Leucovorin rescue (10 mg/m^2 orally every 6 hours for 6 doses) was begun 24 hours after methotrexate. Treatment was given on days 1 and 8 of a 21 day cycle. The overall response rate was superior for simultaneous therapy (62%) compared with sequential therapy (38%). This study, therefore, demonstrated that one-hour sequential methotrexate/5-FU was not superior to simultaneous treatment with these two drugs.

Laboratory studies have suggested that biochemical modulation of 5-FU with methotrexate requires a 24 to 30 hour interval between the administration of both agents. Therefore, in a second randomized study the authors treated 118 patients with methotrexate 250 mg/m^2 IV and 5-FU at 600 mg/m^2 with leucovorin rescue (10 mg/m^2 for 6 doses) at 36 hours. Methotrexate and 5-FU were administered either simultaneously or 18 hours apart on days 1 and 8 of a 21-day treatment cycle. After excessive toxicity was noted in the first 11 patients, the dose of methotrexate was decreased to 200 mg/m^2. 100 patients had newly diagnosed locally advanced disease and 13 patients had recurrent disease. The response rate was 47% for simultaneous versus 45% for 18 hour sequential therapy, excluding a 20% difference in response rate favoring sequential therapy. Survival was also identical on both arms. However, gastrointestinal toxicity including stomatitis and diarrhea was increased with sequential therapy. The authors concluded that no advantage of sequential over simultaneous administration of methotrexate and 5-FU was apparent in head and neck cancer while toxicity was increased. Similar results were reported from a nonrandomized study by Lindelov and Hansen (21). The lack of increased activity with sequential methotrexate and 5-FU is consistent with similar clinical observations in other disease sites that have not supported the laboratory evidence of increased cytotoxicity with sequential methotrexate and 5-FU.

Browman et al also investigated modulation of the antitumor effect and toxicity of methotrexate by leucovorin (22). This randomized trial was based on observations that high-dose methotrexate with leucovorin rescue had failed to show an advantage to low dose methotrexate in head and neck cancer as well as other adult solid tumors (1,23). 61 patients received methotrexate at 40 mg/m^2 weekly with either placebo or leucovorin "rescue" 24 hours later. The response rate in patients receiving leucovorin was 17% versus 37% in patients receiving placebo. Similarly, toxicity was higher in the placebo arm. This study, therefore, confirmed that leucovorin modulates both the toxicity and antitumor efficacy of methotrexate.

Methotrexate is widely considered to be a standard therapy for recurrent head and neck cancer. However, only a minority of patients (<30%) respond and the response duration is short (2-3 months) due to the rapid emergence of drug resistance. Several analogues of methotrexate have been tested with the goal of increasing response rates and/or response duration.

Edatrexate has similar preclinical activity as methotrexate but may be clinically superior since it can enter cells more easily, is a better substrate for polyglutamation and is a more potent inhibitor of the target enzyme dihydrofolate reductase (24,25). Braakhuis et al (26) and Brown et al (27) demonstrated that the drug was active in laboratory head and neck cancer models. Schornagel et al (28) conducted a phase II study of edatrexate in 47 patients with advanced or recurrent disease. Edatrexate was administered as 80 mg/m^2 weekly with two dose increments of 10% if no toxicity was observed after two weeks of treatment. The overall response rate was 24% (95% confidence interval 11-35%) with 12% each CR and PR. Median response duration was 17 weeks (10 to 56 weeks). The toxicity pattern consisted of stomatitis and dermatitis observed in 73% and 25%, respectively. Dose increments were performed in 36% of patients. However, a significant proportion of patients also underwent dose reduction and the average weekly dose administered was 72 mg/m^2. This study suggested similar activity for edatrexate as for methotrexate. Subsequently, a randomized trial was conducted that directly compared edatrexate with methotrexate in recurrent disease. In a preliminary report, no significant difference in response rates was observed (29).

Trimetrexate, another folate antagonist, has also been investigated in recurrent head and neck cancer. Robert et al (30) treated 38 evaluable patients and reported a 26% PR rate with a median response duration of 12 weeks. Myelosuppression and mucositis were the most common toxicities. These results do not suggest that this compound is superior to methotrexate.

Another methotrexate analogue is piritrexim (31-33). It is a lipid soluble folate antagonist that crosses the cell membrane by carrier independent diffusion. Since piritrexim is not polyglutamated intracellularly efflux from the cell also occurs rapidly. Uen et al (34) conducted a phase II study of this drug in 33 evaluable chemotherapy-naive patients. Three patients had a CR and 6 a PR for an overall response rate of 27% (95% confidence interval 13% to 46%) and a response duration of 162 days (36 to 360+ days). Leukopenia, thrombocytopenia and stomatitis were the most frequent toxicities.

Since methotrexate and piritrexim differ in their biochemical properties, we postulated that the two drugs could be given in sequence and that tumor cell populations resistant to one drug might be eradicated by the other. Specifically, cells able to transport and polyglutamate methotrexate might be more sensitive to this drug than to piritrexim, and cells with defective transportation or decreased polyglutamation might be more sensitive to piritrexim. Based on this rationale, a phase II trial was conducted in which patients were treated with methotrexate at 50 mg/m^2 on day 1 and piritrexim at 75 mg/m^2 orally on days 8 through 12 (35).

Dose increments were made for both drugs to achieve grade I toxicity with each agent on each cycle. Five patients (17%, 95% confidence 4-30%) had a PR and time to progression in responding patients ranged from 2 to 6 months. The median survival was 7 months. Mild to moderate myelosuppression was the most common toxicity. This trial did not suggest enhanced response rates with antifolate chemotherapy using these two agents in sequence. However, observed toxicities were, generally, mild to moderate only suggesting suboptimal dose intensity. Furthermore, the treatment schedule may have been suboptimal in that it didn't allow the two drugs to work against tumor cells simultaneously. A subsequent trial of more rapid sequencing of the two drugs has been completed and awaits final analysis. The above trials have attempted to increase response rates in patients with recurrent disease. Studies attempting 5-FU modulation with methotrexate have also been conducted in the neoadjuvant setting. At the University of Chicago, we have utilized the cisplatin and 5-FU combination as basis of our clinical investigations in head and neck cancer. When initially studying cisplatin and 5-FU as induction chemotherapy for 3 cycles in 51 patients, we found a clinical CR-rate of 43% and PR rate of 47% for an overall response rate of 90% (15). This was followed by standard surgery and radiotherapy and 3 cycles of adjuvant chemotherapy. Despite the high initial response rate, the median survival was only 22 months and the 5-year survival 25%. Thus, our experience suggested at best a marginal impact of this regimen on the survival rate of patients with locoregionally advanced head and neck cancer as also confirmed by randomized studies (8-16).

In our subsequent study, we attempted to increase the CR-rate of cisplatin and 5-FU through the sequential addition of methotrexate (36). Chemotherapy consisted of methotrexate 120 mg/m^2 followed 24 hours later by cisplatin at 100 mg/m^2 and a five day continuous infusion of 5-FU at 1000 mg/m^2/day. Leucovorin rescue was given at 25 mg/m^2 every 6 hours for 6 doses 24 hours after administration of methotrexate. Thus, this regimen added a third active drug to cisplatin and 5-FU at a schedule that would also allow modulation of 5-FU. Thirty-eight patients with previously untreated, locoregionally advanced head and neck cancer received 3 cycles as induction chemotherapy followed by local therapy and 3 additional cycles of adjuvant therapy. Nine patients (24%, 95% confidence interval 10% to 38%) achieved a CR and 21 patients (55%) a PR to induction chemotherapy. At a follow-up to 39 months, the median survival was 20 months, with the majority of patients dying of locoregional recurrence. Chemotherapy-related toxicities consisted mainly of mucositis, requiring a dose reduction of 5-FU in the majority of patients. Mucositis was graded as moderate in 49% of patients and severe in 30%. Thus, mucositis appeared increased in severity compared with cisplatin and 5-FU alone. That regimen had resulted in 16% moderate and only 4% severe mucositis.

In a subsequent study, we increased the number of induction chemotherapy cycles with methotrexate, cisplatin and 5-FU from 3 to 4 (37). 10/29 (34%) patients had a CR following 4 cycles. While this was higher than the 24% noted in the previous study following 3 cycles with the same regimen, it was no higher than the 43% CR-rate observed with cisplatin and 5-FU alone and the 95% confidence intervals of CR-rates in all three studies overlap. Therefore, we concluded that the addition of methotrexate to cisplatin and 5-FU had increased toxicity but had not increased the CR rate.

Based on the available information from our own institution and from other groups of investigators, it seems fair to conclude that 5-FU modulation with methotrexate in head and neck cancer has not resulted in increased response or survival rates. However, continued investigations of the methotrexate analogues is warranted given their different pharmacologic characteristics and their potential for interaction with methotrexate, leucovorin, 5-FU and other drugs.

(b) Hydroxyurea (HU)

As single agent HU has limited activity in head and neck cancer (38). However, like other antimetabolites, HU has been used as a radiation enhancer in an attempt to increase local control and cure rates following radiotherapy. Clinical studies in cervical cancer and in malignant gliomas support the use of HU in this context (17). Its exact mechanism of radiation enhancement is unknown, but is postulated to be decreased cellular repair mechanisms of radiation damage due to depletion of nucleotide pools and/or cell cycle syndronization (17,39,40). In addition, it has specific activity against cells in the S-phase of the cell cycle which are less responsive to radiation.

Studies utilizing HU at our institution have focused on its use with 5-FU and radiation. A synergistic interaction of HU with 5-FU has been demonstrated (41). It is felt to be due to depletion of cellular deoxyuridine monophosphate (dUMP) pools thus increasing binding of 5-FdUMP to thymidylate synthase (42). In addition, 5-FU has also been demonstrated to enhance radiation (17,18,43).

In a phase I-II study, we developed a regimen consisting of 5-FU administered as continuous infusion at 800 mg/m^2/day for 5 days, with HU 1000 mg orally given for 11 doses every 12 h starting 6 to 12 hours prior to the 5 FU infusion (44,45). Radiotherapy was administered at 180 to 200 cGy daily during chemotherapy administration. Five days of therapy with this regimen (FHX) were followed by a treatment break on days 6 to 14. Treatment cycles were repeated until completion of a full course of radiotherapy. Eligible patients had locoregionally recurrent disease, metastatic disease in need of palliative locoregional therapy, or had failed to respond to induction chemotherapy. The dose-limiting toxicities of this regimen were mucositis and myelosuppression. High complete and overall response rates in patients with far advanced disease were identified. In addition, the locoregional recurrence rate in previously unirradiated patients was low, suggesting a potential role for this combination in previously untreated patients (45). These high response rates in poor prognosis patients have been confirmed by Gandia et al (46).

Weppelmann et al (47) investigated a similar regimen of 5-FU (300 mg/ m^2/d x5 as IV bolus), HU 1.5 or 2.0 gm/day x5 and simultaneous radiotherapy for 5 days. Eleven patients received 200 cGy once daily, and 10 patients received 120 cGy twice daily for total doses of 40 and 48 Gy, respectively. Cycles were repeated every other week for up to 4 courses. 21 previously irradiated patients with recurrent disease were treated; nine achieved a CR and six a PR and the one year survival was 56%. In this study, neutropenia was the major toxicity. Recommended doses for further investigations with this regimen were 1.5 gm/day of HU and radiotherapy at the twice daily schedule.

(c) Allopurinol

Allopurinol has been investigated as a modulator of 5-FU in the neoadjuvant setting. Greenberg et al (48) administered cisplatin 100 mg/m^2, continuous infusion 5-FU at 1500 mg/m^2/day for 5 days with 900 mg/day of Allopurinol beginning one week before the initiation of chemotherapy and continued for one week after completion of the 5-FU infusion. At this dose of 5-FU, stomatitis was dose-limiting and was severe in 32% of patients. Dose escalation of 5-FU to 2000 mg/m^2/day as originally planned was performed in only two patients. Both patients developed severe toxicity, and this dose was not felt to be feasible. Of 37 patients entered on study, 33 were evaluated for response. The CR rate was 45% and the PR rate 55%. Following local therapy with radiotherapy, the median survival for all 33 patients was 21 months. This study suggests that allopurinol modulation of 5-FU allows for escalation of 5-FU to a maximum tolerated dose (MTD) of 1500 mg/m^2/day. Whether this modulation results in increased activity remains unanswered.

No additional studies investigating allopurinol as a modulator in head and neck cancer have been published. However, allopurinol has been used in an attempt to reduce mucositis following 5-FU chemotherapy with no clear evidence of a benefit to date (49).

(d) Leucovorin

Leucovorin is currently the most frequently used biochemical modulator of 5-FU in solid tumor therapy. Following reports of encouraging activity of the 5-FU/leucovorin combination in colorectal cancer, we initiated a phase I-II study in patients with recurrent and/or metastatic head and neck cancer at the University of Chicago in 1985, investigating the addition of leucovorin to cisplatin and 5-FU (PFL) (50). 100 mg/m^2 of cisplatin were followed by a 5 day continuous infusion of 5-FU at 600 mg/m^2/day which was escalated in cohorts of patients to 800 and 1000 mg/m^2/day. Based on reports of preferential absorption of the l-stereoisomer of leucovorin following its oral administration (51), we chose to investigate the oral administration of this drug at 50 mg/m^2 every 6 h (200 mg/m^2/day) during the entire duration of chemotherapy administration. In a second phase of the study, the dose of leucovorin was increased to 50 mg/m^2 every 48 hours (300 mg/m^2/ day). Since absorption of leucovorin is saturable (51), we chose to increase the frequency of leucovorin administration rather than the amount per dose.

The MTD of 5-FU was 800 mg/m^2/day with leucovorin administered every 6 hours. In these previously irradiated patients, the dose-limiting toxicity was mucositis with mild to moderate myelosuppression also being observed. Similar toxicities were seen when administering 800 mg/m^2/day of 5-FU with leucovorin every 4 h. Of 18 patients evaluated for response, one had a pathologically confirmed CR, and nine had a PR for an overall response rate of 56%. Response rates to cisplatin and 5-FU without leucovorin in patients with recurrent disease have ranged from 11 to 79% (6) and thus overlap with the response rate reported here. The mean peak and trough plasma leucovorin concentrations were 2.61 ($\pm$1.07) μmol/L and 2.46 ($\pm$0.95) μmol/L with leucovorin administration every 6 h, and 2.75 ($\pm$2.15) μmol/L and 2.52 ($\pm$1.48) μmol/L with administration every 4 h. Thus, the more frequent administration of leucovorin appeared to result in somewhat higher plasma concentrations, although no statistically significant difference was found, possibly due to the small number of specimens tested.

Given the encouraging response rate, we decided to continue the investigation of PFL with the more frequent leucovorin administration in previously untreated patients in the neoadjuvant setting. Since we had observed high locoregional control rates with the FHX combination as described above (44,45), we decided to also incorporate this regimen into the trial to enhance locoregional therapy. 64 patients with locoregionally advanced disease were treated with two cycles of induction chemotherapy consisting of either cisplatin, bleomycin and methotrexate (PBM, 33 patients) or the PFL combination (31 patients) for patients with poor pulmonary function tests. Locoregional therapy consisted of surgery (for resectable disease) and concomitant chemoradiotherapy. In this study, we also added leucovorin to the FHX combination in an attempt to further increase the activity of this regimen. The PFL regimen was modified to increase the 5-FU dose to 1000 mg/m^2/day in these previously untreated patients. This resulted in frequently severe mucositis, necessitating a dose reduction of 5-FU during cycle 2 in the majority of patients. These toxicity data confirmed the dose recommendations previously established in patients with recurrent disease. Pharmacokinetic measurements of leucovorin revealed total reduced folate plasma concentrations of 5.3 ($\pm$2.9) and 6.7 ($\pm$3.4) μmol/L on days 2 and 4 of the 5-FU infusion, respectively (52). The sum of the biochemically active l-leucovorin and its metabolite 5-methyltetrahydrofolate exceeded the concentration of d-leucovorin. This was felt to be consistent with selective absorption of the biologically active l-stereoisomer from the gastrointestinal tract (51).

Following the administration of two cycles of chemotherapy, the complete and overall response rates were 21% and 79%, respectively, for PBM and 29% and 81% for PFL. Subsequent local therapy consisted of surgery (32 patients) and/or FHX-L (52 patients). The addition of leucovorin to FHX resulted in a marked increase of severe mucositis. Grade 3 or 4 mucositis was seen in 64% of patients. This led to subsequent dose reductions of 5-FU and the majority of patients received an average of 300-500 mg/m^2/day of 5-FU. This reflects a dose reduction of approximately 50% from the initially targeted dose of 800 mg/m^2/d as administered in the FHX regimen without leucovorin (53).

With a median follow-up of 35 months, the median survival and time to progression for patients treated with PBM was 22 and 17 months, respectively. For patients treated with PFL, the median survival and time to progression had not been reached. The locoregional recurrence rate was 30% with PBM and 26% with PFL. This compared favorably to prior studies conducted at our institution (15,36,37). Interestingly, the distant disease progression (outside the head and neck region) was 24% for PBM and only 3% for PFL (53).

We concluded that the sequencing of induction chemotherapy and concomitant chemoradiotherapy was feasible. The time to progression and survival seen with PFL was encouraging. The high distant failure rate with PBM suggested insufficient systemic activity for that combination. Finally, the high locoregional control rate seen on both arms of the study suggested that concomitant chemoradiotherapy with FHX may improve regional control rates. With improved locoregional control effective systemic therapy to control micrometastatic disease may be needed if overall survival is to be improved. Our study suggests that PFL, but not PBM, is able to accomplish that goal.

Dreyfuss et al (54) pursued a similar strategy of modulating the cisplatin/5-FU regimen with leucovorin in head and neck cancer. 35 patients with locoregionally advanced head and neck cancer were treated with two to three cycles of cisplatin at 25 mg/m^2/day on days 1 to 5, 5-FU 800 mg/m^2/day on days 2 to 6 and intravenous leucovorin at 500 mg/m^2/day on days 1 through 6. In this trial, all three drugs were administered by continuous intravenous infusion. Cycles were repeated every 28 days. Overall, 80% of patients responded; 66% had a CR and 14% a PR as maximum response to induction chemotherapy. When assessing response after two cycles, 26% of patients had a CR. Thus, the activity of PFL following two cycles appeared similar to that seen in our study. The addition of a third cycle of induction chemotherapy has previously been demonstrated to result in an increased CR-rate (12).

The toxicity profile again was dominated by mucositis which was graded as moderate to severe in 94% of patients. Leucovorin pharmacokinetics were determined in 7 patients. At 18 hour of the continuous infusion, the mean leucovorin plasma concentration was 34.3$\pm$1.5 μmol/L of which 8.0$\pm$1.5% was the l-leucovorin isomer. The mean 5-methyltetrahydrofolate concentration was 9.2$\pm$0.6 μmol/L. Survival data from this study following local therapy with surgery and radiotherapy have not been reported to date.

Loeffler et al (55) treated 58 patients with locally advanced or recurrent head and neck cancer with cisplatin 20 mg/m^2/day followed by leucovorin 100 mg/ m^2/day IV bolus and 1 hour later with 5-FU at 400 mg/m^2/day IV bolus, all administered daily for 5 consecutive days on an outpatient basis. Cycles were repeated every 21 to 28 days. 45 patients were previously untreated and 13 had received prior chemotherapy and/or radiotherapy. Following three cycles of induction chemotherapy, 23/45 (51%) patients had a CR and 20/45 (44%) had a PR for an overall response rate of 95%. Updated information on survival following local therapy in these patients has not been published. Of 13 previously treated patients, four had a CR and 6 a PR. Hematological and gastrointestinal toxicity was reported as dose-limiting. This study suggest high activity for PFL in this schedule with the advantage of a more convenient outpatient administration.

Finally, Merlano et al (56) performed a phase II study of leucovorin as 500 mg/m² administered over 2 hours with 5-FU 600 mg/m² as intravenous bolus 1 hour into the leucovorin administration. In 27 patients with recurrent disease, one CR and 7 PRs were observed, for an overall response rate of 30%. Mucositis and diarrhea were the most prevalent side effects. This response rate compares favorably to that reported with 5-FU as single agent in recurrent disease, including infusional 5-FU (57).

Wendt et al (58) pursued a different strategy by incorporating leucovorin into a concomitant chemoradiotherapy regimen. In their phase II study, 62 patients received cisplatin 60 mg/m², 5-FU 350 mg/m² and leucovorin 50 mg/m² as IV bolus, followed by a 4-day continuous infusion of 5-FU at 350 mg/m²/day and leucovorin at 100 mg/m²/day. Radiotherapy was delivered twice daily at 180 cGy on days 2-4 of the infusion and days 7-10 (total dose 2340 cGy over 9 days). This regimen was repeated on days 22 and 44 for a cumulative radiotherapy dose of 7020 cGy. Of 59 evaluable patients 48 (81%) achieved a CR and 11 (19%) a PR. At a mean follow-up of 29 months the projected 2 year survival rate was 52%. Toxicities consisted mainly of mucositis which was graded as severe in 34% of patients.

These studies suggest that modulation with leucovorin holds promise in head and neck cancer. Pertinent examples are the PFL regimen as induction chemotherapy (52-54) as well as the concomitant regimen described by Wendt et al (58). Therefore, we currently continue to study the biochemical modulation of 5-FU in head and neck cancer at the University of Chicago. Recent efforts have focused on the addition of methotrexate and piritrexim to the PFL regimen which did not appear to result in a further increase in activity (59), and on the addition of interferon alfa-2ß (IFN). In this phase I study, we identified 2×10^6 Units/ m²/day for 6 doses as MTD for IFN when administered with PFL (at a reduced 5-FU dose of 640 mg/m²/day) (60). A study investigating the addition of IFN to cisplatin and 5-FU (without leucovorin) is currently being conducted by Bensmaine et al (61). A full report of these trials will need to be awaited to more clearly assess the possible contribution of IFN as a biochemical modulator in head and neck cancer. Finally, pharmacokinetic and pharmacodynamic analyses may help to reduce the incidence of severe mucositis which is the dose-limiting toxicity of all these trials. This has already been shown to be feasible (62) and might result in an improved therapeutic index for these combinations in the future.

REFERENCES

1) Vokes, E.E., 1992, Head and neck cancer, In: Perry MC, ed. Chemotherapy Source Book. Baltimore: Williams and Wilkins, 918.

2) Hong, W.K. and Bromer, R., 1983, Current Concepts: Chemotherapy in head and neck cancer, *N Engl J Med* 308:75.

3) Clark, J.R. and Frei, E. III, 1989, Chemotherapy for head and neck cancer: Progress and controversy in the management of patients with M0 disease, *Sem Oncol* 16(Suppl 6):44.

4) Cooper, J.S., Pajak, T.F., Rubin, P., et al, 1989, Second malignancies in patients who have head and neck cancer: Incidence, effect on survival and implications based on the RTOG experience, *Int J Radiat Oncol Biol Phys* 17:449.

5) Hong, W.K., Lippman, S.M., Itri, L.M., et al, 1990, Prevention of second primary tumors with isotretinoin in squamous cell carcinoma of the head and neck, *N Engl J Med* 323:795.

6) Urba, S.G. and Forastiere, A.A, 1989, Systemic therapy of head and neck cancer: Most effective agents, areas of promise, *Oncology* 3:79.

7) Vokes, E.E., Awan, A.M., and Weichselbaum, R.R., 1991, Radiotherapy with concomitant chemotherapy for head and neck cancer, *Hematol/Oncol Clin North Am* 5:753.

8) Jacobs, C. and Makuch, R., 1990, Efficacy of adjuvant chemotherapy for patients with resectable head and neck cancer: A subset analysis of the head and neck contracts program, *J Clin Oncol* 8:838.

9) Schuller, D.E., Metch, B., Mattox, D., et al, 1988, Preoperative chemotherapy in advanced resectable head and neck cancer: Final report of the Southwest Oncology Group, *Laryngoscope* 98:1205.

10) The Department of Veterans Affairs Laryngeal Cancer Study Group, 1991, Induction chemotherapy plus radiation compared with surgery plus radiation in patients with advanced laryngeal cancer, *N Engl J Med* 324:1685.

11) Laramore, G.E., Scott, C.B., Al-Sarraf, M., et al, 1992, Adjuvant chemotherapy for resectable squamous cell carcinomas of the head and neck: Report on Intergroup Study 0034, *Int J Radiat Oncol Biol Phys* 23:705.

12) Rooney, M., Kish, J., Jacobs, J., et al, 1985, Improved complete response rate and survival in advanced head and neck cancer after three-course induction therapy with 120-hour 5-FU infusion and cisplatin, *Cancer* 55:1123.

13) Ervin, T.J., Clark, J.R., Weichselbaum, R.R., et al, 1987, An analysis of induction and adjuvant chemotherapy in the multidisciplinary treatment of squamous-cell carcinoma of the head and neck, *J Clin Oncol* 5:10.

14) Spaulding, M.B., Lore, J.M., Sundquist, N., 1989, Long-term follow-up of chemotherapy in advanced head and neck cancer, *Arch Otolaryngol Head Neck Surg*, 115:68.

15) Vokes, E.E., Mick, R., Lester, E.P., et al, 1991, Cisplatin and fluorouracil chemotherapy does not yield long-term benefit in locally advanced head and neck cancer: results from a single institution, *J Clin Oncol* 9:1376.

16) Ensley, J., Jacobs, J., Weaver, A., et al, 1984, Correlation between response to cisplatinum-combination chemotherapy and subsequent radiotherapy in previously untreated patients with advanced squamous cell cancers of the head and neck, *Cancer*, 54:811.

17) Vokes, E.E. and Weichselbaum, R.R., 1990, Concomitant chemoradiotherapy: Rationale and clinical experience in patients with solid tumors, *J Clin Oncol* 8:911.

18) Lo, T.C., Wiley, A.L. Jr., Ansfield, F.J., et al, 1976, Combined radiation therapy and 5-fluorouracil for advanced squamous cell carcinoma of the oral cavity and oropharynx: A randomized study, *Am J Roentgenol* 126:229.

19) Browman, G.P., Archibald, S.D., Young, J.E.M., et al, 1983, Prospective randomized trial of one-hour sequential versus simultaneous methotrexate plus 5-fluorouracil in advanced and recurrent squamous cell head and neck cancer, *J Clin Oncol* 12:787.

20) Browman, G.P., Levine, M.N., Goodyear, M.D., et al, 1988, Methotrexate/fluorouracil scheduling influences normal tissue toxicity but not antitumor effects in patients with squamous cell head and neck cancer: Results from a randomized trial, *J Clin Oncol* 6:963.

21) Lindelov, B., Hansen, H.S., 1989, The effect of sequential methotrexate and 5-fluorouracil in patients with recurrent head and neck cancer, *Acta Oncol* 28(2):227.

22) Browman, G.P., Goodyear, M.D.E., Levine, M.N., et al, 1990, Modulation of the antitumor effect of methotrexate by low-dose leucovorin in squamous

cell head and neck cancer: A randomized placebo-controlled clinical trial, *J Clin Oncol* 8:203.

23) Ackland, S.P. and Schilsky, R.L., 1987, High-dose methotrexate: A critical reappraisal, *J Clin Oncol* 5:2017.

24) Sironak, F.M., DeGraw, J.I., Schmid, F.A., et al, 1984, New folate analogs of the 10-Deaza-Aminopterin series. Further evidence for markedly increased antitumor efficacy compared with methotrexate in ascitic and solid murine models, *Cancer Chemother Pharmacol* 12:26.

25) Moccio, D.M., Sironak, F.M., Samuels, L.L., et al, 1984, Similar specificity of membrane transport for folate analogues and their metabolites by murine and human tumor cells. A clinically directed laboratory study, *Cancer Res* 44:352.

26) Braakhuis, B.J., van Dongen, G.A., Bagnay, M., et al, 1989, Preclinical chemotherapy on human head and neck cancer xenografts grown in athymic nude mice, *Head-Neck* 11(6):511.

27) Brown, D.H., Braakhuis, B.J., van Dongen, G.A., et al, 1989, Activity of the folate analog 10-ethyl, 10-deaza-aminopterin (10-EdAM) against human head and neck cancer xenografts, *Anticancer Res* 9(6):1549.

28) Schornagel, J.H., Verweij, J., Cognetti, F., et al, for the EORTC Head and Neck Cancer Cooperative Group, 1991, A randomized phase III trial of methotrexate vs 10-ethyl-10-deaza-aminopterin in patients with advanced and/or metastatic squamous cell carcinoma of the head and neck, *Eur J Cancer* 27(2):138 (Abstract #825).

29) Schornagel, J.H., Verweij, J., de Mulder, P.H.M., et al, 1992, A phase II trial of 10-ethyl-10-deaza-aminopterin, a novel antifolate, in patients with advanced or/or recurrent squamous cell carcinoma of the head and neck, *Ann Oncol* 3:223.

30) Robert, F., 1988, Trimetrexate as a single agent in patients with advanced head and neck cancer, *Semin Oncol* 15(2):22.

31) Duch, D.S., Edelstein, M.P., Bowers, S.W., Nichol, C.A., 1982, Biochemical and chemotherapeutic studies on 2,4-diamino-(2,5-dimethoxybenzyl)-5-methylpyrido[2,3-d] pyrimidine (BW 301U), a novel lipid-soluble inhibitor of dihydrofolate reductase, *Cancer Res* 42:3987.

32) Sedwick, W.D., Hamrell, M., Brown, O.E., Laszlo, J., 1982, Metabolic inhibition by a new antifolate, 2,4-diamino-6-(2,5-dimethoxybenzyl)-5-methyl-pyrido[2,3-d] pyrimidine (BW301U), an effective inhibitor of human lymphoid and dihydrofolate reductase-overproducing mouse cell lines. *Mol Pharmacol* 22:766.

33) Taylor, I.W., Slowiaczek, P., Friedlander, M.L., et al, 1985, Selective toxicity of a new lipophilic antifolate, BW301U, for methotrexate-resistant cells with reduced drug uptake, *Cancer Res* 45:978.

34) Uen, W.-C., Huang, A.T., Mennel, R., et al, 1992, A phase II study of piritrexim in patients with advanced squamous head and neck cancer, *Cancer* 69:1008.

35) Vokes, E.E., Dimery, I.W., Jacobs, C.D., et al, 1991, A phase II study of piritrexim in combination with methotrexate in recurrent and metastatic head and neck cancer, *Cancer* 67:2253.

36) Vokes, E.E., Moran, W.J., Mick, R., et al, 1989, Neoadjuvant and adjuvant methotrexate, cisplatin, and fluorouracil in multimodal therapy of head and neck cancer, *J Clin Oncol* 7:838.

37) Vokes, E.E., Panje, W.R., Mick, R., et al, 1990, A randomized study comparing two regimens of neoadjuvant and adjuvant chemotherapy in multimodal therapy for locally advanced head and neck cancer, *Cancer* 66:206.

38) Vokes, E.E., Haraf, D.J., Panje, W.R., et al, 1992, Hydroxyurea with concomitant radiotherapy for locally advanced head and neck cancer, *Semin Oncol* 19(9):53.

39) Kinsella, T.J., 1992, Radiosensitization and cell kinetics: Clinical implications for S-phase-specific radiosensitizers, *Semin Oncol* 19(9):41.

40) Vokes, E.E., 1992, Interactions of chemotherapy and radiation. *Semin Oncol*, (in press).

41) Moran, R.G., Danenberg, P.V., Heidelberger, C., 1982, Therapeutic response of leukemic mice treated with fluorinated pyrimidines and inhibitors of deoxyuridylate synthesis. *Biochem Pharmacol* 31:2929.

42) Schilsky, R.L., Ratain, M.J., Vokes, E.E., et al, 1992, Laboratory and clinical studies of biochemical modulation by hydroxyurea, *Semin Oncol* 19(9):84.

43) Byfield, J.E., Sharp, T.R., Frankel, S.S., et al, 1984, Phase I and II trial of five-day infused 5-fluorouracil and radiation in advanced cancer of the head and neck, *J Clin Oncol* 2:406.

44) Vokes, E.E., Panje, W.R., Schilsky, R.L., et al, 1989, Hydroxyurea, fluorouracil, and concomitant radiotherapy in poor-prognosis head and neck cancer: A phase I-II study, *J Clin Oncol* 7:761.

45) Haraf, D.J., Vokes, E.E., Panje, W.R., et al, 1991, Survival and analysis of failure following hydroxyurea, 5-fluorouracil and concomitant radiation therapy in poor prognosis head and neck cancer, *Am J Clin Oncol* 14(5):419.

46) Gandia, D., Wibault, P., Guillot, T., et al, Simultaneous chemoradiotherapy as salvage treatment in locoregional recurrences of squamous head and neck cancer patients, *Head and Neck*, (in press).

47) Weppelman, B., Wheeler, R.H., Peters, G.E., et al, 1992, Treatment of recurrent head and neck cancer with 5-fluorouracil, hydroxyurea, and reirradiation, *Int J Radiat Oncol Biol Phys* 22:1051.

48) Greenberg, B., Ahmann, F., Garewal, H., et al, 1987, Neoadjuvant therapy for advanced head and neck cancer with allopurinol-modulated high dose 5-fluorouracil and cisplatin: A phase I-II study, *Cancer* 59:1860.

49) Loprinzi, C.L., Cianflone, S.G., Dose, A.M., et al, 1990, A controlled evaluation of an allopurinol mouthwash as prophylaxis against 5-fluorouracil-induced stomatitis, *Cancer* 65(8):1879.

50) Vokes, E.E., Choi, K.E., Schilsky, R.L., et al, 1988, Cisplatin, fluorouracil, and high-dose leucovorin for recurrent or metastatic head and neck cancer, *J Clin Oncol* 6:618.

51) Straw, J.A., Szapary, D., Wynn, W.T., 1984, Pharmacokinetics of the diastereoisomers of leucovorin after intravenous and oral administration to normal subjects, *Cancer Res* 44:3114.

52) Vokes, E.E., Schilsky, R.L., Weichselbaum, R.R., et al, 1990, Induction chemotherapy with cisplatin, fluorouracil, and high-dose leucovorin for locally advanced head and neck cancer: A clinical and pharmacologic analysis, *J Clin Oncol* 8:241.

53) Vokes, E.E., Weichselbaum, R.R., Mick, R., et al, 1992, Favorable long-term survival following induction chemotherapy with cisplatin, fluorouracil,

and leucovorin and concomitant chemoradiotherapy for locally advanced head and neck cancer, *J Natl Cancer Inst* 84:877.

54) Dreyfuss, A.I., Clark, J.R., Wright, J.E., et al, 1990 Continuous infusion high-dose leucovorin with 5-fluorouracil and cisplatin for untreated stage IV carcinoma of the head and neck, *Ann Int Med* 112:167.

55) Loeffler, T.M., Lindemann, J., Luckhaupt, H., et al, 1988, Chemotherapy of advanced and relapsed squamous cell cancer of the head and neck with split-dose cisplatinum, 5-fluorouracil and leucovorin, *Adv Exp Med Biol* 244:267.

56) Merlano, M., Bacigalupo, A., Benasso, M., et al, 1990, 5-fluorouracil and high-dose folinic acid as second-line chemotherapy in head and neck cancer, *Am J Clin Oncol* 13(1):1.

57) Jacobs, C., Lyman G., Velez-Garcia, E., et al, 1992, A phase III randomized study comparing cisplatin and fluorouracil as single agents and in combination for advanced squamous cell carcinoma of the head and neck, *J Clin Oncol* 10:257.

58) Wendt, T.G., Hartenstein, R.C., Wustrow, T.P.U., and Lissner, J., 1989, Cisplatin, fluorouracil with leucovorin calcium enhancement, and synchronous accelerated radiotherapy in the management of locally advanced head and neck cancer: A phase II study, *J Clin Oncol* 7:471.

59) Vokes, E.E., Haraf, D.J., McEvilly, J.-M., et, 1992, Neoadjuvant PFL augmented by methotrexate and piritrexim followed by concomitant chemoradiotherapy for advanced head and neck cancer: A feasible and active approach, *Ann Oncol* 3:79.

60) Vokes, E.E., Ratain, M.J., Mick, R., et al, 1992, A clinical and pharmacologic phase I-II study of PFL with interferon alfa-2B for head and neck cancer, *Proc Am Soc Clin Oncol* 11:243 (Abstract #782).

61) Bensmaine, A., Azli, N., Soulie, P., et al, 1992, CDDP-5FU Modulation by alpha IFN2B in metastatic and or recurrent head and neck squamous cell carcinoma, *Proc AACR* 33:223 (Abstract #1338).

62) Santini, J., Milano, G., Thyss, A., et al, 1989, 5-FU therapeutic monitoring with dose adjustment leads to an improved therapeutic index in head and neck cancer, *Br J Cancer* 59:287.

BIOMODULATION IN HEAD AND NECK CARCINOMAS:

THERAPEUTIC APPROACHES IN EUROPE

Jan Eskandari

Oncology
Marseille, France

INTRODUCTION

Biomodulation, especially in head and neck carcinomas (H & N Ca.), refers to both cytotoxic drugs and ionizing radiations activities. Due to the heterogeneity of the tumor cells, modulation would address just as well to hypoxic cells as to therapeutically induced resistant cells.

MODULATION IN CHEMOTHERAPY

Chemotherapy in H & N Ca. is still investigational whether in its neoadjuvant form where survival goals have not been reached but where organ preservation is more commonly achieved or in advanced disease where complete remission (CR) is the challenge.

Modulation concerns mainly two drugs, Cisplatin (P) and 5-FU (F), and here Leucovorin(L) is the most studied modulator.

PFL associations[1,2,3,4] give around 50% CR (table 1), and corroborate those results obtained by Dreyfuss[5] and Vokes[6] in the same setting, no matter the mode of administration. Adding drugs does not seem to be advantageous.

Associations including Bleomycine(BLM), Hydroxyurea(HU) or Methotrexate (MTX)[7,8,9] without other modulation give generally results inferior to PFL (10 to 23% CR).

Investigative studies now include Cytokines and the number of studies including Interferon (IFN alpha 2b) or IL_2 is growing every year.

In H & N Ca. we can distinguish between the local adoptive Immunotherapy setting and the systemic utilization of Cytokines.

The first derives among others from Forni et al.[10,11] works showing that peritumoral inoculation of low doses of

Novel Approaches to Selective Treatments of Human Solid Tumors: Laboratory and Clinical Correlation Edited by Y. M. Rustum, Plenum Press, New York, 1993

209

Table 1. Induction Chemotherapy. PFL based regimens.

Authors (Ref.)	N	Stage	Protocol drug:mg/m^2/d	RR	CR
Loeffler et al. Germany, 1988 (1)	45	III, IV	P:20 x5d F:400 x5d L:100 x5d	95%	51%
Caty et al. France, 1992 (2)	30	III, IV	P:100 xd1 F:600 x5d L:200 x5d	88%	48%
Guaraldi et al. Italy, 1992 (3)	33	III, IV	P:30 x5d F:500 x5d L:200 x5d BLM:15 x5d	58%	12%
Bensmaine et al. France, 1992 (4)	28	IV	P:100 xd1 F:600 x5d L:150 x4d VDS:0.8 x4d	52%	15%
Schneider et al. France			PFL ongoing study		

P=Cisplatin ; F=5-FU ; L=Leucovorin ; BLM=Bleomycin ; VDS=Vindesine.

recombinant IL$_2$ with spleen lymphocytes from sarcoma bearing BALB/c mice leads to a total inhibition of tumor growth in these same mice. H & N Ca., representing the best human model for evaluation of a locoregional Immunotherapy, series of clinical studies were undertaken, first initiated by Cortesina et al.[12,13,14,] with cervical perilymphatic injections of natural IL$_2$ for 10 days in recurrent inoperable patients, and reported up to 65% RR unfortunately not lasting. These results were partially confirmed by Squadrelli-Saraceno et al.[15] but not by Matjissen et al.[16] who observed a lack of clinical response in non pretreated patients associated with the absence of lymphoid infiltration or tumor necrosis as usually described[17,18] and contrasted with Melioli et al. study[19] which in the same conditions showed an activation of T cells and a potentiation of NK activity in the peripheral blood.

Experience with systemic administration of Cytokines is presented in Table 2. Interesting results are obtained in relapsed patients by Toma et al.[20] (2/10 CR, 2/10 PR) with P-IFN regimen and by Bensmaine et al.[21] (2 CR and 5 PR/11 pts) with PF-IFN. However these results are lower than those of Vokes et al.[22] PFL+IFN association (60% CR, 32% PR).

Martin Gore initiated a still ongoing randomized study comparing PF plus IFN-alpha-2b vs PF and achieved a phase I study[23] with Interleukin (IL$_2$) administered intra arterially up to 3.10^7 iu/24 hrs in continuous infusion for 10 days. Interestingly, tumor heavy lymphocytic infiltration was associated with extensive tumor necrosis and was predictive of response (2 responders/11 patients).

Fiorentino et al.[24] evaluated in advanced malignancies the immune effects of a combination of IFN alpha 2b ($3MU/m^2$/day) in the first week and IL_2 during the second week with increasing doses up to $2,4MU/m^2$/day subcutaneously then repeating this cycle for a total of 6 weeks. 4/12 stabilization only but a significant enhancement of natural killer activities were noted.

Table 2. Induction Chemotherapy with Cytokines.

Authors (Ref.)	N	Stage	Protocol drug:mg/m²/d	RR	CR
Toma et al. Italy, 1991 (20)	10	recur.	P:20 x5d IFN:3.10⁶x5d	4/10	2/10
Bensmaine et al. France, 1992 (12)	11	recur.	P:100 xd1 F:1000 x4d IFN:3MUx5d	7/11	2/11
Gore et al. UK, 1992	20	recur.	PF+IFN vs PF	ongoing random. study	
Gore et al. UK, 1992 (13)	12		IL_2: 3.10⁷U	2/11	
Fiorentino et al. Italy, 1991 (24)	12	adv. malign.	IFN:3MU wks1,3,5 IL_2:2MU wks2,4,6	4	2

P=Cisplatin ; F=5-FU ; IFN=Interferon alpha-2b ; IL_2=Interleukin

MODULATION IN IONIZING RADIATIONS

Radiotherapy (RT) still remains a standard in the treatment of H § N Ca., and we must not forget that we can modulate tumor cell as well as normal cell response through variations of its different parameters.

Variations in Time-Dose Factors

Clonogenic Assays, labelling index based Tpot calculation and DNA content evaluated by flow cytometry showed that we could influence cell survival by altering either overall treatment time (OTT) or fractionation (Fx).

H & N tumors seem to express low clonogenic fraction around 0,71% according to Geara et al.[25], but in vitro and vivo observations made by Fowler et al.[26,27], Bentzen et al.[28], Trott et al.[29] and others assess the fact that a faster compensatory proliferation occurs after the onset of radiation with a lag of 1 to 4 weeks. This pattern of so called delayed acceleration of repopulation, though controversial in its origin, provides the basis for altering OTT and/or fractionation either homogeneously or by accelerating the dose delivery only at the end of the radiotherapy as tried by Sanguinetti et al.[30] with 76% CR (19/25 pts).

According to Bentzen et al.[31] increasing OTT would decrease tumor control if the total dose is not increased in the range of 0.68 Gy/day.

But a British Institute of Radiology study, including 611 patients recently reported an increase in late effects when longer OTT was associated with higher total doses[32].

An EORTC randomized trial[33] (Table 3) showed an advantage in DFS with increased fractionation and dose delivery in the same OTT. This was corroborated by a Brazilian study[34] and a Spanish study[35], this latter incidently showing that the hyperfractionation arm is equivalent to 5-FU combination arm.

Table 3. Clinical Trials with altered Time-Dose Factors

Authors (Ref.)	N	Protocol Gy/Frac/wks	DFS	Surv.	Tox.
Horiot et al. EORTC,1990 (Randomized) (33)	356	70Gy/34/7 vs 80,5Gy/70/7	38% 5 yrs(s) 56%		ns
Sanchiz et al. Spain,1990 (Randomized) (35)	859	60Gy/30/6 vs 70,4Gy/64/6,4 vs 60Gy/30/6 +5FU=250mg/m²eod	38 mths s 84 mths ns 85 mths		ns
Pinto et al. Brazil, 1991 (Randomized) (34)	98	70Gy/64/6,5 vs 66Gy/33/6,5	25% ns 7%	27% 42mths(s) 8%	ns
Saunders et al. UK, 1991 (38)	92	54Gy/36/12d (CHART)	49% (95% CR)	63% 2yrs	4 mye- litis

s=significant ; ns=not significant

Begg et al.[36] (EORTC) suggested that tumors with low Tpot (below 4 days) would show resistance to conventional but not to accelerated RT. And more recently Geido et al.[37] demonstrated a better progression free survival in patients whose tumor expressed a Tpot superior to 5 days (67% vs 31% at 2 years).

CHART experience[38] shows indeed very high response rates with 3 fractionated RT in a decreased OTT but 4 cases of myelitis are reported probably due to insufficient lag between the fractions.

Therefore we should be very careful in this modulation and the debate is still open and very promising.

Radiosensitization

Which is to interact with radiations by inhibiting the cellular repair capacities or to fix more tightly the radiation induced damage.

This chapter will mainly address oxymimetic agents represented by Misonidazole and analogs, which are electron affinic compounds, trapping electrons migrating within intracellular DNA, thus increasing the number of free radicals and which after the positive results of the Danish DAHANCA[39] studies are integrated in large Phase I (RTOG)[40] or Phase III (Chassagne)[41] trials. Preliminary results do not show survival improvement except for Niromazole (Overgaard)[42] in advanced supraglottic carcinomas when combined with RT (at 4 years 52% vs 29% with RT alone).

MODULATION WITH COMBINED MODALITIES

In vitro and in vivo studies regularly suggest at least a potentiation if not a sensitization of ionizing radiation by several well known drugs. The most frequently involved are Cisplatin and 5-FU which for H & N Ca. represent a real advantage.

Cisplatin and analogs appear to be rather radiosensitizing in hypoxic cells and best results are obtained at low radiation doses which are closer to clinical use. Mechanisms do not seem to involve cell cycle (Skov)[45] nor repair of X-ray induced DNA damage as shown recently by Lambin, Scalliet et al.[46] .

Clinical trials are not yet conclusive whether we deal with additivity or synergism[47,48,49,50,51,52] although showing a high response rate and an advantage of combined modalities with Platinum compounds.

5-FU alone does not seem to be supra-additive with ionizing radiation although its enhancement of radiation effects has been shown in a randomized study by Lo et al.[53] in advanced H & N Cancer patients where 2 years NED survival was 48.5% vs 17.6% respectively for RT + 5-FU thrice weekly and RT alone.

It can be reasonably expected that Leucovorin would enhance 5-FU radiosensitization activity by shifting its cytotoxicity towards DNA synthesis thus altering the cellular repair capacities.

Lawrence et al.[54] yielded series of in vitro studies showing that preincubation with Leucovorin increases the effectiveness of FdUrd as a radiosensitizer. Using neutral elution there was no increase in the radiation induced DNA double strand breaks (DSB) but a significant decrease in the rate of repair of DSB which was potentiated by Leucovorin. Another Fluoro-Pyrimidine modulator, Dipyridamol, was tested which as a potent inhibitor of nucleoside transport and particularly of Thymidine influx, could prevent DNA synthesis. But it failed to show any 5-FU mediated radiopotentiation.

On the other hand Scanlon et al.[55] provided data suggesting that Cisplatin potentiation of 5-FU, apart its specific cytotoxicity, is due to an increase of intracellular reduced folates via endogenous synthesis of Methionine, leading to a similar final situation as with Leucovorin.

We therefore proposed and achieved jointly with Y. RUSTUM a Phase I-II study combining weekly 5-FU-LV, without Cisplatin to conventional radiotherapy[56]. The only toxicity was mucous which was dose limiting and the recommended dose of 5-FU is 500mg/m². Response rate was 88% with 52% CR and at 2 years 30% of patients were alive and NED.

To end this section are multidrug combinations that presently give way to numerous clinical trials in H & N Ca. (Table 4). Either with conventionally fractionated radiotherapy where CR rates vary from 33% to 56% (to note is the utilization of MMC as a bioreductive drug in several studies and the Gandia study involving Vokes' scheme with HU on recurrent patients with 38 % CR). Or with altered fractionation where Wendt et al.[60] obtained exceptionally good results concerning CR rates (81%) as well as DFS (60% at 2 years). But the question remains whether these results are due to the combination of PFL with RT or to the choice of a hyperfractionated RT when looking back to the CHART experience with very similar results.

Table 4. Chemoradiotherapy - Multidrug Association

Authors (Ref.)	N	Stage	Protocol	CR	DFS	S
Dobrowski et al. Austria, 1989 (57)	41	III IV	RT+F-MMC	56%		63% 18mths
Hanauske et al. Germany, 1992	ongoing	III IV inop.	RT+F-MMC Surg. RT+F-MMC	Preliminary 80% RR Prior.to surg.		
Gandia et al. France, 1992 (58)	35	recur	RT+F-HUeowk	13/34	7/35 (20 mths)	1/35
Merlano Italy, 1991 (59)	116 Random	III, IV Inop	RT+VLB-BLM MTX-Lrescue vs RT	33% 14%		22% 4yrs (s) 10%
Wendt Germany, 1989 (60)	59	III, IV	RTHF+PFLx3 q21d	81%	60% (24 mths)	

RT=Conventional RT	P=Cisplatin	HU=Hydroxyurea
RTHF=Hyperfractionated RT	F=5-FU	BLM=Bleomycin
L=Leucovorin	MMC=Mytomicin	CMTX=Methotrexate

SCHEDULE MODULATION

To conclude we have to look for new scheduling of treatment modalities. Schedule modulation of LV and 5-FU have been already extensively reviewed and discussed as future directions.

Concerning H & N Ca. it is well-known that a strong correlation exists between resistance to CDDP and radiotherapy and this has been suggested by Ensley et al.[64]. What underlines this cross resistance was the object of several recent in vitro studies :

De Pooter, Scalliet et al.[65] reported that cell lines from ovarian Ca. (AOvC) rendered resistant to CDDP show resistance to radiation and this pattern was stable. Contrastingly, the same cell lines when rendered resistant to ionizing radiations by chronic exposure, not only did not show resistance to CDDP but even demonstrated an enhanced sensitivity to the drug transiently for six months and this pattern was associated with proportionally increased formation of Platinum-DNA adducts.

Similarly Dempke et al.[66] very recently demonstrated hypersensitivity not only to CDDP but also to MTX and 5-FU of ovarian Ca. cell lines pre-exposed to fractionated irradiation. Moreover in these pre-treated cell lines Thymidylate Synthase (TS) activity was increased (but not DHFR activity) and DNA Polymerase beta was decreased (but not DNA Polymerase alpha). A decrease in repair capacities is then suggested especially for 5-FU which is known to be inactive when its target enzyme TS activity is enhanced.

The authors conclude that all these data provide the evidence, first that the depletion of a specific DNA repair enzyme by fractionated radiation could be associated with enhanced toxicity to certain drugs, and second that activities of key enzymes of the folate metabolism in tumor cells can be modulated not only by exposure to MTX or 5-FU but also to fractionated radiation.

Maybe as a clinical illustration there is a very recently issued study from Institut Curie[67] which has nothing to do with biomodulation but which could indirectly suggest that the use of Cisplatinum based regimens prior to radiotherapy may induce resistance to the latter. It is a summation of two randomized studies involving two Platinum based induction regimens followed by RT vs RT alone. As it is now established there is no survival benefit from either, but when we look to detailed response patterns we note that aside the lack of difference in local control (around 75% at 6 years), between patients in CR after RT alone and those in CR after chemotherapy, those patients who do not respond to Chemotherapy but are rendered disease free after RT, do very badly and all recur before 2 years.

Of course, we can see here the prognostic value of chemotherapy but this latter group of patients which can achieve a CR after RT maybe should have not been pre-treated with a Cisplatin based regimen.

These series of data if confirmed may prove relevant to optimal clinical design of combinations of radiotherapy and chemotherapy in H & N Ca.

REFERENCES

1. T.M. Loeffler, J. Lindemann, H. Luckhaupt et al.,Chemotherapy of Advanced and Relapsed Squamous Cell Cancer of the Head and Neck with Split-dose Cisplatinum, 5-Fluorouracil and Leucovorin, Adv.Exp.Med.Biol. 244:269(1988)   .

2. A. Caty, J. Lefebvre, X. Mirabel et al., Induction Chemotherapy by a Combination of 5-FU-Cisplatinum-Folinic Acid in Advanced Head and Neck Squamous Cell Carcinoma, Pro.ASCO 11 Abst.793(1992).

3. M. Guaraldi, A. Martoni, A. Tononi et al., 5-Fluorouracil + Folinic Acid with Cisplatinum and Bleomycin in the Treatment of Advanced Head and Neck Squamous Cell Carcinoma, Ann. Onc.2:379(1991).

4. A. Bensmaine, E. Tellez-Bernal, T. Guillot et al., Chimiothérapie Néoadjuvante par CDDP, 5-FU, Acide Folinique et Vindésine (Perfusion Continue) dans les Carcinomes ORL localement avancés, Bull.Cancer 79:558(1992).

5. A. Dreyfuss, J.R. Clark, J.E. Wright et al., Continuous Infusion High-Dose Leucovorin with 5-Fluorouracil and Cisplatin for Untreated Stage IV Carcinoma of the Head and Neck, Ann.Int.Med. 112:167(1990).

6. E.E. Vokes, R.L. Schilsky, R.R. Weichselbaum et al., Induction Chemotherapy with Cisplatin, Fluorouracil and High-Dose Leucovorin for Locally Advanced Head and Neck Cancer : A Clinical and Pharmacologic Analysis, J.Clin.Oncol. 8:241(1990).

7. G. Fountzilas, J.Daniilidis, K.S. Sridhar et al., Induction Chemotherapy with a New Regimen Alternating Cisplatin, Fluorouracil with Mitomycin, Hydroxyurea and Bleomycin in Carcinomas of Nasopharynx or Other Sites of the Head and Neck Region, Cancer 66:1453(1990).

8. G. Fountzilas, P. Kosmidis, P. Makrentonakis et al., Carboplatin Continuous Infusion 5- Fluoro uracil and Mid-Cycle High-Dose Methotrexate as Initial Treatment in Patients with Locally Advanced Head and Neck Cancer, Tumori 77:426(1991).

9. H. Boussen, E. Cvitkovic, J.L. Wendling et al., Chemotherapy of Metatstatic and/or Recurrent Undifferenciated Nasopharyngeal Carcinoma with Cisplatin, Bleomycin and Fluorouracil, J.Clin.Oncol. 9:1675(1991).

10. G. Forni, M. Giovarelli, A. Santoni, A Lymphokine-Activated Tumor Inhibition in vivo. The Local Administration of Interleukin-2 Triggers Nonreactive Lymphocytes from Tumor-bearing Mice to Inhibit Tumor Growth, J.Immunol. 134:1305(1985).

11. G. Forni, H. Fujiwara, F. Martino et al., Helper Strategy in Tumor Immunology : Expansion of Helper Lymphocytes and Utilization of Helper Lymphokines for Experimental and Clinical Immunotherapy, Cancer Met. Rev. 7:289(1988).

12. G. Cortesina, A. de Stefani, M. Giovarelli et al., Treatment Recurrent Squamous Cell Carcinoma of the Head and Neck with Low Doses of Interleukin-2 Injected Perilymphatically, Cancer 62:2482(1988).

13. G. Cortesina, A. de Stefani, E. Galeazzi et al., The Effect of Preoperative Local Interleukin-2(IL-2) Injections in Patients with Head and Neck Squamous Call Carcinoma, Acta Oto-Lar. 111:428(1991).

14. G. Cortesina, A. De Stefani, E. Galeazzi et al., Interleukin-2 Injected around Tumor-Draining Lymph Nodes in Head and Neck Cancer, Head-Neck 13/2:125(1991).

15. M. Squadrelli-Saraceno, L. Rivoltini, G. Cantu et al., Local Adoptive Immunotherapy of Advanced Head and Neck Tumors with Lak Cell and Interleukine-2, Tumori 76:566(1990).

16. V. Mattijssen, P. H. De Mulder, J. H. Schornagel et al., Clinical and Immunopathological Results of a Phase II Study of Perilymphatically Injected Recombinant Interleukin-2 Locally for Advanced, Nonpretreated Head and Neck Squamous Cell Carcinoma, J.Imm. 10:63(1991).

17. P. Musiani, E. De Campora, S. Valitutti, Effect of Low Doses of Interleukin-2 Injected Peri-lymphatically and Peritumorally in Patients with Advanced Primary Head and Neck Squamous Cell Carcinoma, J.Biol.Resp.Mod 8:571(1989).

18. P.J. Cohen, M.T. Lotze, J.R. Roberts et al., The Immunopathology of Sequential Tumor Biopsies in Patients Treated with Interleukin-2, Am.J.Pathol. 129:208(1987).

19. G. Melioli, G. Margarino, M. Scala et al., Perilymphatic Injections of Recombinant Inter-leukin-2 (rIL-2) Partially Correct the Immunologic defects in Patients with Advanced Head and Neck Squamous Cell Carcinoma, Laryngo.102/5:572(1992).

20. S. Toma, M. Benasso, M. Merlano et al., Concomittant Cisplatin and Recombinant Interferon alpha-2b in Head and Neck Cancer, Drug Invest. 3:341(1991).

21. A. Bensmaine, N. Azli, F. Janot et al., Etude de la faisabilité de l'Association 5-FU-CDDP-Interféron (IFN alpha 2b) dans les Récidives et/ou Métastases des Carcinomes Epidermoïdes de la Tête et du Cou, Bull.Cancer 79:559(1992).

22. E.E. Vokes, M.J. Ratain, R. Mick et al., A Clinical Pharmacologic Phase I-II Study of PFL with Interferon alpha-2b (IFN) for Head and Neck Cancer (HNC), Pro.ASCO 11 Abst.782(1992).

23. M.E. Gore, P. Riches, K.A. MacLennan et al., Intra-Arterial Interleukin-2 in Squamous Cell Carcinoma of the Head and Neck, Pro. ASCO 11 Abst.814(1992).

24. B. Fiorentino, C. Amatetti, P. di Stefano et al., Weekly Sequential Administration of Interferon-alpha-2b (IFNa-2b) and Interleukin-2 (IL-2) in Patients with Advanced Malignancies, Pro.ASCO. 11 Abst.835(1992).

25. F. Geara, T.A. Girinski, N. Chavaudra et al., Estimation of Clonogenic Cell Fraction in Primary Culture Derived from Human Squamous Cell Carcinomas, Int.J.Rad.Oncol.Biol.Phys. 21:661(1991).

26. J.F. Fowler, The Phantom of Tumor Treatment-Continually Rapid Proliferation Unmasked, Rad.Oncol 22:156(1991).

27. J.F. Fowler, Apparent Rates of Proliferation of Acutely Responding Normal Tissues during Radiotherapy of Head and Neck Cancer, Int.J.Rad.Oncol.Biol.Phys.21:1451(1991).

28. S.M.Bentzen, H.D. Thames, Clinical Evidence for Tumor Clonogen Regeneration : Interpretations of the Data, Rad.Oncol. 22:161(1991).

29. K.R. Trott, J. Kummermehr, Accelerated Repopulation in Tumours and Normal Tissues, Rad.Oncol. 22:159(1991).

30. G. Sanguinelli, R. Corvo, E. Accomando et al., Accelerated Hyperfractionated (Concomitant Boost) Radiotherapy for Head and Neck Carcinomas : Preliminary Results, 3rd Int.Conf.on H & N Ca., San Francisco, California (July 26-30 1992).

31. S.M. Bentzen, L.V Johansen, J. Overgaard et al., Clinical Radiobiology of Squamous Cell Carcinoma of the Oropharynx, Int.J.Rad.Oncol.Biol.Phys. 20:1197 (1991).

32. G. Wiernick, C.J. Alcock, T.D. Bates et al., Final Report on the Second British Institute of Radiology Fractionation Study : Short versus Long overall Treatment Times for Radiotherapy of Carcinoma of the Laryngo-Pharynx, Br.J.Radiol. 64:232(1991).

33. J.C. Horiot et al.,Hyperfractionated compared with Conventional Radiotherapy in Oropharyngeal Carcinoma : an EORTC Randomized Trial, Int.J.Radiat.Oncol.Biol.Phys. 26:779(1990).

34. L.H. Pinto, P.C.V. Canary, C.M.M. Araujo et al., Prospective Randomized Trial Comparing Hyperfractionated versus Conventional Radiotherapy in Stages III and IV Oropharyngeal Carcinoma, Int.J.Rad.Oncol.Biol.Phys. 21:557(1991).

35. F. Sanchiz, A. Milla, J. Torner et al., Single Fraction per Day versus Two Fractions per Day versus Radiochemotherapy in the Treatment of Head and Neck Cancer, Int.J.Rad.Oncol. Biol. Phys. 19:1347(1990).

36. A.C. Begg, I. Hofland, M. Van Glabbeke et al., Predictive Value of Potential Doubling Time for Radiotherapy of Head and Neck Tumor Patients : Results from the EORTC Cooperative Trial 22851, Sem.Radiat.Oncol. 2:1(1992).

37. E. Geido, W. Giaretti, R. Corvo et al., Cell Kinetics by in vivo Bromodeoxyuridine and Flow Cytometry for the Radiotherapy Planning of Head and Neck Tumors, 3rd Int.Conf. on H & N Ca., San Francisco, California (July 26-30 1992).

38. M.I. Saunders, S. Dische, E.J. Grosch et al., Experience with CHART, Int.J.Radiat.Oncol.Phys. 21:871(1991).

39. J. Overgaard, H. Sand, A.P. Andersenet al., Misonidazole Combined with Split-course Radiotherapy in the Treatment of Invasive Carcinoma of Larynx and Pharynx. Report from the DAHANCA 2 Study, Int.J.Radiat.Oncol.Biol.Phys. 16:1065(1989).

40. C.N. Coleman, L. Noll, N.Riese et al., Final Report of the Phase I Trial of Continuous Infusion Etanizadole (SR 2508) : a Radiation Therapy Oncology Group Study, Int.J.Radiat.Oncol.Biol.Phys. 22:577(1992).

41. D. Chassagne, I. Charreau, H. Sancho-Garnier et al., First Analysis on Tumor Regression for the European Randomized Trial of Etanizadole Combined with Radiotherapy in Head and Neck Carcinomas, Int.J.Radiat.Oncol.Biol.Phys. 22:581(1992).

42. J. Overgaard, H. Sand-Hassen, B. Lindelov et al., Nimorazole as a Hypoxic Radiosensitizer in the Treatment of Supraglottic, Larynx and Pharynx Carcinoma. First Report from the DAHANCA protocol 5-85, Radiother.Oncol. 20:143(1990).

43. D.J. Honess, N.M. Bleehen, Effects of Calcium Channel Blockers on Renal Function in Mice, Int.J.Radiat.Oncol.Biol.Phys. 22:443(1992).

44. M.R. Horsman, P.E.G. Kristjansen, M. Mizuno et al., Biochemical and Physiological Changes Induced by Nicotinamide in a C3H Mouse Mammary Carcinoma and CDF1 Mice, Int.J.Radiat.Oncol.Biol.Phys. 22:451(1992).

45. K. Skov, S. MacPhail, Interaction of Platinum Drugs with Clinically Relevant X-Ray Doses in Mammalian Cells : a Comparison of Cisplatin, Carboplatin, Iproplatin and Tetraplatin, Int.J.Radiat.Oncol.Biol.Phys. 20:221(1991).

46. P. Lamblin, P. Scalliet, B. Coster et al., Influence of Cisplatinum on Intestinal Tolerance to Photon and Neutron Irradiation in Mice, (to be published 1992).

47. J.M. Bachaud, J.M. David, G.Boussin et al., Combined Postoperative Radiotherapy and Weekly Cisplatin Infusion for Locally Advanced Squamous Cell Carcinoma of the Head and Neck : Preliminary Report of a Randomized Trial, Int.J.Radiat.Biol.Phys. 20:243(1991).

48. M. Busch, E. Dühmke, Longtime Impact of Low Dose Cisplatinum and Accelerated Fractionation of Radiotherapy of Head and Neck Cancer, Pro;ASCO. 11 Abst.789(1992).

49. P. Volling, S. Starr, Carboplatin Plus Radiation Therapy in Head and Neck Cancer, Sem.Oncol. 18:17(1991).

50. M. Airoldi, V. Brando, G. Cortesina et al., Simultaneous Radiation Therapy (RT) and Chemotherapy (CT) with Carboplatin (CBDCA) for Locally Unresectable Stage III-IV Head and Neck Cancer (HNC), Pro.ASCO. 11 Abst.805(1992).

51. R. Orecchia, G.L. Sannazzari, M. Airoldi et al., Daily Carboplatin (CBDCA) and Standard Radiation Therapy (RT) in Inoperable Head and Neck Cancer (HNC) : a Dose-Finding Study, Pro.ASCO. 11 Abst. 795(1992).

52. A. Testolin, F. Pozza, F. Bagatella et al., Combined Treatment for Locally Advanced Carcinoma of Head and Neck. Preliminary Results of a Randomized Trial : Cisplatin (CP) vs Carboplatin (CBP) and Concomittant Radiotherapy (RT), Pro.ASCO. 11 Abst. 794(1992).

53. T.C. Lo, A.L. Wiley, F.J. Ansfield, Combined Radiation Therapy and 5-Fluorouracil for Advanced Squamous Cell Carcinoma of the Oral Cavity and Oropharynx : a Randomized Study, Am.J.Roentgenol. 126:229(1976).

54. T.S. Lawrence, D.K. Heimburger, D.S.Shewach, The Effects of Leucovorin and Dipyridamole on Fluoropyrimidine-Induced Radiosensitization, Int.J.Radiat.Oncol.Biol.Phys.20:377(1991).

55. K.J. Scanlon, M. Kashani-Sabet, Elevated Expression of Thymidylate Synthase Cycle Genes in Cisplatin-Resistant Human Ovarian Carcinoma A2780 Cells, Proc.Natl.Acad.Sci.USA 85:650(1988).

56. J. Eskandari,H. de Muizon, D. Bonnet et al., 5-Fluorouracil-Leucovorin and Concomittant Radiotherapy in Advanced Head and Neck Carcinomas : a Phase I Study, Pro.ASCO. 11 Abst.791(1992).

57. W. Dobrowsky, E. Dobrowsky, H. Strassl et al., Response to Preoperative Concomittant Radiochemotherapy with Mitomycin C and 5-Fluorouracil in Advanced Head and Neck Cancer, Eur.J. Cancer.Clin.Oncol. 25:845(1989).

58. D. Gandia, P. Wibault, P. Marandas, Radiochimiothérapie Simultanée(RS) dans les récidives Locorégionales des Cancers Epidermoïdes de la Tête et du Cou (CETC), Bull.Cancer 79:558(1992).

59. M. Merlano, M. Benasso, M. Cavallari et al., Combined Chemotherapy and Radiation Therapy in Advanced Inoperable Squamous Cell Carcinoma of the Head and Neck, Cancer 67:915(1991).

60. T.G. Wendt, R.C. Hartenstein, T.P.U. Wustrow, Cisplatin, Fluorouracil with Leucovorin Calcium Enhancement, and Synchronous Accelerated Radiotherapy in the Management of Locally Advanced Head and Neck Cancer : a Phase I Study, J.Clin.Oncol.7:471(1989).

61. M.J. Evans, C.J. Kovacs, J.M. Gooya et al., Interleukin-I alpha Protects against the Toxicity Associated with Combined Radiation and Drug Therapy, Int.J.Radiat.Oncol.Biol.Phys. 20:303(1991).

62. C.J. Kovacs, J.M. Gooya, J.P. Harrell et al., Altered Radioprotective Properties of Interleukin I alpha (IL-1) in Non-Hematologic Tumor-Bearing Animals, Int.J.Radiat.Oncol.Biol.Phys. 20:307(1991).

63. G.J. Peters, C.L. van der Wilt, F. Gyergyay et al., Protection by WR-2721 of the Toxicity Induced by the Combination of Cisplatin and 5-Fluorouracil, Int.J.Radiat.Oncol.Biol.Phys. 22:785(1992).

64. J.F. Ensley, J.R. Jacobs, A. Weaver et al., The Correlation between Response to Cisplatinum Combination Chemotherapy and Subsequent Radiotherapy in Previously Untreated Patients with Advanced Squamous Cells Cancers or the Head and Neck, Cancer 54:811(1984).

65. C.M.J. De Pooter, P.G. Scalliet, H.J. Elst et al.,Resistance Patterns between Cisdiamminedichloroplatinum(II) and Ionizing Radiation, Cancer Research 51:4523(1991).

66. W.C.M. Dempke, L.K. Hosking, B.T. Hill, Expression of Collateral Sensitivity to Cisplatin, Methotrexate, and Fluorouracil in a Human Ovarian Carcinoma Cell Line Following Exposure Fractionated X-Irradiation in vitro, Sem.Oncol. 19:66(1992).

67. C. Jaulerry, J.Rodriguez, F. Brunin et al., Induction Chemotherapy in Advanced Head and Neck Tumors : Results of two Randomized Trials, Int.J.Radiat.Oncol.Biol.Phys. 23:483(1992).

DISCUSSION OF DR. VOKE'S/DR. ESKANDARI'S PRESENTATION

Audience: Regarding the choice of FUra/leucovorin regimens in which you used are platinum and biochemical modulators in head and neck cancer, given the high incidence or higher incidence of oral mucositis that you'd expect with the continuous infusion 5 day FUra/leucovorin regimen with head and neck cancer, has anyone, to your knowledge, looked at a weekly Roswell Park type FUra with high dose leucovorin with platinum in this disease?

Dr. Vokes: When I was at the University of Pennsylvania, Dr. Haller and I initiated a pilot trial of that regimen of FUra/leucovorin and platinum in a variety of diseases and in a small group of patients it appears to us at this point, and this trial is still going on, that toxicity attributable to platinum is not synergistic in terms of the mucosal. So that the weekly schedule may be a reasonable direction to go in the future with head and neck cancers.

Dr. Eskandari: I agree. We have used the weekly schedule of RPCI of FUra/CF/cisDDP in patients with advanced head and neck cancer and results are encouraging with mangageable toxicity.

Audience: Dr. Vokes, have you tried growth factors in relation to reducing mucosites?

Dr. Vokes: In one trial we are doing that. We have a regimen of cisplatin/FUra and hydroxyurea with concomitent radiation and that is based on the initial 5-FU/hydrea regimen and if you will it's an attempt of combining the new adjuvant part with the concomitent part. When adding cisplatin to FUra hydrea the dose limiting toxicity was myelosuppression at fairly low doses of cisplatin and in that trial we have now added GCSF in the off weeks. So it's a week of chemotherapy with radiation followed by a a week of GCSF. It seems to ameliorate at least a short-term myelosuppression. We do have chronic thromocytopenia. As far as the mucositis is concerned, there is anecdotal, since this was not a parallel investigation, initial evidence suggest decreased incidence of mucositis.

Audience: How about local regional?

Dr. Eskandari: Local regional I don't know if a faster response is observed in the primary than the neck. There could be differential in the tumor volume. The neck nodes are usually a bit larger than the primary sites but I don't know.

Audience: In the interferon study, how did you verify the complete responses? Were they surgically re-biopsied or were they clinically restaged?

Dr. Eskandari: As I reported here, the reported responses were documented. Patients did go for subsequent local therapy and whenever possible we had at least a biopsy of these but 56% response rate was clinically determined. It's our experience, however, when surgery is carried out, residual tumor is generally found.

Dr. Frei: At the Dana Farber, about 50% of patients are confirmed in CR when undergoing surgery. I think our rate would be less I don't have the exact figure.

Dr. Spaulding: I have a comment to make concerning the weekly x6 FUra/CF cisplatinum in head and neck. In 6 patients treated, no mucositis was observed, grade I at best so I agree that that's a better regimen. Just, also to comment in the terms of the biopsy, in the VA laryngeal trial, these are patients who had a complete response with biopsy. The clinical correlation is very high with a complete response using a superficial biopsy. Of the 60 or so patients who had a complete response, 50 of them, I think it was, had no tumor in the biopsy specimen. So I think you have to do a complete resection.

Audience: When head and neck tumors are concerned, there are many discussions about the length of therapy, the number of courses that should be done before the local treatment. When the first trials of FUra and cisplatin were used, people remarked that relapses were earlier. What do you think about that? Is there some data in order to try to say what's the optimum duration of the chemotherapy?

Dr. Vokes: I don't think so. I think it's clear that you can go from 2 to 3 cycles and increase your complete response rate if you go from 3 to 4, and again this is partially Dana-Farber information although we had a similar experience, the incidence of CR was not increased. Whether increased survival can be observed when the duration of treatment was increased from 2 to 3 cycles is not clear. So, I cannot truly answer this, I don't know what the optimum cycle number is. Depending on the endpoint of response I think it's fair to say that 3 is better than 2.

Audience: Dr. Eskandari, what is your future direction for the treatment?

Dr. Eskandari: As I mentioned, we started the trial of FU/CF without cisplatin weekly RPCI schedule along with the radiotherapy. With the interesting data obtained, we are planning to keep the same modality of FUra/CF and add cisplatin to this weekly regimen.

Dr. Meropol: One more comment in response to the question by Dr. Hines regarding the use of growth factors with these chemotherapy regimens. We conducted, in the North Central Group, a trial of GCSF in patients receiving 5-FU and low dose leucovorin with oral mucositis as the rate limiting toxicity. Initially we scheduled the GCSF concurrently with the chemotherapy beginning on day 1 of each cycle and treating through day 14 with the GCSF. Our observation with that schedule was that there was actually augmented myelosuppression associated, we feel, with the concurrent administration of chemotherapy and a colony stimulating factor. With that observation, we made a protocol revision to begin the growth factor on day 6, 24 hrs after the last dose of chemotherapy and found that myelosuppression was not observed. So, just a cautionary note in terms of scheduling of growth factors with chemotherapy.

Dr. Frei: Again, a comment. The issue of the number of courses to be delivered was raised. I'm not sure that we would cure anybody with Hodgkin's disease or non-Hodgkin's lymphoma with 2 or 3 or 1 course of chemotherapy. With the rapidity of achieving high response in the order of 60 to 70%, at least initially, head and neck tumors appear to be as sensitive as some of the lymphomas or hematological malignancies which is a very important thing. It's possible that if we were to deliver 4, 5 or 6 courses of something like PFL, that is highly effective, we could achieve the same thing. I remember in 1973-74 when we introduced just 1 course of neoadjuvant chemotherapy at that time with methotrexate only it was sort of a revolution and getting in more courses which is essential for the control of other sensitive diseases is something we should I think work towards in head and neck cancer.

RATIONALE FOR THE COMBINATION THERAPY OF 5FU AND CDDP

Nagahiro Saijo[1] and Yoshikazu Sugirnoto[2]

[1]Pharmacology Division
National Cancer Center Research Institute
Tsukiji 5-1-1 Chuo-ku Tokyo
[2]Cancer Research Laboratory, Hanno Research Center
Taiho Co., Ltd., 216-1
Nakayashita, Yaoroshi, Hanno-city, Saitama 357

INTRODUCTION

Fluorinated pyrimidines such as 5FU, ftoraful and UFT are widely used in Japan and have a biggest share in the market of anticancer drugs and they have been mainly used for the treatment of gastrointestinal malignancies such as stomach cancer and colon cancer.

5FU is metabolized within cells to FdUMP. FdUMP can covalently bind to TMP synthase in the presense of 5, 10 methylene tetrahydrofolate and inhibit DNA synthesis by depleting the cells of dTMP. 5FU is also metabolized to 5FUTP, which is incorporated into RNA and cause the dysfunction of RNA. One or both of these 5FU metabolites is believed to account for the antineoplastic activity of 5FU in vitro and in vivo experimental studies (Chabner 1981; Heiderburger et al., 1983; Moran et al., 1979). (Figure 1)

Several combinations or biochemical modulations involving 5FU have been demonstrated to show the better antitumor activity not only in preclinical studies but also in the clinical trials. Leucovorin, methotrexate, levamisol, interferon and PALA have improved the therapeutic efficacy of 5FU in human disease (Houghton et al., 1982). The combination chemotherapy including 5FU and CDDP arowses interest not only of basic pharmacologists but also of medical oncologist because the combination has been demonstrated to be active against various solid tumors such as stomach, head and neck and non small cell lung cancers (O' Dwyer et al., 1990; Vokes et al., 1988, 1990, 1991 & 1992). In the present study, the experimental basis will be presented about why the combination of 5FU and LV is not active against non-small cell lung cancer although the combination is demonstrated to show high response rate against colon cancer. The mechanism of collateral sensitivity to 5FU in CDDP-resistant cell hurnan lung cancer cell line, which may be one of the rationale of the combination effect of 5FU and CDDP.

Novel Approaches to Selective Treatments of Human Solid Tumors: Laboratory and Clinical Correlation Edited by Y. M. Rustum, Plenum Press, New York, 1993

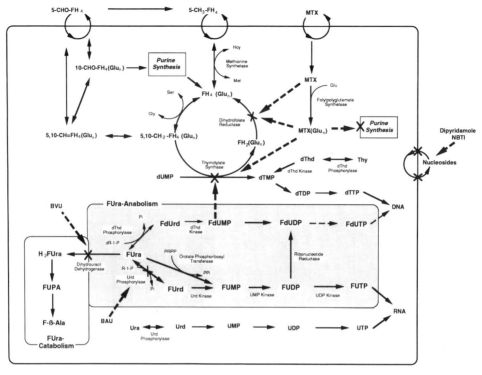

Figure 1.   The mode of action of 5FU and biochemical modulation of 5FU by leucovorin, MTX and etc.

Phase II Study of 5FU with Leucovorin in Non-small Cell Lung Cancer

In our phase II study of 5FU with high dose leucovorin, fourteen patients with inoperable or recurrent non-small cell lung cancers were treated with 5FU+high dose leucovorin.   The administration schedule was followed by Roswell Park schedule, 2hr infusion of LV at a dose of 500mg/m^2 and 30 min infusion of 5FU at a dose of 600mg/m^2 given lhr after the start of LV infusion.   This regimen was followed weekly six times. Table I showe the patient characteristics and response.   Although all the patients have good PS and no prior chemotherapy, no responder was observed among 14 patients. From these data it could be concluded that the schedule of 5FU with high dose LV therapy employed could not be expected to produce a response rate ≥20% against NSCLC (Ohe et al., 1990).

Table 1.   Negative phase II study of 5FU+LV in non-small cell lung cancer without prior chemotherapy

No. of patient	14
Age: median (range)	63 (47–75)
Sex: male/female	9/5
Histology: adeno/sq	9/5
PS: 0–1/2	13/1
Stage: IIIA/IIIB/IV	2/4/8
Prior chemotherapy: +/−	0/14
Response : PR	0
NC	10
PD	4

In Vitro Enhancement of Fluoropydimide Induced Cytotoxicity by Leucovorin

To study the difference in the efficacy of the combination against different tumors, we compared the effect effect of l-LV(20µM) on the cytotoxity of FU, FdUrd and FUrd in vitro against cell lines of 5 colorectal carcinomas, 5 gastric carcinomas and 4 non-small cell lung carcinomas using colony forming assay. The cell lines were maintained in RPMI 1640 medium supplemented with 10 % heat-inactivated dialyzed fetal bovine serum and penicillin and streptomycin. Figure 2 shows the dose response curve of l-LV on the cytotoxicity of FdUrd to LoVo colon adenocarcinoma cell line. The sensitizing effect of l-LV on FdUrd cytotoxity was observed at approximately 0.003µM of l-LV concentration, and reached a plateau at about 0.3µM. At the concentration used in this experiment, the colony formation was not inhibited in any cell lines by l-LV alone. Based on these data, we selected 20µM of l-LV concentration as a concentration to detect the maximum effects of l-LV-modulation.

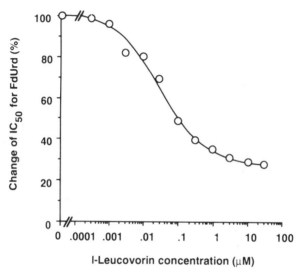

Figure 2.   Sensitization of 5FU effect by LV

The sensitivity to 5FU was slightly higher in gastric carcinoma cell lines than in colorectal and NSCLC cell lines. LV sensitization of FUra-cytotoxicity was observed in colorectal (COLO201) and gastric (TMK-1, KATO III) carcinoma cell lines, and in no NSCLC cell lines if the ratio of IC_{50} with LV / IC_{50} without LV more than 2 was considered to be positive sensitization. Table 2 shows the cytotoxicity of FdUrd with or without LV. Cellular sensitivity to FdUrd was significantly higher in colorectal and gastric carcinoma cell lines than that in NSCLC cell lines. LV enhanced the FdUrd cytotoxicity in all colorectal carcinoma cell lines and some gastric carcinoma cell lines, but not in the NSCLC cell lines. Cellular sensitivity of FUrd was higher in order of gastric, NSCLC and colorectal carcinoma cell lines. There is a significant difference in IC_{50} of FUrd between colorectal carcinoma and gastric carcinoma. In FUrd, which is thought to be mainly metabolized to FUTP inducing RNA damage, LV modulated only one cell line in gastric carcinoma, KATOIII (Sugimoto et al., 1992b). These data demonstrated that 1) The responses to three fluorinated pyrimidines differed in the different tumor cell lines and that 2) The response to LV modulation is different in tumor types.

Table 2.   Effect of 1-LV on the cytotoxicity of FdUrd in human carcinoma cell lines

| | Cell line Ratio[a] | IC$_{50}$ values of FdUrd (μM) | | |
		-LV	+LV	
Colorectal carcinoma	WiDr	0.0125 ± 0.005	0.0040 ± 0.0015*	3.09
	DLD-1	0.1295 ± 0.052	0.0370 ± 0.0113*	3.50
	LoVo	0.0344 ± 0.014	0.0089 ± 0.0033***	3.85
	COLO201	0.1160 ± 0.016	0.0215 ± 0.0092***	5.40
	COLO320DM	0.0805 ± 0.009	0.0175 ± 0.0064***	4.60
Gastric carcinoma	TMK-1	0.0860 ± 0.0320	0.0230 ± 0.0106*	2.40
	KATO III	0.5000 ± 0.2100	0.0580 ± 0.0198*	4.52
	MKN 28	0.0880 ± 0.0260	0.0300 ± 0.0156*	2.93
	MKN 45	0.0285 ± 0.0097	0.0138 ± 0.0069	2.07
	MKN 74	0.3200 ± 0.1267	0.4200 ± 0.0980	0.76
Non-small cell lung carcinoma	PC-7	4.30 ± 2.62	4.60 ± 1.58	0.93
	PC-9	0.73 ± 0.21	0.40 ± 0.26	1.83
	PC-13	1.30 ± 0.09	0.93 ± 0.31	1.40
	PC-14	2.02 ± 1.36	1.70 ± 0.87	1.19

a) ; Data are represent as means ± SD for triplicate assays.
b) ; (Ratio)=(IC$_{50}$ value of FdUrd without LV / IC$_{50}$ value of FdUrd with LV)
*, *** ; Significant difference from IC$_{50}$ value of FdUrd without LV by unpaired Student's t-test, p< 0.05 and p < 0.0001, respectively.

We attempted to determine the ternary complex formation of FdUMP-TS-mTHF in the LV sensitizing cell lines TMK-1 and LoVo and in the LV refractory cell lines PC-7 and PC-9.   Figure 3 shows ^{3}H-FdUMP binding to TS which shows the ternary complex formation with FdUMP-TS-mTHF.   The result demonstrates that LV enhanced ternary complex formation in LV sensitizing cell lines, but not in LV-refractory cell lines.   When the cells were treated with FdUrd alone,   the amount of ternary complex formation in FdUrd sensitive colorectal and gastric carcinoma cell lines was also greater than that of FdUrd resistant NSCLC cell lines (Sugimoto et al., 1992).   These data are corresponded to the results of colony forming assay.   These in vivo and in vitro data corresponded well with the data of clinical trials.

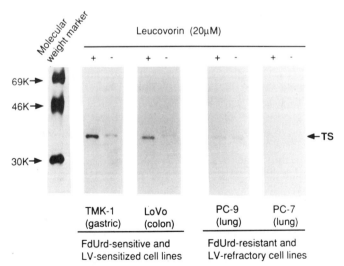

Figure 3.   Ternary complex formation in gastric colon and lung cancer cell lines

The Rationale for the Combination Therapy for CDDP and 5FU

There seems to be various rationales for the combination of 5FU and CDDP. The subjects of discussions are as follows: 1. In vitro and in vivo combination effect,   2. Mechanistic analysis of the combination,   3. Collateral sensitivity to 5FU in CDDP resistant cell lines,   4. Clinical trials of combination therapy.

In vitro and in vivo combination effect

Scanlon showed that in vitro A2780 cell growth was synergistically inhibited by the combination of cisplatin and 5FU and the effect was reversed by adding dThd. Yamada demonstrated that the combination of cisplatin and UFT, the mixture of uracil and ftoraful, could inhibit the in vivo growth of xenografts such as KM 12C, LX-1 and Lu-24 tumors.   Other authors also reported the supraadditive and synergictic effect of cisplatin and 5FU against varieties of tumors not only in vitro but also in vivo in human as well as animal tumors.

The mechanistic analysis of the combination of 5FU and CDDP

Cisplatin decreases the uptake of methionine.   In order to supply the decreased methionine, folate pools are increased.   As a results the formation of ternary complex consisted from 5 ,10-CH_2FH_4, TS and FdUMP was increased (Figure 4).   Scanlon reported that the folate pools in A2780 cells including CH_2-H_4 folates and H_4 folates, were significantly increased in the presence of cisplatin (Scanlon et al., 1983 & 1986). They also found that the formation of ternary complex was significantly increased by the treatment with 10mM of cisplatin.

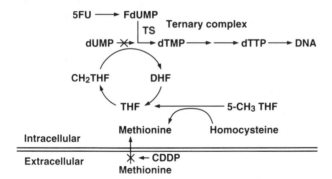

Figure 4.   Possible sites of interaction between 5FU and CDDP
(biochemical modulation of 5FU by CDDP)

In the experiment of Shirasaka, similar phenomenon was observed in Yoshida ascites carcinoma (YAC).   The combination of 5FU and CDDP strongly inhibited the growth of the tumor compared with each drug alone.   The uptake of methionine was evaluated in YAC cells.   Each rat was given various doses of CDDP 8 days after inoculation of YAC.   Tumor cells obtained 6hr after i. P. injection of CDDP were incubated with lmM L-methionine.   The uptake of methionine was inhibited dose dependently. They observed the reduced folate pool in mice and rats inoculated with P388 and YAC, respectively.   In the groups of animals given CDDP, the reduced folate pool was significantly increased in P388 and Yoshida ascited carcinoma (Shirasaka et al.). These results suggest that CDDP could modulate the metabolism of 5FU and the antitumor activity of 5FU was augmented by the increased formation of ternary complex. Yamada reported the similar phenomenon in other tumor types by combining
UFT with CDDP.

On the other-hand antimetabolites and inhibitors of signal transduction have demonstrated to sensitize the effect of CDDP.   In the case of 5FU, the decreased nucleotide levels induced by 5FU is considered to influence the repair capacity of DNA damaged by CDDP (Bungo et al., 1990).   However, the details has not yet been clarified.

The Colleteral Sensitivity to 5FU of a CDDP-resistant Human Non-small Cell Lung Cancer Cell Line

We have developed several CDDP resistant cell lines (Hong et al., 1988). Almost all the cell lines showed collateral sensitivity to 5FU (Ohe et al., 1990).   PC-7/CDDP cells were about 4.7 times as resistant to CDDP than PC-7 cells in a colony forming assay.   On the other hand, PC-7/CDDP cells were more sensitive to 5FU than PC-7 cells.   IC$_{50}$ of FUra in PC-7/CDDP cells was about four times lower than that in PC-7 cells.   The effect of dThd and Urd on 5FU cytotoxicity was evaluated to find out whether FUra acts mainly by inhibiting DNA synthesis or by alternating RNA function dThd is thought to protect against the reduction in dTTP pools and Urd is thought to prevent the incorporation of FUTP into RNA.   Urd prevented 5FU cytotoxicity in PC-7 cells,   but only a little prevention was observed in PC-7/CDDP cells.   It was suggested that the altered RNA function is not a main cause of collateral sensitivity to 5FU in PC-7/CDDP.   On the other hand, dThd prevented 5FU cytotoxicity in both cell lines.   However, a highr concentration of dThd was necessary for the prevention of 5FU-induced cytotoxicity in PC-7/CDDP cells indicating that the function of the salvage pathway of DNA synthesis is decreased.   The effect of leucovorin on the cytotoxicity of 5FU was evaluated by a colony forming assay.   This reduced folate is known to enhance the inhibition of TS by FdUMP as previously presented.   In this study leucovorin enhanced the cytotoxicity of FUra in PC-7/CDDP but not in PC-7 cells (Figure 5).   These data suggest that 5FU acts mainly deoxyribonucleotide synthesis in PC-7/CDDP cells.

Next we measured the cellular accumulation of 5FU and its incorporation into nucleic acid in each cell lines by using ^{14}C-5FU.   Total accumulation of 5FU in PC-7/CDDP cells was decreased to 10% of that in PC-7 cells.   The incorporation of 5FU into RNA was parallel with the total accumulation in each cell line.   Corresponding to

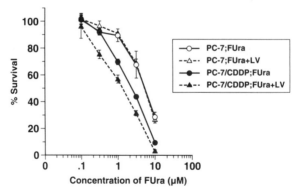

PC-7 and PC-7/CDDP cells were treated by continuous exposure to various concentrations of FUra in the presence or absence of 20µM of leucovorin and then assayed for colony formation.

Figure 5.   Effect of leucovorin on the cytotoxicity of FUra in PC-7 and PC-7/CDDP cells

the inhibitory effect of Urd on 5FU-induced cytotoxicity, the amount of 5FU incorporated into RNA in PC-7/CDDP cell was 17% of that in PC-7 cells. The incorporation of 5FU into the DNA fraction was very small in PC-7 and PC-7/CDDP cells. The amounts of intracellular metabolites of 5FU were measured by TLC. Fluoro ribonucleotides such as FUMP, FUDP and FUTP production in PC-7/CDDP cells was decreased to less than 18% of that in PC-7 cells. FdUMP, which interacted with TS, was present at higher level in PC-7/CDDP cells than the fluoro-ribonucleotide, although the amount of FdUMP in PC-7/CDDP cells was 65% of that in PC-7 cells. There was no enhanced degradation of FUra in PC-7/CDDP cells in comparison with that in PC-7 cells. These data further suggest that alteration of RNA function is not a cause of collateral sensitivity to 5FU in PC-7/CDDP (Sugimoto et al., 1992a). Inhibition of TS activity by FdUMP results in a reduction in dTTP levels. TS activity by exposure of PC-7 and PC-7/CDDP cells to 1, 5 and 10pg of 5FU per ml for 6hr was determined by FdUMP binding activity. There was a concentration dependent inhibition of total TS by 5FU. Unexpectedly, the TS activity of the cisplatin-sensitive PC-7 cells was inhibited more by 5FU than that of the cisplatin resistant PC-7/CDDP cells (Ohe et al., 1990). The level of dTTP was measured after the treatment with 5FU for 6hr at 37C . 5FU produced greater reduction in dTTP level in CDDP resistant cells after 6hr 5FU treatment by the alkaline elution techniques. More DNA single strand breaks were observed in PC-7/CDDP cells. These data suggest that the toxicity of 5FU in PC-7/CDDP may be mainly due to the inhibition of synthesis of substrate for DNA replication (Sugimoto et al., 1992a).

The degree of inhibition of TS activity was not correlated with the degree of reduction in dTTP level. PC-7/CDDP cells incorporate much less exogenous dThd in to DNA than PC-7 cells. Based on these data, it was speculated that salvage synthesis of dTMP might be different between these cell lines. The membrane transport of dThd was examined, which was the initial process of the dThd salvage pathway. The shows short term uptake of dThd at 25C was examined by the rapid sampling technique. Initial uptake of dThd by PC-7/CDDP cells was lower than that by PC-7 cells after treatment with 5mM dThd. However, the amount of dThd taken up by PC-7/CDDP cells was close to that by the parental cells at a high concentration of dThd (Figure 6).

From these data, the decreased uptake of dThd may be responsible for the decreased dTTP production in PC-7/CDDP cells. The rate of dThd transport was determined. As the process of dThd transport was very rapid at 25C, we decreased the temperature to determine the initial rate of dThd uptake. Although the initial rate

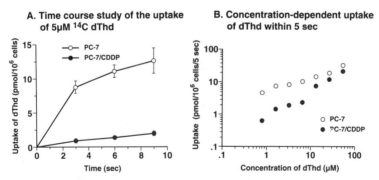

Figure 6. Short term uptake of thymidine (dThd) in PC-7 and PC-7/CDDP cells at 25 °C

of dThd uptake by PC-7/CDDP cells became also lower than that by PC-7 cells at 15C, the difference in dThd-uptake disappeared with the dicrease in assay temperature. An inhibitor of facilitated diffusion of nucleoside, dipyridamole (DP) inhibited the dThd uptake by both cell lines to a similar extent.   These data suggested that the factor associated with temperature-dependent and DP-insensitive transport of dThd may be different in PC-7/CDDP cells (Sugimoto et al., 1992a).

From these data, it was suggested that 5FU-induced cytotoxicity in PC-7/CDDP cells is associated with the inhibition of dTTP synthesis and the decreased uptake of dThd is a possible mechanism of the collateral sensitivity to 5FU in PC-7/CDDP cells. All the data presented so far suggested the favorable effect of the combination of CDDP with 5FU.

Clinical trials and conclusion

There are several clinical reports of combination therapy using CDDP and 5FU. This combination could produce the favorable response rate in colon, stomach and head & neck cancers.   In addition there are numerous trials combining other modulators to 5FU and CDDP.

The Japanese clinical oncology group (JCOG) is now conducting the randomized controlled trial including 5FU+ CDDP regimen against stomach cancer. From this study, the superiority of this combination could be demonstrated in the treatment of advanced stomach cancer.

Acknowledgement

This work was supported in part by a Grant-in Aid from the Ministry of Health and Welfare for a Comprehensive 10-year Strategy for Cancer Control and from the Minatory of Education, Science, and Culture, Japan

References

M. Bungo, Y. Fujiwara, K. Kasahara, K. Nakagawa, Y. Ohe, Y. Sasaki, S. Irino and N. Saijo, Decreased accumulation as a mechanism of resistance to cisdiamminedichloroplatinum(II) in human non-small cell lung cancer cell lines: relation to DNA darnage and repair., Cancer Res., 50: 2549, (1990).

B. A. Chabner, Pyrimidine antagonists. In pharmacologic basis of Cancer Treatment, B. A. Chabner(ed) ppl83-212. The W. B. Saunders CO.: Philadelphia, (1981).

C. Heiderberger, P. V. Danenberg, and R. G. Moran, Fluorinated pyrimidines and their nucleosides. In advances in enzymology and related areas in molecular biology. A. Meister(ed.) pp57-119 John Wiley & Sons: New York. (1983).

W. S. Hong, N. Saijo, Y. Sasaki, K. Minato, H. Nakano, K. Nakagawa, Y. Fujiwara, K. Nomura, and P. R. Twentyman, Establishment and characterization of cisplatin resistant sublines of human lung cancer cell lines., Int. J. Cancer., 41: 462, (1988).

J. Houghton, C. Schmidt, and P. J. Houghton, The effect of derivates of folic acid on the fluorodeoxyuridylate-thymidylate symthase covalent complex in human colon xenografts., Eur. J. Clin. Oncol., 18: 347. (1982).

R. G. Moran, C. P. Spears, C. Heidelberger, Biochemical determination of tumor sensitivity to 5-fluorouracil: ultrasensitive methods for the determination of 5 fluoro-2'-deoxyuridate, 2'-deoxyuridate, and thymidylate synthase., Proc. Natl. Acid. Sci, 76: 1456, (1979).

P. J. O'Dwyer, M. J. Comfeld, R. Peler, and R. L. Comis, Phase I trial of 5-fluorouracil, leucovorin and cisplatin in combination., Cancer Chemother. Phannacol., 27: 131, (1990).

Y. Ohe, Y. Sugimoto, and N. Saijo, Collateral sensitivity of cisplatin-resistant human non-small lung cancer cell lines to thymidylate synthase inhibitors., Cancer J., 3: 332, (1990).

Y. Ohe, T. Shinkai, K. Eguchi, Y. Sasaki, T. Tamura, K. Nakagawa, A. Kojima, K. Yamada, F. Oshita, T. Miya, and N. Saijo, Nagative phase Il study of S-fluorouracil and high dose leucovorin in non-small cell lung cancer., Jpn. J. Clin. Oncol., 20: 364, (1990).

K. J. Scanlon, R. L. Safirstein, H. Thies, R. B. Gross, S. Waxman, and J. B. Guttenplan, Inhibition of amino acid transport by cis-diamminedichloroplatinurn derivatives in L1210 murine leukemia cells., Cancer Res., 42: 4211, (1983).

K. J. Scanlon, E. M. Newman, Y. Lu, and D. G. Priest, Biochemical basis for cisplatin and 5-fluorouracil synergism in human ovarian carcinoma cells., Proc. Natl. Acid. Sci., 83: 8923, (1986).

T. Shirasaka, Y. Shimamoto, H. Ohshimo, H. Saito, and M. Fukushima., Metabolic basis of the synergistic antitumor activities of 5-fluorovracil and cisplatin in rodent tumor models in vivo., Personal comrnunications.

Y. Sugimoto, Y. Ohe, K. Nishio, T. Ohmori, T. Morikage, Y. Fujiwara, and N. Saijo, Mechanism of collateral sensitivity to fluorouracil of a cis-diamminedichloroplatinum(II)-resistant human non-small cell lung cancer cell line., Br. J. Cancer, 65: 857, (1992-a).

Y. Sugimoto, Y. Ohe, K. Nishio, T. Ohmori, Y. Fujiwara, and N. Saijo, In vitro enhancement of fluoropyrimidine-induced cytotoxicity by leucovorin in colorectal and gastric carcinoma cell lines but not in non-small-cell lung carcinoma cell lines., Cancer Chemother. Pharmacol., 30: 417, (1992-b).

E. E. Vokes. K. E. Choi, R. L. Schilsky, W. J. Moran, C. M. Guarnieri, R. R Weichselbaum, and R. R Ranje, Cisplatin, fluorouracil, and high dose leucovorin for recurrent or metastatic head and neck cancer., J. Clin. Oncol., 6: 618, (1988).

E. E. Vokes, R. L. Schilsky, R. R. Weichselbaum, M. F. Kazloff, and W. P. Panje, Induction chemotherapy with CDDP, 5FU and high-dose leucovorin for locally advanced head and neck cancer: a clinical and pharmacologic analysis., J. Clin. Oncol., 8: 241, (1990).

E. E. Vokes, M. Rosemarie, E. P. Lester, W. R. Panje, and R. R. Weichselbaum, Cisplatin and fluorouracil chemotherapy does not yeild long-term benefit in locally advanced head and neck cancer: Results from a single institution., J. Clin. Oncol., 9: 1376, (1991).

F. E. Vokes, R. R. Weichselbaum, R. Mick, J-M. McEvilly, D. J. Harof, and W. R. Panje, Favorable long-term survival following induction chemotherapy with cisplatin, fluorouracil, and leucovorin and concomitant chemoradiotherapy for locally advanced head and neck cancer., J. Natl. Cancer Inst., 84: 877, (1992).

BIOCHEMICAL MODULATION OF FLUOROPYRIMIDINES: THE "GISCAD" STUDIES

R. Labianca, G. Pancera, S. Barni, S. Cascinu, G. Comella, P. Foa, G. Martignoni, A. Zaniboni, G. Giaccon, G. Luporini for GISCAD (Italian Group for the Study of Digestive Tract Cancer)

c/o Division of Medical Oncology, San Carlo Borromeo Hospital via Pio II, n.3 - Milan (Italy)

INTRODUCTION

GISCAD was established in July 1990, following the positive experience of the Medical Therapy Group of FONCAD (Italian Task Force against Digestive Tract Cancer). <u>Aims</u> of the group are:

- to promote the clinical research in digestive tract cancers (with emphasis on medical systemic and locoregional therapy, both in adjuvant setting and in advanced disease) by means of policentric Phase II-III trials.

- to perform educational activity through Symposia and Courses concerning diagnosis, treatment and follow-up of these tumors.

- to pursue a liaison with other cooperative groups, in order to organize, when indicated, Intergroup studies.

- The organigram of the group is as follows:

*President:	G. Luporini
*Supervisor Committee:	E. Ascari, G. Beretta, B. Cesana, G. Cetto, N. Kemeny, M. Marangolo
*Secretary:	R. Labianca
*Scientific Committee:	S. Barni, G. Comella, P. Foa, G. Martignoni, A. Zaniboni, S. Cascinu
*Operative Office:	G. Giaccon, M. Vinci, R. Valsecchi
*Data Manager:	G. Pancera
*Statistician:	G. Dallavalle

Since the beginning of its activity, GISCAD was particularly involved in the clinical evaluation of biochemical modulation of fluoropyrimidines.

Novel Approaches to Selective Treatments of Human Solid Tumors: Laboratory and Clinical Correlation Edited by Y. M. Rustum, Plenum Press, New York, 1993

ADVANCED COLORECTAL CANCER

a) <u>The first study</u> performed by the group was a randomized Phase III trial (<u>GISCAD C-00</u>) comparing 5fluorouracil (5FU) + Folinic Acid (FA) versus equidose 5FU alone. The scheme of treatment was: FA 200 mg/mq days 1-5 + 5FU 400 mg/mq days 1-5 (every 28 days) versus 5FU 400 mg/mq days 1-5 (every 28 days). Over a period of 2 years (March 1987 - March 1989) 182 patients consecutively observed in 16 Institutions were randomized between these 2 regimens: the results indicated a significant (p=0.046) increase in Response Rate (20.6% versus 10%) for the combination, without a prolongation of survival (11.5 and 11 months, respectively)[1]. No difference between the 2 treatments was detected in terms of palliative effect on Performance Status (PS) and on pain; overall toxicity was acceptable and lower in comparison with other Phase II-III trials, without any significant difference between the 2 arms. We concluded that this real, although modest, improvement of 5FU activity by the modulation with FA could justify the evaluation of this regimen in the adjuvant setting, while in advanced disease new attempts at increasing the activity of the 2 drugs, through the addition of other modulators, were warranted. Our study was included in the overview recently published by the Advanced Colorectal Cancer Meta-Analysis Project[2] which confirmed, pooling the data of 9 randomized trials, the advantage of 5FU plus FA over 5FU alone in terms of objective tumor response, while survival was not improved suggesting that tumor response should no longer be considered a valid surrogate end-point for survival in patients with advanced colorectal cancer.

b) The <u>following studies</u> conducted by GISCAD explored the possibility of increasing the activity of 5FU + FA through the addition of α2b-Interferon (IFN) as a second modulator: these studies were stimulated by the exciting results obtained by Wadler[3] in a small group of patients with 5FU + IFN (62% Partial Responses - PR - in previously untreated patients). A pilot trial, in which high doses of IFN (10 x 10^6 IU on alternate days) were added to 5FU + FA (scheme as above) was performed at the Division of Medical Oncology of S. Carlo Borromeo Hospital in Milan (DOM-OSCB): the results[4] were disappointing, with Response Rate (25%) and survival (9.5 months) similar to those observed with 5FU + FA alone and a sharp increase of toxicity (fever, fatigue, neurotoxicity, stomatitis and diarrhea). Due to the unfavorable cost/benefit ratio the study was closed and a new Phase II trial, with different doses and schedule of IFN, was started by the group. This trial (<u>GISCAG C-01</u>) moved from experimental data[5] suggesting that low doses of IFN can achieve an optimal inhibition of thymidilate synthase (TS) and that the drug should be administered also before the beginning of 5FU + FA in order to optimize the mechanism of biochemical modulation. So, the evaluated regimen was: FA 200 mg/mq day 1-5 (every 28 days) + 5FU 400 mg/mq day 1-5 (every 28 days) + IFN 3 x 10^6 IU on alternate days, starting the week before the beginning of 5FU + FA and with intensification of administration (i.e.: 3 x 10^6 IU daily) during the 5 days of chemotherapy. In one year (November 1990 - November 1991) 63 patients from 15 Institutions were enrolled: objective Response Rate was 24% with a median duration of 9+

months and an overall survival of 12 months (paper in press). Even though toxicity was much lower in comparison with that observed with higher doses of IFN, also this trial failed to obtain an improvement of activity over 5FU + FA. Further studies with IFN (±FA) as a modulator of 5FU must rely on a deeper knowledge of IFN action on the basis of experimental (preclinical) studies.

c) The "third generation" studies focused on 2 points: the role of the laevogyrous[l] stereoisomer of the racemic FA and the question of the optimal dose of FA. As far as the first point is concerned, a Phase II trial (GISCAD C-02) was started in order to assess the role of oral FA, capable of selecting the l-form in experimental and early clinical studies: unfortunately, we were compelled to close this study after the entry of the first 7 patients, due to the trading of the sole l-FA in Italy in April 1991. Since June to October 1991, DOM-OSCB participated, together with other 5 Italian Centers, in a Phase II evaluation of l-FA as a modulator of 5FU: the dose employed was 50% (=100 mg/mq) of the racemic compound. The data (paper in press) indicated an activity and toxicity strictly similar to those observed for the classic 5-days regimen: the results agree with the data of French and Canadian experiences.

The problem of low doses of FA was raised by 2 NCCTG studies[6,7], in which 20 mg/mq of FA were found to be equiactive, less expensive and possibly less toxic than 200 mg/mq (5 days regimen) and 500 mg/mq (weekly regimen); however, these results were not re-evaluated in other studies and we deemed of interest to conduct a confirmatory phase III trial (GISCAD C-03), comparing l-FA at 2 different dose levels (10 mg/mq versus 100 mg/mq) days 1-5 in combination with 5FU (370 mg/mq days 1-5). In less than one year (November 1991 – September 1992) 120 patients from 17 Centers were randomized: a sample size of 398 cases is expected in 3 years accrual. Of course, no data of activity are still available, while toxicity proved acceptable, without significant difference between the 2 arms and without deaths related to treatment.

d) Future Studies of the group will concern, for example, a deeper evaluation of a modification of the weekly schedule for FA + 5FU: on the basis of experimental data, indicating that for an optimal inhibition of TS 4 (and not 2) hours of FA infusion could represent the best duration, we performed, at DOM-OSCB, a pilot study on 20 patients with such a schedule. Although the Response Rate was, one again, 25%[8], toxicity was much lower than expected, indicating the possibility of an increase of dose.

Another field of priority interest concerns the definition of the best treatment for unresectable, but not extensive (<50%) liver metastases: the DOM-OSCB experience, in a feasibility study, indicated the possibility, without heavy toxicity, of combining i.a. FUDR (0.25 mg/kg/day – day 15-28) and i.v. 5FU (400 mg/mq day 1-4) + l-FA 100 mg/mq (day 1-4) (recycle every 28 days). In the first 17 patients so treated, we observed not only a high Response rate (~70%) but also a possible reduction in extrahepatic progression (in 4 patients only)[9]. These data deserve a further evaluation in a large Phase III (GISCAD C-04) starting in January 1993, in which the combination of locoregional plus systemic chemotherapy will be compared to locoregional treatment only.

OTHER DIGESTIVE TRACT CANCER (ADVANCED DISEASE)

In liver and biliary tract cancers (not amenable of resection or other locoregional treatments, such as alcoholization or chemoembolization) and in advanced gastric and pancreatic carcinomas, a Phase II evaluation of 5FU (370 mg/mq day 2-6) + 1-FA (100 mg/mq day 2-6), both recycled every 28 days, plus IFN (3 x 10^6 IU day 1-7) as ongoing: these 2 trials were activated in June 1992 and less than 20 patients have been so far treated. The rationale of such a treatment comes from the modest, but established, activity of 5FU in these cancers and from the possibility, demonstrated by Grem[10] and Cascinu[11], of achieving an effective double modulation with a schedule similar or equal to that above reported. We scheduled a duration of administration of 1-FU of 2-hours on the basis of the interesting results (low toxicity and possibly enhanced activity) reported this year by Machover[12]. Of course, at least 1 year accrual (and 50-60 patients) will be necessary in order to achieve enough data.

COLORECTAL CANCER (ADJUVANT SETTING)

Due to the absolute need of performing large-scale trials on this matter, the policy of GISCAD is to induce its members to participate in Intergroup studies.

Since January 1989 until December 1991, the SITAC trial recruited 900 patients (Dukes B2-C): the protocol planned a randomization between 5FU 370 mg/mq day 1-5 + FA 200 mg/mq (or 100, if the 1-form was used) day 1-5 every 28 days x 6 courses and a comparable group of control. These patients will be analyzed together with other 600 patients from Canadian and French Institutions, with the first preliminary data available at the end of 1992 (a presentation at 1993 ASCO Meeting is foreseen).

In April 1992 a new trial (SMAC study) started in Italy: patients are randomized among 3 treatments (5FU + FA as above, a short course of post-operative intraportal 5FU and the combination of the 2 therapies). An accrual time of 3 years with 1200 patients, is planned.

At the end, we must mention a study in which patients with resected liver metastases will be randomized between 5FU + FA (usual regimen, as above reported) and observation only. This study (based on the promising result of a retrospective Italian study[13] has been proposed by GISCAD and by other Italian Institutions (II Surgical Clinic of Padua University, Surgical Pathology of Genoa University and M. Negri Institute in Milan) to EORTC Gastrointestinal Cancer Cooperative Group: the PRC (Protocol Review Committee) approvel is pending. The trial will be conducted, on an Intergroup basis, together with the National Cancer Institute of Canada.

REFERENCES

R. Labianca, G. Pancera, E. Aitini, S. Barni, A. Beretta, G.D. Beretta, B. Cesana, G. Comella, L. Cozzaglio, M. Cristoni, P. Spagnolli, L. Frontini, O. Gottardi, G. Martignoni, R. Scapaticci, F. Smerieri, M. Vinci, A. Zadro, A. Zaniboni, and G. Luporini: "Folinic Acid + 5-Fluorouracil (5FU) Versus Equidose 5FU in Advanced Colorectal Cancer. Phase III Study of GISCAD (Italian Group for the Study of Digestive Tract Cancer". Ann. Oncol. 2: 673-679 (1991).

P. Piedbois, M. Buyse, Y. Rustum, D. Machover, C. Erlichman, R.W. Carlson, F. Valone, R. Labianca, J.H. Doroshow and N. Petrelli: "Modulation of Fluorouracil by Leucovorin in Patients with Advanced Colorectal Cancer: Evidence in Terms of Response Rate". J. Clin. Oncol. 10: 896-903 (1992).

S. Wadler and P.M. Wiernik: "Clinical Update on the Role of Fluorouracil and Recombinant Interferon-alpha 2a in the Treatment of Colorectal Carcinoma". Semin. Oncol. 17: 16-21 (1990).

R. Labianca, G. Pancera, L. Tedeschi, G. Dallavalle, and G. Luporini: "High-dose Alpha 2b Interferon + Folinic Acid in the Modulation of 5-Fluorouracil. A Phase II Study in Advanced Colorectal Cancer with Evidence of an Unfavorable Cost/Benefit Ratio". Tumori, 78: 32-34 (1992).

C. Allegra: "Clinical Drug Resistence". ASCO Editorial Booklet, 197-229 (1990).

M.A. Poon, M.J. O'Connell and H.S. Wieand: Biochemical Modulation of Fluorouracil with Leucovorin. Confirmatory Evidence of Improved Therapeutic Efficacy in Advanced Colorectal Cancer". J. Clin. Oncol. 9: 1967-1972 (1991).

J. Gerstner, M.J. O'Connell, H.S. and H.S. Wieand: "A Prospectively Randomized Clinical Trial Comparing 5FU Combined with Either High or Low Dose Leucovorin for the Treatment of Advanced Colorectal Cancer". Proc. ASCO 404 (1991).

G. Pancera, R. Labianca, Y.M. Rustum, M. Clerici and G. Luporini: "Biochemical Modulation of 5-Fluorouracil with 4-hours Infusion of Folinic Acid: A Pilot Study in Advanced Colorectal Cancer". Proc. ASCO 494 (1991).

G. Pancera, R. Labianca, S. Samori, G. Mortara, M. Pirovano, G. Giaccon, A.C. Luporini, D. Tabiadon, G. Dallavalle and G. Luporini: "Chemioterapia Locoregionale e Sistemica nelle Metastasi Epatiche da Carcinoma del Colon-Retto". X Riunione AIOM, Pordenone, 4-7 Novembre (1992).

J.L. Grem, N. McAtee, R.F. Murphy: "A Pilot Study of Interferon Alpha 2a in Combination with Fluorouracil Plus High-Dose Leucovorin in Metastatic Gastrointestinal Carcinoma". J. Clin. Oncol. 9: 1811-1917 (1991).

S. Cascinu, A. Fedeli, S. Luzi Fedeli and G. Catalano: "Double Biochemical Modulation of 5-Fluorouracil by Leucovorin and Cyclic Low-dose Interferon Alpha-2b in Advanced Colorectal Cancer Patients". Ann. Oncol. 3: 489-491, (1992).

D. Machover, X. Grison, E. Goldschmidt, J. Zittoun, J. Plotz and G. Metzger:"Fluorouracil Combined with the Pure (65) Stereoisomer of Folinic Acid in High-dose for Treatment of Patients with Advanced Colorectal Carcinoma: A Phase I-II Study". J.N.C.I. 5: 321-327, 1992.

G. Pancera, D. Nitti, D. Civalleri, S. Marsoni, R. Labianca, M. Lise, V. Bachi and G. Luporini: "A Retrospective Analyis of 119 Patients with Resected Metastases from Colorectal Cancer: Is There a Role for Adjuvant Chemotherapy?". Proc. ASCO 524, 1992.

GENERAL DISCUSSION

Dr. Chabner: Until the activity of platinum/5-FU with esophageal cancer was demonstrated, we had pretty much thought that platinum was not going to be a very useful agent particularly for colon, rectal cancer, pancreatic cancer and lower GI tumors. I'd like to propose the first question. Does the experience with head and neck cancer and the possible interaction of platinum with 5-FU and folates augmenting 5-FU action, does this change the thinking of those people who were interested in GI cancer about the usefulness of cisplatin or carboplatin? We have a panel of about 6 or 7 people and I would just ask anyone of them to respond to this particularly those of you who are involved with treating colorectal cancer. Does this change your thinking about the possiblity or the potential of cisplatin in these diseases?

Dr. Arbuck: I think the difference really between head and neck and colon is that platinum is a very active agent for head and neck cancer and not so, unfortunately, for colon cancer. Certainly there have been a lot of phase II studies of 5-FU and platinum combinations in colon cancer not terribly impressive I think in colon cancer I could toss it pretty easily. Gastric cancer though is another issue.

Dr. Chabner: Are there any ongoing randomized trials looking at 5-FU regimens with and without platinum in gastric cancer?

Dr. Arbuck: 5-FU/platinum randomized trials. Off hand I can't think of anything specific, I'd be surprised if we couldn't find some data in the literature. I can certainly say that with 5-FU/LV in gastric cancer that issue really hasn't been addressed satisfactorily although we have leucovorin now in the intergroup adjuvant study in gastric cancer. There is some conflicting data from phase II studies in the literature on gastric cancer and there hasn't been a phase III trial.

Dr. Chabner: I guess the answer to the question would then be since no one seems to be willing to test the idea that platinum is simply a modulator of folate metabolism and for that reason it should be tried more extensively in GI tumors. What you really are going back to is the idea that it depends on the sensitivity of the tumor to platinum. There has to be some demonstration of activity of platinum in that setting. I don't recall whether Dr. Scanlon actually looked at platinum resistant tumors and tried to see whether there was modulation of 5-FU activity in a platinum resistant tumor. That would be an interesting question. Is platinum interaction with 5-FU through its effects on folates rather than DNA repair or other action?

Dr. Arbuck: I think Dr. Scanlon's work was in 2780 cells is that right? These cells are sensitive to platinum.

Dr. Chabner: Dr. Abad did you want to comment on that?

Dr. Abad: I have a comment concerning colorectal cancer and cisplatin treatment. We have compared 5-FU and cisplatinum with 5-FU alone and we don't achieve any difference. We don't have difference but on the other hand Dr. Kemeny shows superiority of the combination versus the 5-FU alone. It's possible that the difference lies in the schedule of drug administration. Dr. Kemeny used 5 days cisplatinum administered together with 5-FU and we use it by a short i.v. push of platinum and 5 days administration of 5-FU.

Dr. Arbuck: I don't believe Dr. Kemeny's trial demonstrated significant improvement on the platinum arm by the addition of FU. There was some additional toxicity and I don't believe that Dr. Kemeny recommends 5/FU and platinum for colon cancer.

Audience: That was the same experience with the ECOG. Cisplatinum added considerable toxicity, which I'm sure Dr. Chabner remembers from the last phase III trial, that we had to drop the cisplatinum. It really added terrific toxicity and no increase in response.

Dr. Palmeri: We had little experience with colorectal cancer using the RPCI schedule of FU/LV in combination with cisplatinum. we obtained an overall response rate of over 21%. What was interesting in our experience was that when we looked at the site of disease, the totality of the response rate was obtained only in rectal cancer not in colon cancer.

Audience: I wonder if Dr. Vokes could clarify something for me. It seems to me I've been hearing that oral leucovorin hasn't been very effective in the colon case and yet you were using oral leucovorin for the head and neck. Why do you think that works so well?

Dr. Vokes: I can't answer that. I think there hasn't been a comparison of the oral versus the intravenous but when you compare our data with that of Dana Farber the toxicity and response data are very similar. The initial reason for choosing the oral form was select absorption and we tied in pharmacological and pharmacokinetic parameters of measuring leucovorin absorption into our initial trial. But I can't tell you which of the two is better. In our current trial, we have substituted oral leucovorin with the pure L form and that trial is still ongoing given intravenously at 300 mg/m^2/d. We've treated about 36 patients so far. The toxicity and response again seems to be very similar to what we had previously which is consistent with the observations made in colorectal cancer.

Dr. Hines: I don't know if you got the impression from Dr. Priest's data but our oral study did show a 48% overall response rate in untreated colorectal cancer metastatic disease using oral schedule which was hourly x4 with the RPCI schedule, 500 mg/m^2/wk dose of leucovorin given orally weekly with 600 mg/m^2 of 5-FU. That study is now part of the large ECOG study. It's one of the 5 arms that you saw yesterday that Dr. O'Dwyer showed and it's getting the same responses that the other arms are getting in that study as of now.

Dr. Hines: Of interest was that the amount of polyglutamate folate in tumor after the oral administration of dL LV was almost 5x higher than the level in tumor when the same dose of dL leucovorin was given as a 2 hr i.v. infusion.

Audience: Are we giving cisplatin/5-FU in head and neck cancer, for instance, by the exact schedule? I ask that because there's some in vitro data, I believe, which suggests that platinum given after 5-FU induces greater cytotoxicity than platinum given before or during 5-FU. But I'm not aware of any clinical studies which would support that. Does anyone?

Dr. Rustum: We published some data somewhere about 3 or 4 years ago when we looked at the schedule dependency for the interaction between 5-FU and cisplatin in cell lines in vitro indeed if you gave cisplatin first and 5-FU second in vitro one does get a higher cytotoxicity than when you give the two drugs together. But, in vivo, greater therapeutic selectivity was obtained when cisplatin was administered 24 hrs after 5-fluorouracil. One could not rule out the possibility that cisplatin is obviously inducing an increased level of folate, but probably the major effect is at the DNA level by increased DNA damage and perhaps delayed repair.

Audience: I would like to comment on that. We have recently completed some studies on the combination of cisplatinum and 5-fluorouracil in vivo in mice. Based also on Dr. Rustum's paper which was with L1210 cells I believe, we looked at colon tumor cells and administered 5-FU 24 hrs after cisplatinum and also we reversed the schedule. There was not a real significant difference between both schedules so we actually continued giving both compounds together. The other question we ask ourselves is whether cisplatinum has been given at a level high enough to produce any antitumor effect because it has a rather steep dose response so if you are too low with your dose then you will not see anything. So, that's something which has to be considered. For that purpose, we added WR2721 to the schedule and we were able to increase the cisplatinum dose and increase more of the antitumor effects. So, maybe that's, I wouldn't say whether WR2721 would be the ideal agent. It might be, at least in our hands it worked. But it at least demonstrated, in my point of view, that you have increase the dose of cisplatinum to get some effect. In addition to that there was also some effects on thymidylate synthase inhibition.

Audience: When you add WR2721 are you trying to mitigate the renal toxicity or the leukopenia or what?

Audience: When we looked at this, the overall toxicity, GI toxicity which was less, we also looked at leukopenia which was also somewhat reduced. In another study in our laboratory it was more focused on renal toxicity and it was also reduced but it was just in combination with cisplatinum and WR2721 and also carboplatin.

CLINICAL EXPERIENCE WITH UFT IN JAPAN

Minoru Kurihara

Department of Internal Medicine
Toyosu Hospital, Showa University
Tokyo, Japan

OUTLINE OF UFT

UFT is an anticancer drug combining Tegafur and uracil in a molar ratio of 1 to 4. Tegafur is absorbed well not only by oral route but also by intrarectal administration, then the Tegafur is gradually converted to 5-FU mainly in the liver microsomes[1] in vivo, and certain level of 5-FU in blood is maintained for a longer period. Furthermore, the incidence of side effects with Tegafur is very low, therefore it can be administered for long period, and from such reasons it has been widely used in clinical practice.

Fujii[2] and his co-workers found out the fact that uracil inhibits degradation of 5-FU (Figure 1). An idea came to them that the combination of Tegafur and uracil could elevate 5-FU level in tumor tissue.

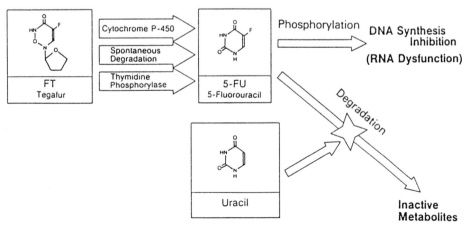

Figure 1. Metabolic schema of UFT.

Novel Approaches to Selective Treatments of Human Solid Tumors: Laboratory and Clinical Correlation Edited by Y. M. Rustum, Plenum Press, New York, 1993

Based on this idea, an attempt was made to study 5-FU levels in tumor tissue and blood after co-administration of Tegafur and uracil in AH130 bearing rats[3]. This study revealed that 5-FU levels in tumor and blood were maximum when ratio of Tegafur and uracil was 1 : 4. Then, similar results were obtained in clinical trials[4]. According to these experiences, oral UFT, the combination of Tegafur and uracil was developed.

After that, various clinical trials were carried out to confirm these findings above mentioned. 5-FU levels [5] in tumor tissue were measured after UFT, 3 capsules (Tegafur:300mg) was orally administered to 49 patients with stomach cancer, colonic cancer, breast cancer etc. In 36 cases (73.5%), concentration of 5-FU was highter than $0.05 \mu g/g$. Out of detectable 8 cases, 6 cases showed 5-FU levels at more than $0.05 \mu g/g$ in tumor tissue even 12 hours after UFT administration. In order to confirm the difference in 5-FU levels between blood, normal and tumor tissues, 5-FU levels in them were measured 4-5 hours after 2 capsules of UFT were orally administered to patients with stomach cancer[6]. The following 5-FU levels were obtained: $0.011 \mu g/ml$ in blood; $0.026 \mu g/g$ in normal gastric wall; $0.09 \mu g/g$ in tumor tissue. As described above, clinical usefulness of UFT was also suggested from the point of clinical pharmacology.

CLINICAL TRIALS IN JAPAN[7]

Ota et al carried out phase II study of UFT at 104 institutions from April 1979 to September 1980. Table 1 shows partially the results. UFT was orally administered at a daily dose of 300-600 mg for more than 4 weeks. For example, as to gastric cancer, 3 cases of CR and 49 cases of PR were obtained in 188 evaluable cases, and the response rate was 27.7%. However, extra-mural review was not done in this investigation

Table 1. Clinical results of UFT therapy.

Tumor	Eligible cases	Evaluable cases	Response					Response rate CR+PR(%)
			CR	PR	NC	(MR)	PD	
Stomach	286	188	3	49	96	(12)	40	27.7
Colon & rectum	80	56		14	30	(5)	12	25.0
Brest	78	50	1	15	28	(1)	6	32.0

To evaluate the effectiveness of UFT, comparative study with Tegafur is very important. Strictly speaking, a randomized controlled study is required, however, in this study a historically comparative analysis of UFT was performed with the results of Phase II study of Tegafur. Clinical efficacy was compared between two drugs by collected data from the same institutions using the same evaluation criteria. For stomach cancer, the response rate of UFT (15/50,30.0%) was higher than that of Tegafur (14/61,23.0%). There was no significant difference between two groups in the efficacy. However, extra-mural review was not done.

On the other hand, a comparative analysis of the side effects by UFT and
Tegafur was performed with 551 cases received UFT and 1502 cases received Tegafur
respectively. There were significantly lower gastrointestinal symptoms with UFT
than Tegafur, and the incidence of hematological disturbance was low in UFT,
though no significant difference between them was observed. Because of the
excellent selective toxicity of UFT against tumor tissue, the antitumor activity
increased, and the side effect decreased due to a half daily dose of Tegafur.

EVALUATION OF ANTITUMOR EFFECT

More than 10 years ago, I compared two evaluation methods (X-ray findings and
palpation) of anti-tumor effects on gastric cancer chemotherapy. Namely, only 7
(6.4%) out of 109 patients who received chemotherapy showed tumor reduction of
over 50% based on X-ray findings. Out of these 109 patients, intra-abdominal
masses were found by palpation in 68 (62.4%) patients. More than 50% of tumor
reduction according to palpation was recognized in 8 (11.8%) patients out of 68
ones. Therefore, when we evaluate the antitumor effects of a certain drug, we
must carefully examine what evaluation method has been used.

Table 2. The Criteria for Evaluating of Efficacy of Chemotherapy and
RadiationTherapy in the Treatment of Gastric Cancer.

Type of Primary Lesion	Measurable lesion (a)	Not measurable, but evaluable lesion(b)	Diffusely infiltrated lesion(c)	
Evaluating Scale	Tumor shrinkage rate	Macroscopic change Margin:flatten Ulcer:decrease	extention rate of affected area	
CR	not detected(aCR)	not detected(bCR)	not detected(cCR)	≧ 4wks
PR	≧ 50% (aPR)	≧ 50% evaluated(bPR)	≧ 100% (cPR)	
NC	< 50% (aNC)	< 50% evaluated(bNC)	< 100% (cNC)	
MR	≧ 25% < 50% (aMR)	≧ 25% < 50% (bMR)	≧ 100%(<4wks)(cMR)	
PD	≧ 25% increase(aPD)	progression(bPD)	progression(cPD)	

Established by Japanese Research Society for Gastric Cancer
(The General Rules for the Gastric Cancer Study, March 1985, 11th Edition)

Because of great advances of diagnostic technique for gastric cancer in
Japan, recently antitumor effects by drugs have been evaluated also by radiology,
endoscopy or CT scan in terms of primary foci and metastatic sites. Table 2
shows the Criteria for Evaluating Efficacy of Chemotherapy and Radiation Therapy
in the Treatment of Gastric Cancer established by The Japanese Research Society
for Gastric Cancer. The criteria classify the primary foci of inoperable gastric
cancer into the following three subtypes by X-ray or endoscopic findings:
measurable lesion (a-lesion), not measurable but evaluable lesion (b-lesion) and
diffusely infiltrated lesion (c-lesion). Complete Response (CR) is defined as
disappearance of tumor for a minimum of 4 weeks. CR of each lesion is described
as aCR, bCR and cCR respectively. For measurable lesion, aPR is similar to WHO's

criteria. That is, shrinkage of tumor is more than 50% for PR. bPR requires a marked regression and flattering of elevated or ulcerated lesion, namely decrease of more than 50%. When the affected area enlarges more than 100% in the X-ray film, this result is defined as cPR. Each PR also needs the period of a minimum for 4 weeks without growing of any lesion or the appearance of new lesions. As shown in this table aNC and bNC, aMR and bMR, aPD and bPD are easily established. cNC is defined as less than 100% expansion of the affected area.

RANDOMIZED COMPARATIVE STUDY

The clinical result[8] obtained in 10 institutions in Japan, which was carried out based on each own protocol, and the result was evaluated on the criteria previously mentioned. Extra-mural review revealed that effective cases were most frequent in the combination of Tegafur or UFT with Mitomycin C (MMC). The combination efficacy of UFT and MMC was confirmed by the data concering the nude mice transplanted a strain of human cancer[9]. Based on these results, we conducted a randomized controlled study in the treatment of inoperable and advanced gastric cancer by two arms. That is, Regimen A consisted of Tegafur and MMC, and Regimen B involved UFT and MMC.

Table 3. 50% survival period by tumor spreading type (month)

	No.of Cases	Localized Type	Liver Metastatic Type	Ascitic Type	Distant Metastatic Type
Kimura et al (1967)	85	7.5	3.7	3.5	3.1
Kurihara et al (1980)	100	10.0	4.5	4.0	3.5

On the other hand, as shown in Table 3, we have to consider that prognosis of patients is mainly influenced by not therapy but cancer spread of patients. Therefore, patients were stratified by tumor spreading type into the following three groups before entry into the study: abdominal localized type, liver metastatic or ascitic type and distant metastatic type. They were randomly assigned by a central office to therapy regimens according to the tumor spreading type, using telephone randomization.

In Regimen A, patients were treated with 5 mg/m² of MMC intravenously on a weekly basis and 500 mg/m²/day of Tegafur (enteric granules) orally. In Regimen B, patients were treated with 5 mg/m² of MMC intravenously on a weekly basis and 375 mg/m²/day of oral UFT. Dose modifications were made based on blood analysis: for WBC between 3,000 and 3,500/mm³, platelets— 80,000 to 100,000/mm³, bilirubin — 1.2-3× N (normal value), GOT or GPT— 2-3× N and urea nitrogen— 1.2-1.5× N, the dose of MMC and/or UFT was decreased by 25% of the initial dose; for WBC between 2,500 and 3,000/mm³ and platelets— 60,000 to 80,000/mm³, the dose of MMC and/or UFT was decreased by 50% of the initial dose. When WBC counts were less than 2,500/mm³, platelets— less than 60,000/mm³, bilirubin— more than 3× N, GOT or GPT more than 3× N and urea nitrogen more than 1.5× N, MMC and/or UFT were discontinued.

In the period between January 1985 and October 1988, patients had been confirmed by central office and 186 patients were considered to meet the eligibility criteria for the study. Among them three were excluded from the study as ineligible and 183 (98.4%) were evaluated as eligible. Fourteen cases were judged as incomplete. Thus there were 169 evaluable patients consisting of 90 for Regimen A and 79 for Regimen B respectively.

We examined the background factors of the eligible patients, according to treatment regimen A or B. There were no differences in the following factors between them: sex, age, performance status, tumor spreading type, macroscopic or histologic classification, and primary lesion subtype. As mentioned before, these main background factors in both Regimens had no significant bias. We also examined the dosage status of Tegafur, UFT or MMC. There was difference between Tegafur and UFT in total dose due to different daily dose. As to MMC in total dose, there was no significant difference.

Table 4. Antitumor Effect.

	Tegafur+ MMC		UFT+ MMC		
	CR+PR/No.of cases	Response rate (%)	CR+PR/No.of cases	Response rate (%)	Chi-square test
Total	7/90	7.8	20/79	25.3	P=0.004
Stomach a lesion	3/26	11.5	11/27	40.7	P=0.036
b lesion	3/33	9.1	7/28	25.0	P=0.185
c lesion	1/31	3.2	2/24	8.3	P=0.819
Liver	1/32	3.1	10/32	31.3	P=0.008
Lymphnodes	3/20	15.0	4/13	30.8	P=0.518
	Effective/No.of cases	Efficacy (%)	Effective/No.of cases	Efficacy (%)	
Ascites	1/31	3.2	2/9	22.2	P=0.679

Table 4 shows clinical efficacy of this treatment with the Regimen A or Regimen B. Clinical efficacy in total cases was as follows ; For regimen A, the response rate was 7.8%. For Regimen B, that was 25.3%. P value such as 0.004 was revealed by Chi-square test. Therefore, UFT administered group, that is, Regimen B showed significantly higher response rate than Regimen A. According to the gastric lesion subtype, Regimen B was effective in the classification of a-lesion. Moreover, we evaluated clinical efficacy according to evaluable tumor type. The response rate for Regimen B (6/28, 21.4%) was higher than that for Regimen A (1/31, 3.2%) in localized type. Similarly, Regimen B (10/37, 27.0%) was surperior to Regimen A (3/42, 7.1%) in liver metastatic or ascitic type.

EXAMINATION ON SURVIVAL

Figure 2 shows the survivals of the patients. The survival rate of patients for Regimen B was higher than that for Regimen A at approximate 1 year point. However, there was no significant difference in distribution of survival duration between the two Regimens.

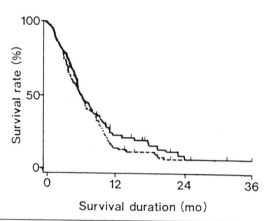

Regimen	No. of Case	50% Survival	Survival Rate (%)			
			1yr	1.5yr	2yr	3yr
A	97	180 days	13.9	5.8	5.8	5.8
B	85	180 days	22.4	14.8	5.3	5.3
Logrank test :		p=0.306				
Generalized Wilcoxon :		p=0.402				

Figure 2. Survival curves of patients received Regimen A (·····) and Regimen B (—).

There was not significant difference both Regimens in prognostic factors. However prognostic factors influence so much upon survival. Then, using prognostic factors mentioned above, we corrected survival rate curve by proportional hazard method. Figure 3 shows that Regimen B was better than Regimen A.

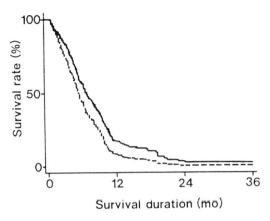

Variable	Beta	Standard Error	Chi-Square	P	R	Z:PH
Regimen	-0.34871717	0.16960301	4.23	0.0398	-0.041	-0.83
PS	-0.02460966	0.00514746	22.86	0.0000	-0.126	1.01
Localized Type	-1.00637083	0.18760806	28.77	0.0000	-0.143	1.91
a lesion	-0.51472768	0.18321442	7.89	0.0050	-0.067	0.24

Figure 3. Survival curves of patients received Regimen A (····) and Regimen B (—) corrected by proportional hazard method.

We studied survival curves for patients by classification of tumor spreading type: abdominal localized, liver metastatic or ascitic and distant metastatic type. This examination revealed the difference in survival curves among tumor spreading type. (median survival period; 295 days, 165 days and 136 days. abdominal localized type vs liver metastatic or ascitic type p=0.0001, abdominal localized type vs distant metastatic type p=0.0001 (generalized Wilcoxon test)). Furthermore survival curves for patients by overall response rate generated the same tendency. (median survival period; PR − 312 days, NC− 198 days and PD− 97 days. PR vs NC p=0.01, NC vs PD p=0.0001 (generalized Wilcoxon test)). Evaluation of antitumor effect according to more detailed classification of primary foci, that is, a-lesion, b-lesion and c-lesion revealed more correct results. In other words, there was a clear correlation between antitumor effect and survival duration by this evaluation.

AN EFFECTIVE CASE BY UFT + MMC THERAPY

This patient was diagnosed as Borrmann type 3 gastric cancer at posterior wall of gastric upper body. Furthermore, multiple liver metastasis and Virchow metastasis were observed. Therefore, we started the combination therapy of UFT with MMC. After 19 weeks of the chemotherapy, we judged that primary gastric focus was bPR, liver metastatic foci were PR, Virchow lymph node was CR, therefore overall efficacy was considered to be PR. At 27 weeks after the therapy, antitumor effect in primary gastric focus and liver metastatic foci were much improved than at the time of 10 weeks, clinical efficacy including against Virchow metastases. The overall efficacy was judged PR, because these effects continued for more than 4 weeks. (Table 5)

Table 5. Clinical course of gastric cancer with liver and Virchow metastases.(37y.♂)

NEW COMBINATION THERAPY (UFT+CDDP+MMC)

Recently, multi-drug combination therapy including CDDP has been tried in the treatment of gastric cancer[10]. This multi-drug combination consisting of UFT has been conducted in Japan[11]. We are conducting UFT+ CDDP+ MMC therapy against unresectable gastric cancer. Treatment method is as follows: In one course; 60 mg/m^2 of CDDP on day 1, 5.75 mg/m^2 of MMC on day 2 and 267 mg/m^2 of UFT from day 8 to 28. Our target is that this therapy should be done more than 2 courses.

Table 6. Effective cases by UFT+CDDP+MMC therapy.

Case	Primary	Metastases		Ascites	Antitumor effect	Effective duration (days)	Survival duration (days)
1	bPR	Liver	PR	—	PR	102+	559+
2	bPR	Lymph node	PR	—	PR	41	137
3	bPR	Lymph node Virchow	MR CR	disappear	PR	66	245
4	bPR	Liver	CR	—	PR	75	290+

As shown in Table 6, four PR cases have been obtained to date. There are many problems to be solved such as dosage and administration of CDDP or necessity of MMC, therefore, we suppose that it is necessary to evaluate usefulness of this kind of therapy including UFT+CDDP therapy.

As mentioned before, UFT, which was developped in Japan, has a great role as a drug that is to be introduced to cancer chemotherapy.

REFERENCES

1. H. Toide, H. Akiyoshi, Y. Minato, H. Okuda and S. Fujii, Comparative Studies on the Metabolism of 2-(Tetrahydrofuryl)-5-fluorouracil and 5-Fluorouracil, *Gann*. 68:553-560(1977).
2. S. Fujii, K. Ikenaka, M. Fukushima and T. Shirasaka, Effect of Uracil and its Derivatives on Antitumor Activity of 5-Fluorouracil and 1-(2-Tetrahydrofuryl)-5-fluorouracil, *Gann*. 69:763-772(1978).
3. S. Fujii, S. Kitano, K. Ikenaka and T. Shirasaka, Effect of Coadministration of Clinical Doses of 1-(2-Tetrahydrofuryl)-5-fluorouracil and Level of 5-Fluorouracil in Rodents, *Gann*. 70:209-214(1979).
4. Y. Fukui, N. Imabayashi, M. Nishi, K. Majima, M. Yamamura, K. Hioki and M. Yamamoto, Clinical Study on the Enhancement of Drug Delivery into Tumor Tissue by Using UFT, *Jpn. J. Cancer Chemother.* 7(12):2124-2129(1980).
5. K. Kimura, S. Suga, T. Shimaji, M. Kitamura, K. Kubo, Y. Suzuoki and K. Isobe, Clinical Basis of Chemotherapy for Gastric Cancer with Uracil and 1-(2-Tetrahydrofuryl)-5-flurouracil, *Gastroenterologia Japonica*. 15(4):324-329(1980).
6. M. Maeta, A. Izumi, R. Hamazoe, Y. Osaki, N. Shimazu and S. Koga, Intra-tumorous 5-FU Consentration after Coadministration of FT-207 with Uracil, *Igaku No Ayumi*. 116:97-100(1981).
7. K. Ota, T. Taguchi and K. Kimura, Report on Nationwide Pooled Data and Cohort Investigation in UFT Phase II Study, *Cancer Chemother. Pharmacol.* 22:333-338(1988).
8. M. Kurihara, T. Akiya, K. Futatsuki et al, Evaluation of Chemotherapeutic Effect on Advanced Gastric Cancer Cases with Primary Focus by the Criteria of Chemotherapeutic Effects on Gastric Cancer, *Oncologia*. 21(2):93-97(1988).
9. Y. Takahashi, R. Kikuchi, M. Ueno and M. Mai, Effect of Combination of UFT and MMC (UFT-M Thrapy) on Human Colonic Cancer Xenotransplanted in Nude Mice, *Jpn. J. Cancer Chemother.* 14(5):1345-1347(1987).
10. P. Preusser, H. Wilke, W. Achterrath et al, Advanced Gastric Carcinoma: A Phase II Study with Etoposide(E), Adriamycin(A) and Spilit Course Cisplatin(P)=EAP, *Proc. of Amer. Soc. Clin. Oncol.* 6:292(1987).
11. M. Hayakawa, K. Morise, T. Sakai et al, Combination Chemotherapy with UFT · Etoposide · CDDP · Adriamycin(FEPA) in Advanced Gastric Cancer, *Jpn. J. Cancer Chemother.* 16(10):3393-3398(1989).

CLINICAL STUDIES OF THE MODULATION OF FTORAFUR

Patrick J. Creaven[1], Youcef M. Rustum[2], Nicholas J. Petrelli[3] and Vera A. Gorbunova[4]

Division of Investigational Therapeutics[1], Department of Medicine, Department of Experimental Therapeutics[2] and Department of Surgery[3], Roswell Park Cancer Institute (RPCI), Buffalo, NY 14263 and Cancer Research Center (CRC) RAMS[4], Moscow, Russia

Biochemical modulation of fluoropyrimidines has now been evaluated clinically for more than a decade in the treatment of colorectal carcinoma and more recently in other tumors. Although real progress has been made in terms of increased response rate[1-3] there has been little, if any, effect on survival. Several approaches have been used in an attempt to improve on response rates and impact on survival with fluoropyrimidine modulation. Some of these are listed in Table 1.

Table 1. Some Approaches to Improve Results in Fluoropyrimidine Modulation

Approach	Example	Reference
Change in schedule and dose of FUra/LV	10 day CI FUra, intermittent LV.	4
	24h CI FUra/LV.	5
	High dose 24h CI LV, 3h infusion FUra.	6
Use of 6S-LV/FUra	Daily x 5 FUra/5.5 day CI 6S-LV	7
	Daily x 5 FUra/6S-LV	8
	Weekly FUra/6S-LV 2h infusion	9
Use of other modulators with FUra	PALA	10
	Interferon	11
Use of other fluoropyrimidines	Ft/LV	12
	FUdR/LV	13
	Ft/U	14-17

(CI - Continuous infusion)

Novel Approaches to Selective Treatments of Human Solid Tumors: Laboratory and Clinical Correlation Edited by Y. M. Rustum, Plenum Press, New York, 1993

253

Ftorafur (Ft) is a fluoropyrimidine with good oral bioavailability which can, therefore, be administered chronically without the necessity of continuous intravenous infusion. Because it requires activation to 5-fluorouracil (FUra), it presents possibilities of selectivity that make it an attractive target for biochemical modulation. In this chapter we shall discuss the background of Ft and its modulation and some recent and ongoing studies of this approach.

Ft is 1-(2-tetrahydrofuranyl)-5-fluorouracil. It was synthesized in 1967[18] and introduced clinically in Russia and in Japan and evaluated by both the intravenous and oral route. Initial studies in the USA often used high dose intravenous regimens, many of which gave unacceptable CNS toxicity[19]. Daily oral treatment was better tolerated and clinically active[7] but Ft failed to achieve wide acceptance in the USA.

Ft by itself has modest antitumor activity. Early results from the Soviet Union, reported by Blokhina et al[20] are shown in Table 2. Some of the US clinical experience has been summarized by Friedman and Ignoffo[19] and is given in Table 3.

Table 2. Clinical Activity of Ftorafur: Russian Experience

Cancer Site	N	PR	%
Stomach	73	7	9.6
Colon/rectum	71	5	7.0
Breast	17	4	23.5
Esophagus	7	7	--

Ref. 20

Table 3. Clinical Activity of Intravenous Ftorafur. U.S. Experience

Dose/Schedule	N	CR	PR	RR (%)	Disease Site
4 g/m^2/week	24	1	0	4	Colon/rectum
2.5 g/day x 5 q 5 weeks	36	1	3	11	Colon/rectum
2.5 g/day x 5 q 3 weeks	84	0	9	11	Colon/rectum
2.25 g/day x 5	14	1	0	7	Head and neck

Ref. 19

Ft is primarily a precursor of FUra. Studies of the pharmacokinetics and metabolism of Ft have shown complete GI absorption and a plasma decay with a terminal phase half-life of $9.2 \pm 1.0 h^{21}$. The drug is converted into FUra but circulating FUra may not account for all of the toxicity and antitumor activity seen[22,23].

Studies of the metabolism of Ft[24-26] indicate two major routes to FUra from Ft. These are splitting of the N-1-C-2' bond, with the formation of FUra and 4-hydroxybutanal and oxidation at the 5' position with the formation of FUra and succinaldehyde (Fig. 1). The first mechanism may proceed by hydrolysis or through the action of thymidine phosphorylase. The second mechanism is mediated by cytochrome P_{450}, mainly in the liver. It is not clear which is the more important mechanism.

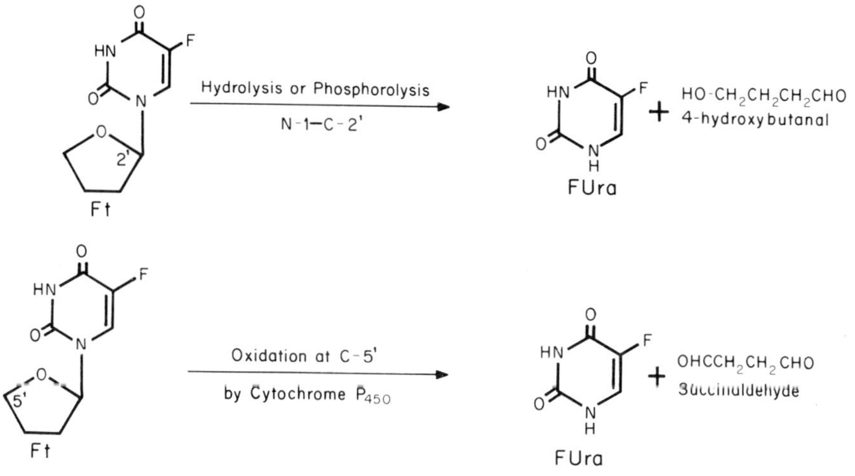

Fig. 1. Metabolic Patterns of Ft

Table 4. Ratio of FUra in Tumor:Blood After Oral Ft and UFt in Rats Bearing AH130

| Drug | Hours After Drug Administration | | | |
	1	2	4	9
Ft	3.43	3.38	4.67	11.0
UFt	10.38	5.77	23.25	11.25

Ref. 27

In 1978, Fujii and co-workers[26,27] reported the effect of co-administration of uracil (U) with F (UFt) to tumor bearing animals. They showed that the FUra levels in the tumor were increased disproportionately as compared with the levels in the blood (Table 4).

They also showed that the co-administration of uracil could increase the therapeutic efficacy of ftorafur against an experimental rodent tumor. Evaluation of the optimal molar ratio of Ft to U showed this to be 1:4.

Uracil acts by inhibiting the reduction of FUra to dihydroFUra, the first step in the catabolism of FUra. It may also inhibit the pathway to incorporation into RNA, thus directing more of the activity of FUra to inhibition of the DNA biosynthetic pathway (Fig. 2).

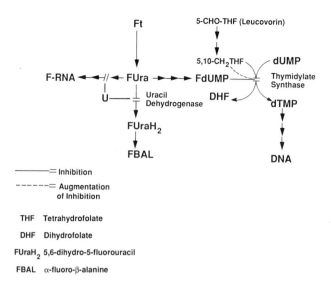

Fig. 2. Biochemical pathways of UFt

The use of this combination was explored clinically in Japan. A report of the pooled Japanese data has been published by Ota et al[28] (Table 5). Patients received 300-600 mg/day, subdivided into 2 or 3 daily doses, for more than 4 weeks.[1] Responses of 25% or more were seen in a number of tumor types if evaluable cases are used as the denominator. If all cases are used, the response rates are significantly lower. However, these responses are achieved with a low level of toxicity (Table 6).

Table 5. Clinical Activity of UFt: Japanese Experience

Tumor Site	N		RR %			
	A*	B*	CR	PR	b**	a**
Stomach	286	188	3	49	27.7	18.2
Colon/rectum	80	56	-	14	25.0	17.5
Breast	78	50	1	15	32	20.5
Lung	57	43	-	3	7.0	5.3
Liver	45	26	-	5	19.2	11.1
Pancreas	20	16	-	4	25.0	20.0
Gall bladder/bile duct	17	12	-	3	25.0	17.6
Head & neck	17	12	1	2	25.0	17.6
Thyroid	12	10	-	5	50.0	41.7

Ref. 28

* A "Eligible"; B "Evaluable"
** a - Responses x 100/A
** b - Responses x 100/B

[1]In all of the studies discussed in this chapter the doses given are the amount of Ft in the combination.

Table 6. Common Toxicities of UFt - Japanese Experience
(N = 551; Any Toxicity 41.4%; Hematologic Toxicity 6.9%)

Toxicity	Occurrence (%)
Anorexia	24.3
Nausea/Vomiting	12.5
Diarrhea	11.1
Malaise	5.6
Stomatitis	5.3
Skin Pigmentation	5.1
Leucopenia	4.0
All others <4%	

Ref. 28

Interest in this approach in the USA has led to clinical trials in 4 centers, exploring a number of schedules as shown in Table 7. Toxicity seen has included nausea, vomiting, stomatitis, diarrhea, abdominal pain and myelosuppression. Muggia et al[14,15] gave 400 mg/m^2/day for 28 days divided into 3 daily doses given every 8h. Five complete and 2 incomplete cycles were given. Severe toxicity was seen on day 33 after 1 complete cycle; both incomplete cycles were stopped on day 24, one because of gr III or IV diarrhea. Pazdur et al[16] evaluated a daily x 5 and a daily x 28 schedule (with drug given q8h). The data are shown in Table 8.

At RPCI we studied weekly high dose UFt at 3 dose levels, 600, 900 and 1200 mg/m^2/week[17]. Planned treatment was for 6 weeks. At 600 mg/m^2, 3 patients had complete courses. The highest toxicity seen was grade II nausea and vomiting in one patient. At 900 mg/m^2, 4 patients had complete courses; 2 other patients had the drug administration halted when the weekly schedule was abandoned because of toxicity at

Table 7. Phase I Studies of UFt in the USA

Center	Schedule
Kenneth Norris Jr. Cancer Center	1. Daily x 28 at 8 am 2. Daily x 28 at 6 pm q 6 wks 3. Daily x 28 split dose 4. With LV (IV on days 1,8,15 22 or p.o. weekly)
University of Texas M.D. Anderson Cancer Center	q 8h x 5 days q 4 weeks q 8h x 28 days q 6 weeks
Memorial Sloan Kettering Cancer Center	q 8h x 5 days q 4 weeks q 8h x 28 days q 6 weeks
Roswell Park Cancer Institute	Single dose weekly x 6 q 8 wks

Table 8. UFt Phase I Study: University of Texas MD Anderson Cancer Center

Schedule I (q 8h x 5 days q 28 days): Daily doses explored (mg/m^2/dose)

120	n = 3
170	n = 3
266	n = 8
300	n = 5

At 300 mg/m^2/dose, neutropenia gr IV was seen in 4/5 pts

At 266 mg/m^2/dose, toxicities were neutropenia gr IV (1), nausea and vomiting gr II (4), diarrhea gr II (2).

The recommended dose for phase II studies was 266 mg/m^2/dose.

Schedule II (q 8h x 28 days): Doses explored mg/m^2/dose

60	n = 3
120	n = 6
133	n = 8
150	n = 6

Dose limiting toxicity was diarrhea and abdominal pain in 2/8 at 133 and 3/6 at 150 mg/m^2/dose.

Recommended dose for phase II studies 120 mg/m^2/dose.

Ref. 16

1200 mg/m^2 (see below). The highest toxicity seen was grade II in 2 patients. At 1200 mg/m^2/week, six patients were entered. One received only one dose because of an acute reaction and two were discontinued when it became clear that this was an excessively toxic dose. The maximum number of doses administered was 3 because of marked toxicity. The data are shown in Table 9. The MTD is between 900 and 1200 mg/m^2/week. No attempt was made, further to define the MTD, as it was elected not to pursue this schedule for future studies.

Table 9. UFt Phase I Study: RPCI
Single Dose Weekly x 6

	600 mg/m^2 (n=3)		900 mg/m^2 (n=4)		1200 mg/m^2 (n=3*)				
	I	II	I	II	I	II	III	IV	Total
Leucopenia	-	-	2	1	-	-	1	2	3
Thrombocytopenia	-	-	1	-	2	-	-	1	3
Nausea & Vomiting	1	1	3	-	1	1	-	-	2
Diarrhea	2	-	2	-	-	-	-	2	2
Anorexia	-	-	1	-	-	1	1	-	2
Fatigue	1	-	1	1	-	1	2	-	3
Complete courses	3		4		0 (2 doses 2; 3 doses 1)				

* Study was closed early; patients discontinued because of toxicity seen in other patients are not included.

Table 10. Area Under The Plasma Concentration x Time Curve (AUC, mM.h) After UFt

UFt mg/m^2	N	Ft	U	FUra
600	5	0.8 ± 0.1	0.3 ± 0.1	0.16 ± 0.02
900	5	2.0 ± 0.5	1.1 ± 0.2	0.37 ± 0.05
1200	3	8.1 ± 3.8	4.4 ± 1.8	2.17 ± 1.0

Table 11. Plasma Clearance of Ft and U after UFt.

UFt (mg/m^2)	Plasma Clearance (L/h)	
	Ft	U
600	6.7 ± 1.1	62 ± 17
900	4.1 ± 0.9	28 ± 6
1200	1.5 ± 0.8	10.3 ± 5.4

The pharmacokinetic data indicate nonlinear pharmacokinetics of Ft, U and of the FUra produced (Tables 10 & 11).

Ho et al[29] have studied the pharmacokinetics of Ft, FUra and U after UFt in 21 patients. The drug was given every 8 hrs at daily doses of 160-900 mg/m^2/day. Cp_{max} for FUra was linear with dose except for 3 patients who showed high levels of 5-FU >1.2 μg/ml. It thus appears that, at low individual doses of UFt, the pharmacokinetics are linear in most patients, but that, as the dose increases, non-linearity becomes marked with corresponding non-linearity in the toxicity.

Some initial investigations of the effect of further modulation of Ft by the addition of weekly oral leucovorin have been carried out by Muggia et al[15] in a small number of patients. There does not appear to be any change in the toxicity patterns, though there is a suggestion that diarrhea may occur earlier in those patients in whom leucovorin is added to the UFt.

Studies of the modulation of Ft by uracil and daily oral leucovorin are now being conducted in the same four centers who conducted the original UFt studies (see above, Table 7). UFt is given 3 times a day and leucovorin is given with the UFt either in a high or a low dose (150 and 15 mg/day, respectively). These phase I studies are ongoing and no data are available yet.

Modulation of daily oral Ft by LV has been carried out by Manzuik et al in collaboration with RPCI[12]. Twenty patients with metastatic colorectal carcinoma were studied at 3 dose levels, 1200, 1600 and 2000 mg/day of Ft with 495 mg/day of leucovorin. Ft was given at 9 am, 3 pm and 9 pm, LV at 7, 8, and 9 am and at 3 and 9 pm. Toxicity consisted of stomatitis, diarrhea, leucopenia, parasthesias, nausea, vomiting and abdominal pain. The data are summarized in Table 12.

Table 12. Phase I Study of Ft/LV in Colorectal Carcinoma

| Dose (mg/day) | N | Courses | | | Stomatitis | No. of Courses With Toxicity (Severe Toxicity in Parentheses) | | | | |
		C	IC	Total		Diarrhea	Leucopenia	Parasthesias	Nausea/Vomiting	Abdominal Pain
1200	5	9	3	12	3 (1)	3 (1)	2	1	2	1
1600	10	12	15	27	11 (5)	7 (2)	1	1	5	5
2000	5	0	5	5	3 (2)	3	-	-	1 (1)	1
Responses:	1 CR; 4 PR; RR 25%									

Ref. 12

In this small group of patients there was 1 CR and 4 PR for a response rate of 25%. Pharmacokinetics showed a median plasma AUC of Ft of 235 mg/ml.h and FUra of 3.4 mg/ml.h. The study indicated that Ft + LV was well tolerated with an MTD of 1600 mg/day (approximately 900 mg/m^2/day) in divided doses.

In summary, Ft is a precursor of FUra which is activated to FUra by an enzymatic process which presents possibilities of increased antitumor selectivity. Its antitumor activity and selectivity are modulated by the addition of uracil and may also be modulated by the addition of leucovorin. The use of these two modulators in combination is currently being actively explored.

ACKNOWLEDGEMENT

The authors wish to thank Dr. Derek Raghavan for review of the manuscript and Ms. Martha Courtney for manuscript preparation. The assistance of Elmer Berghorn, R.N. and Cheri Frank with the studies carried out at RPCI is gratefully acknowledged. These studies were partially supported by USPHS CA21071 and by the TAIHO Pharmaceutical Co. Ltd.

REFERENCES

1. N. Petrelli, H.O. Douglass, Jr., L. Herrera, D. Russell, D.M. Stablein, H.W., et al. The modulation of fluorouracil with leucovorin in metastatic colorectal carcinoma: A prospective randomized phase III trial. J. Clin. Oncol. 7: 1419-1426, 1989.

2. P.J. Creaven. 5-Fluorouracil and folinic acid: Summary of clinical experience, in: "The Expanding Role of Folates and Fluoropyrimidines in Cancer Chemotherapy," Y. Rustum, J.J. McGuire, eds., Plenum Press, New York and London 1988, pp. 303-311.

3. Advanced Colorectal Cancer Meta-Analysis Project. Modulation of fluorouracil by leucovorin in patients with advanced colorectal cancer: Evidence in terms of response rate. J. Clin. Oncol. 10: 896-903, 1992.

4. T.M. Loffler, F.W. Weber and T.U. Hausamen. Protracted continuous-infusion 5-fluorouracil with intermittent high-dose leucovorin in advanced and metastatic colorectal cancer: A pilot study. in "Leucovorin Modulation of Fluoropyrimidines: A New Frontier in Cancer Chemotherapy," H.M. Pinedo, Y.M. Rustum, eds., Royal Society of Medicine Services Limited, London and New York 1989, pp. 65-68.

5. B. Ardalan, L. Chua, E. Tian, R. Reddy, K. Sridhar, et al. A phase II study of weekly 24-hour infusion with high-dose fluorouracil with leucovorin in colorectal carcinoma. J. Clin. Oncol. 9: 625-630, 1991.

6. P.J. Creaven, Y.M. Rustum, N.J. Petrelli, M. Rodriguez, C. Frank and J.K. Solomon. A pharmacokinetically directed phase I/II study of 5-fluorouracil/high dose leucovorin in colorectal carcinoma resistant to standard doses. Proc. Am. Assoc. Cancer Res., 33: 218, 1992.

7. E.M. Newman, S.A. Akman, J.S. Harrison, L.A. Leong, K.A. Margolin, et al. Pharmacokinetics and toxicity of continuous infusion (6S)-folinic acid and bolus 5-fluorouracil in patients with advanced cancer. Cancer Res. 52: 2408-2412, 1992.

8. D. Machover, X. Grison, E. Goldschmidt, J. Zittoun, J-P. Lotz, et al. Fluorouracil combined with the pure (6S)-stereoisomer of folinic acid in high doses for treatment of patients with advanced colorectal carcinoma: A phase I-II study. J. Natl. Cancer Inst. 84: 321-327, 1992.

9. P.J. Creaven, N. Petrelli, Y.M. Rustum, L. Herrera, J.W. Cowens, et al. Phase I study of 6S-leucovorin and 5-fluorouracil in colorectal carcinoma. Proc. Am. Assoc. Cancer Res. 32: 174, 1991.

10. B. Ardalan, G. Singh, H. Silberman. A randomized phase I and II study of short-term infusion of high-dose fluorouracil with or without N-(phosphonacetyl)-L-aspartic acid in patients with advanced pancreatic and colorectal cancers. J. Clin. Oncol. 6: 1053-1058, 1988.

11. S. Wadler, B. Lembersky, M. Atkins, J. Kirkwood and N. Petrelli. Phase II trial of fluorouracil and recombinant interferon alfa-2a in patients with advanced colorectal carcinoma: An Eastern Cooperative Oncology Group Study. J. Clin. Oncol. 9: 1806-1810, 1991.

12. L.V. Manzuik, N.I. Perevodchikova, V.A. Gorbunova, A.S. Singin, G.C. Gerasimova, et

al. Initial clinical experience with oral ftorafur and oral 6R,S-leucovorin in advanced colorectal carcinoma. Proc. Am. Soc. Clin. Oncol. 11: 119, 1992.

13. D. Raminski, P.J. Creaven, Y.M. Rustum, S. Perrapato, R. Huben, et al. Phase I clinical trial of floxuridine with leucovorin in patients with advanced genitourinary cancer. Proc. Am. Soc. Clin. Oncol. 11: 206, 1992.

14. D. Spicer, F. Muggia, A. Tulpule, K. Chan, G. Leichman, et al. Phase I circadian dosing of daily oral uracil plus 1-(tetrahydro-2-furanyl)-5-fluorouracil with leucovorin. Proc. Am. Soc. Clin. Oncol. 10: 118, 1991.

15. F.M. Muggia, S. Jeffers, C.G. Leichman, A. Tulpule, R. Hanisch, et al. Potential for uracil + ftorafur to mimic protracted infusions of 5-fluorouracil. Proc. Am. Soc. Clin. Oncol. 11: 135, 1992.

16. R. Pazdur, D.H. Ho, Y. Lassere, B. Bready, I.H. Krakoff, et al. Phase I trial of oral ftorafor and uracil. Proc. Am. Soc. Clin. Oncol. 11: 111, 1992.

17. Y.M. Rustum, P.J. Creaven and N.J. Petrelli. Clinical pharmacokinetics of a uracil-ftorafur combination in patients with advanced solid tumors. Proc. Am. Soc. Clin. Oncol. 11: 110, 1992.

18. S. Hillers, R.A. Zhuk and M. Lidaks. Analogs of pyrimidine nucleosides. I. N-(α-furanidyl) derivatives of natural pyrimidine bases and their antimetabolites. Dokl. Akad. Nauk SSSR 176: 332-335, 1967.

19. M.A. Friedman and R.J. Ignoffo. A review of the United States clinical experience of the fluoropyrimidine, ftorafur (NAC-148958). Cancer Treatment Reviews 7: 205-213, 1980.

20. N.G. Blokhina, E.K. Vozny and A.M. Garin. Results of treatment of malignant tumors with ftorafur. Cancer 30: 390-392, 1972.

21. M.I. Anttila, E.A. Sotaniemi, M.I. Kairaluoma, R.E. Mokka and H.T. Sandquist. Pharmacokinetics of ftorafur after intravenous and oral administration. Cancer Chemother. Pharmacol. 10: 150-153, 1983.

22. C.L. Hornbeck, J.C. Griffiths, R.A. Floyd, N.C. Ginther, J.E. Byfield, et al. Serum concentrations of 5-FU, ftorafur and a major serum metabolite following ftorafur chemotherapy. Cancer Treat. Rep. 65: 69-72, 1981.

23. J.L. Au, A.T. Wu, M.A. Friedman and W. Sadee. Pharmacokinetics and metabolism of ftorafur in man. Cancer Treat. Rep. 63: 343-350, 1979.

24. Y.M. El Sayed and W. Sadee. Metabolic activation of R,S-1-(tetrahydro-2-furanyl)-5-furorouracil (ftorafur) to 5-fluorouracil by soluble enzymes. Cancer Res. 43: 4039-4044, 1983.

25. G.A. Belitsky, V.M. Bukhman and I.A. Konopleva. Changes in toxic and antitumor properties of ftorafur by induction or inhibition of the microsomal enzyme activity. Cancer Chemother. Pharmacol. 6: 183-187, 1981.

26. S. Fujii, K. Ikrenaka, M. Fukushima and T. Shirasaka. Effect of uracil and its derivatives on antitumor activity of 5-fluorouracil and 1-(2-tetrahydrofuryl)-5-fluorouracil. Gann 69: 763-772, 1978.

27. S. Fujii, S. Kitano, K. Ikenaka and T. Shirasaka. Effect of coadministration of uracil or cytosine on the antitumor activity of clinical doses of 1-(2-tetrahydrofuryl)-5-fluorouracil and level of 5-fluorouracil in rodents. Gann 70: 209-214, 1979.

28. K. Ota, T. Taguchi and K. Kimura. Report on nationwide pooled data and cohort investigation in UFT phase II study. Cancer Chemothera. Pharmacol. 22: 333-338, 1988.

DISCUSSION OF DR. KURIHARA'S/DR. CREAVEN'S PRESENTATION

Audience: Dr. Creaven, in your abstract the main point that I found intriguing and wondered if you wanted to amplify on it at all, was the comment that the uracil/triphosphate could also inhibit incorporation of FUTP into RNA thus emphasizing the action of FU via the effect of FdUMP on the thymidylate synthase. Do you want to comment further on that? Is it wishful thinking or are there some data to help out?

Dr. Creaven: I think it's a reasonable postulate. We've always assumed that primary action of uracil was to prevent the breakdown of 5-FU to dihydro 5-FU but there might be a subsidiary action with the uracil being activated to UTP and thus competitively inhibiting the incorporation of FUTP into RNA but I don't have any data to support that.

Audience: Dr. Kurihara, in Japan the mode of administration is usually by a prolonged course of therapy. I wonder if you could comment on how long the average patient receives the drug and whether consideration has been given in Japan to modulation by another chronically administered drug such as leucovorin and perhaps even interferon?

Dr. Kurihara: Yes. Usually the UFt is administered as long as possible. And the second question, the combined use with UFt and interferon. This modulation has not been done in Japan.

THE ROLE OF THE REDUCED-FOLATE CARRIER AND METABOLISM TO INTRACELLULAR POLYGLUTAMATES FOR THE ACTIVITY OF ICI D1694

Ann L. Jackman, William Gibson, Melody Brown, Rosemary Kimbell and
* F. Thomas Boyle

Drug Development Section, The Institute of Cancer Research, 15 Cotswold Road, Sutton, Surrey, UK

*ICI Pharmaceuticals, Mereside, Alderley Park, Macclesfield, Cheshire, UK

INTRODUCTION

ICI D1694 is a quinazoline inhibitor of thymidylate synthase (TS) that was developed to act, at least in part, via metabolism to polyglutamate forms[1]. The original rationale was based on the fact that CB3717, which was active in clinical studies, formed intracellular polyglutamates[2]. These polyglutamates were ~100-fold better as inhibitors of TS and were not readily effluxed from the cell. Provided that the life-threatening and dose-limiting nephrotoxicity of CB3717 (see Clarke et al; this volume) was lost it was felt that a useful antitumour agent could be made. As the nephrotoxicity was thought to be due to the poor water-solubility of CB3717, particularly in acid urine, compounds with increased solubility were synthesised (see Clarke et al, this volume). Many of these compounds also had increased cytotoxicity but were generally poorer inhibitors of isolated TS and it was realised that a number of factors were responsible for these observations. Studies suggested that, unlike CB3717, many of the new analogues utilised the reduced-folate/MTX cell membrane transport carrier (RFC) which improved the rate of uptake and, for those that were substrates for folylpolyglutamate synthetase (FPGS), improved the rate of metabolism to polyglutamate forms (e.g. 2-desamino-2-methyl-N^{10}-propargyl-5,8-dideazafolate; ICI 198583)[3,4]. The combination of good transport via this carrier and very much improved FPGS substrate activity was a feature of a series of benzoyl ring modified quinazolines (5-membered rings) where the N^{10}-substituent was usually methyl[5]. These compounds, although ~20-fold poorer than CB3717 as TS inhibitors were up to 500-fold more cytotoxic. In mice, improved potency over CB3717 was maintained by either single bolus or repeated once daily bolus administration (depending on the mouse model used, see Clarke et al, this volume) even though clearance of the compounds from the plasma was more rapid than CB3717 ($\beta t^{1}/_{2}$ of ~30 mins)[6] (unpublished observations; D.R. Newell and D.I. Jodrell). All these observations suggested a high level of

Novel Approaches to Selective Treatments of Human Solid Tumors: Laboratory and Clinical Correlation Edited by Y. M. Rustum, Plenum Press, New York, 1993

metabolism to polyglutamates which were not only the inhibitory species but also highly retained inside cells. Experiments were beginning to suggest that we were not strictly developing compounds with the same biochemical features as CB3717 because of the relatively poor rate of CB3717 polyglutamate formation and the different transport systems involved. However their high potency and ease of administration allowed for an easy assessment of their therapeutic efficacy. One compound particularly, ICI D1694, was active against a wide range of human tumour xenografts and toxicities were confined to the normal proliferating tissues of the gut and bone-marrow[1,6]. Development to clinical study proceeded and the European Phase I study has confirmed the antiproliferative effects and demonstrated several clinical responses suggesting that the drug will have antitumour activity (see Clarke et al, this volume). ICI D1694 represents the first TS inhibitor to be used clinically that uses the reduced-folate/MTX carrier and acts almost exclusively through its polyglutamate forms. Detailed below is the experimental evidence to support this statement.

RESULTS AND DISCUSSION

Cellular Uptake and Polyglutamation of [5-³H] ICI D1694

Transport and Polyglutamation. ICI D1694 is thought to enter cells via the reduced-folate/MTX cell membrane carrier, for example a cell line (L1210:1565) with a greatly impaired ability to transport reduced-folates or MTX into the cell is highly cross-resistant to ICI D1694[1]. The drug also competes for the uptake of ³H MTX into L1210 cells (data not shown). The uptake of 0.1μM ³H ICI D1694 was measured into L1210 cells suspended in RPMI 1640 tissue culture medium and in 160mM HEPES buffer pH 7.4. In the latter buffer, within 20 mins there was a 15-fold accumulation of ³H intracellularly (Fig. 1a). In RPMI medium uptake was slower and by 40mins a 3-fold

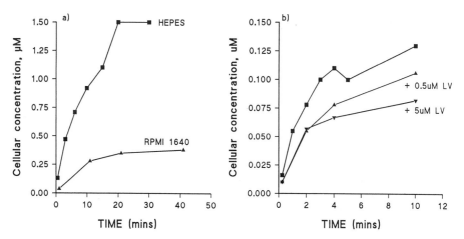

Fig.1. The uptake 0f 0.1μM [5-³H] ICI D1694 into L1210 cells a) in HEPES buffer or RPMI 1640 b) in serum-supplemented RPMI with and without the addition of folinic acid (leucovorin; LV).

L1210 cells at 3-5 x 10^5/ml were resuspended at ~5 x 10^6/ml in either 160mM K⁺ HEPES buffer pH 7.4, RPMI 1640 tissue culture medium or RPMI 1640 with 10% donor horse serum (DHS). At various times, 2 x 1ml samples were added directly to 9mls of ice-cold PBS, spun 5 mins at 600g, washed x 2 with PBS and the cell pellets hydrolysed overnight with 0.5ml 1M NaOH. After neutralisation with HCl, scintillant was added and the radioactivity estimated by liquid scintillation counting.

accumulation was achieved (Fig.1a). Although the rate of uptake slowed after 10mins a steady-state was not achieved even after 60mins (data not shown). The more rapid rate of uptake of ICI D1694 in anion deficient buffer (HEPES) is typical of folate-analogues that utilise the reduced-folate/MTX carrier e.g. MTX[7]. When we examined the level of parent drug we discovered that significant polyglutamation occurred after only a few minutes (Fig 2). After 4 mins incubation in HEPES buffer 30% of the intracellular drug was as polyglutamate forms (principally diglutamate) and by 15 mins 50% was found as the di and triglutamate with even some formation of tetraglutamate. Fifteen mins incubation in the RPMI medium also resulted in synthesis of polyglutamates (~50% of ^{3}H material; mainly di and triglutamates)(data not shown). In the normal conditions of serum containing tissue culture medium containing 0.1μM ^{3}H ICI D1694, there was an ~6-fold accumulation effect and ~85% of the cellular ^{3}H was associated with the di, tri and tetraglutamates at 30mins (Fig.3a). After 4hrs there was an ~25-fold concentration of the drug intracellularly and 97% occurring as polyglutamates (principally tetraglutamate) (Fig.3b). This rate of polyglutamation is higher than that observed with other compounds that use the same carrier mechanism e.g. ICI 198583 or MTX. Indeed almost no polyglutamates could be detected in L1210 cells after 24hrs incubation with 0.1μM MTX (96% as the parent drug) (data not shown). Studies with a variety of human tumour cell lines including lymphoblastoid, ovarian, breast and colon, has demonstrated that ICI D1694 is substantially polyglutamated in all of these lines resulting in an intracellular concentration effect of 1 to 2 orders of magnitude within 4 to 24hrs (W. Gibson et al; submitted). The major polyglutamate form varied between tri- and pentaglutamate.

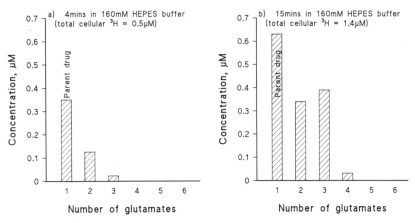

Fig. 2. The formation of polyglutamates of ICI D1694 in L1210 cells after exposure to 0.1μM [5-^{3}H] ICI D1694 in 160mM K$^+$ HEPES buffer pH 7.4 for a) 4mins b) 15mins.
Polyglutamates were extracted and analyzed by ion-pairing HPLC as previously described[8]. Results are the mean of duplicate cultures.

Retention of ^{3}H ICI D1694 Polyglutamates. L1210 cells that were incubated for 4hrs with 0.1μM ^{3}H ICI D1694, and resuspended in drug-free medium for 24hrs lost ~20% of the ^{3}H which was accounted for by the loss of the parent drug and its di and most of its triglutamates (Fig. 3c & d). It is not surprising that this occurred as the di- and even the triglutamate have cytotoxic activity, albeit reduced over the parent drug and therefore probably cross the cell membrane (data not shown). The total level of the higher polyglutamates (greater than tetra) remained the same although further chain elongation continued so that the pentaglutamate predominated with some formation of the hexaglutamate. This suggests that polyglutamates >triglutamate are not lost from the cell, at least in this 24hr time period. In a similar experiment the initial incubation time was reduced to 30mins so that ~90% of the drug was in the mono-triglutamate forms (Fig. 3a & b). The amount of ^{3}H material lost from the cell was only ~30% and the remaining drug underwent substantial chain elongation to give tetra, penta and some hexaglutamates. This indicates that the rate of polyglutamation is faster than the loss of the lower polyglutamates from the cell.

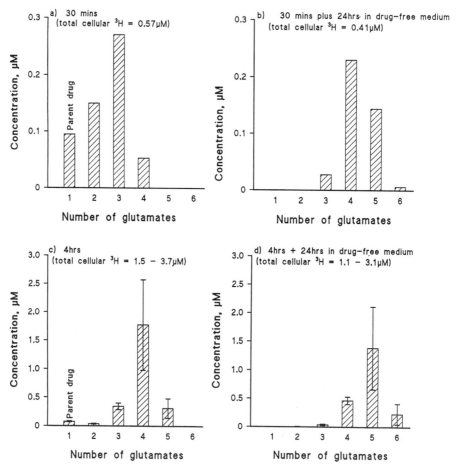

Fig. 3. The formation and retention of ICI D1694 polyglutamates in L1210 cells exposed to 0.1μM [5-^{3}H] ICI D1694 for 30mins or 4hrs.

Cells were grown under normal tissue culture conditions (RPMI 1640 with 10% DHS). Polyglutamates were either estimated immediately after these times or after the cells had been washed and resuspended in drug-free medium for 24hrs. For the drug-free medium experiments only, the total cellular concentration and the level of each polyglutamate has been adjusted to take into account dilution out by cell division. The results are expressed as the means of duplicate cultures. Error bars are the range points for two separate experiments.

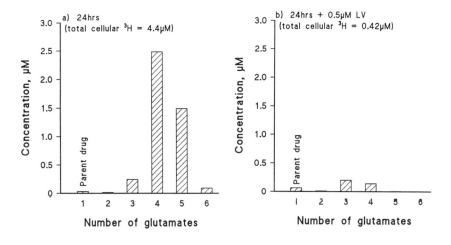

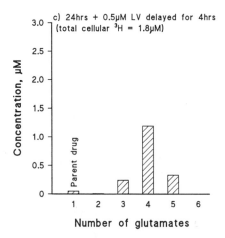

Fig. 4. The effect of $0.5\mu M$ folinic acid (leucovorin; LV) on the formation of ^3H ICI D1694 polyglutamates in L1210 cells. a) $0.1\mu M$ ICI D1694 for 24hrs b) $0.1\mu M$ ICI D1694 plus $0.5\mu M$ LV for 24hrs c) $0.1\mu M$ ICI D1694 plus $0.5\mu M$ LV for 24hrs but the LV was added 4hrs after the addition of ICI D1694. Each result is the mean of duplicate cultures.

The Effect of Folinic Acid on ^3H ICI D1694 Polyglutamation. Fig. 1b shows that 0.1 and $0.5\mu M$ folinic acid can compete for uptake of $0.1\mu M$ ^3H ICI D1694 into cells but in view of the rapid polyglutamation described above, it is probable that the antagonism is at the level of both transport and polyglutamation. Further studies investigated the effect after 24hrs incubation with $0.5\mu M$ folinic acid. Cells treated with folinic acid had substantially less cellular ^3H material, $\sim 15\%$ of the 24hr control. The level of mono, di and triglutamate was not significantly different so that the folinic acid effects were primarily on the formation of the higher chain length polyglutamates (Fig.4a and b). Thus if the cells are exposed to the two agents together, although there may be an initial competition for cellular transport, a steady-state is reached and later effects are primarily due to competition for polyglutamation. If cells were treated with $0.1\mu M$ ^3H ICI D1694 for 24hrs but the $0.5\mu M$ folinic acid was delayed and added after 4hrs the cellular ^3H was now 40% compared with cells treated with ICI D1694 alone (Fig.4c). Although there was a significant reduction in tetra and pentaglutamates, the total level of cellular ^3H and the general pattern of polyglutamates formed was not

269

dissimilar to that of a normal 4hr incubation (Fig.3c) in the absence of folinic acid suggesting that folinic acid interferes with the formation but not the retention of ICI D1694 polyglutamates.

Folinic Acid Protection Experiments in Culture

As might be expected from the experiments described above, folinic acid can effect the growth inhibitory effects of ICI D1694. Folinic acid at $0.5\mu M$ increases the L1210 IC_{50} ~50-fold[1] (Table 3). Folinic acid, when given as a 4hr delayed rescue only increased the ICI D1694 IC_{50} 5-fold, which is consistent with the substantial polyglutamation of the drug in the 4hr incubation period[1]. If the folinic acid concentration was raised there was a remarkable competitive dose effect so that $25\mu M$ made the drug nearly 6000-fold less active than in the absence of folinic acid (IC_{50} = $50\mu M$)[1].

Table 1. The structure of ICI D1694 and related compounds; their L1210 TS inhibition and substrate activity for mouse liver FPGS.

Trivial name	R^1 C^2	R^2 C^7	R^3 N^{10}	aryl	[5]TS inhibition, Ki (nM)	FPGS activity, Km (μM)
ICI D1694	CH_3	H	CH_3	thiophene	[1]60	[1]1.3
2-NH_2 "	NH_2	H	CH_3	thiophene	~40	
7-CH_3 "	CH_3	CH_3	CH_3	thiophene	10	
ICI 198583	CH_3	H	CH_2CCH	benzene	[2]10	[2]40
2-NH_2 " (CB3717)	NH_2	H	CH_2CCH	benzene	[3]3	[3]40
7-CH_3 "	CH_3	CH_3	CH_2CCH	benzene	3	[4]non-sub

[1]Ref.1   [2]Ref.3   [3]Ref.5
[4]Personal communication; R.G. Moran.
[5]L1210 TS; ^{3}H release assay as described in Ref.1

Analogues of ICI D1694 that Illustrate the Importance of the Reduced-Folate Carrier and Polyglutamation for the Potent Activity of ICI D1694

The studies described above show that ICI D1694 is extensively polyglutamated, and in view of these polyglutamates being both concentrated in the cell and being more potent TS inhibitors it would seem that they should be the active drug species. So if the potent cytotoxic activity of ICI D1694 is dependent on both cell entry via the RFC and on polyglutamation it seems likely that analogues with altered activity for either of these processes should be less potent cytotoxic agents. Experience with analogues of 2-desamino-2-methyl-N^{10}-propargyl-5,8-dideazafolate (ICI 198583) suggested that small modifications to ICI D1694 could alter these properties. ICI 198583 itself is a weaker substrate for isolated FPGS and is less rapidly and extensively polyglutamated than ICI D1694[3]. CB3717 is in fact the 2-NH_2 analogue of ICI 198583 and it is this 2-NH_2 that prevents uptake of this drug via the RFC[3,4]. The 2-NH_2 substitution was therefore introduced into the ICI D1694 molecule. Similarly 7-methylation of ICI 198583 renders the compound a non-substrate for isolated FPGS (R.G. Moran, personal communication) and therefore the 7-CH_3 analogue of ICI D1694 was synthesised. The effects of these modifications, to both compounds, on TS and cell growth inhibitory activity are included in Table 2. For both ICI 198583 and ICI D1694 7-methylation (despite improving their TS inhibitory potency) reduces their growth inhibition (2 and 180-fold). The substitution of the 2-CH_3 with NH_2 also reduces growth inhibition of ICI 198583 and ICI D1694, 39-fold and 70-fold respectively.

Table 2. The activity of ICI D1694 and related compounds against two resistant cell lines, the L1210:1565 (impaired RFC) and the L1210:MB3 (polyglutamation defect)

	Inhibition of cell growth, IC_{50} (μM)			Relative resistance	
				$\dfrac{\text{L1210:1565}}{\text{L1210}}$	$\dfrac{\text{L1210:MB3}}{\text{L1210}}$
	L1210	L1210:1565	L1210:MB3		
ICI D1694	0.009	0.92	70	102	7800
2-NH_2 "	0.72	0.5	94	0.7	131
7-CH_3 "	1.6	43	9	27	6
ICI 198583	0.13	8	2.7	62	21
2-NH_2 " (CB3717)	5.5	5.5	13	1	2
7-CH_3 "	0.2	8	0.6	40	3

The L1210:1565 cell line has a greatly impaired ability to transport reduced-folates or MTX across the cell membrane[9]. The L1210:MB3 has acquired resistance to ICI D1694 due to a failure to polyglutamate the drug or related compounds[10]. The conditions for the growth of L1210 and L1210:1565 cells has been described previously[4]. The conditions for the growth of the L1210:MB3 line are identical to those of the L1210 cells except that they are routinely sub-cultured in 5μM ICI D1694. Drug is removed 2 weeks prior to an experiment.

Resistant Cell Lines with Either Defective RFC-Mediated Transport or Polyglutamation. The effect of the RFC and polyglutamation on the growth inhibition seen with these analogues can be examined by a number of methods. Two resistant L1210 cell lines, one deficient in the RFC (L1210:1565)[9] and another with acquired resistance to ICI D1694, unable to polyglutamate ICI D1694 (L1210:MB3)[10], ICI 198583 and related compounds provide a good deal of insight into the importance of the two processes. Thus 2-NH_2-ICI D1694, like CB3717, is equally active against both the L1210 parental and the L1210:1565 cell lines indicating that neither compound use this transport mechanism. Cross-resistance was seen to ICI D1694 and both the 7-CH_3 analogues consistent with their use of the RFC. Against the L1210:MB3 line ICI D1694 was poorly active with a resistance factor of 7,800 ($IC_{50} = 70\mu$M) while ICI

198583 had a resistance factor of 21. The fact that ICI 198583 retained some activity against the L1210:MB3 line must relate to its slower rate of polyglutamation compared with ICI D1694 so that the unmetabolised parent drug, with its potent TS inhibitory activity, still allows a reasonable level of growth inhibition to occur (L1210:MB3 IC_{50} = 2.7μM). However only a very low level of cross-resistance was seen to the 7-CH_3 compounds suggesting that polyglutamation contributes little (or not at all) to the activity of these analogues. It should be noted that a small transport defect in this line results in a low level (3-5-fold) of cross-resistance to compounds that use the RFC but are unable to be polyglutamated because of modifications to the glutamate moiety. Lipophilic analogues that neither use the RFC or are polyglutamated have an L1210:MB3/L1210 ratio of just one. The resistance factor of 2.4 for CB3717 indicates a very low level of dependence on polyglutamation for activity of this drug in a normal 48hr L1210 growth inhibition assay. This is not surprising because even at a 10 x IC_{50} concentration of 50μM CB3717 polyglutamates are slow to form[2].

Folinic Acid Protection Experiments. Under continuous exposure (48hrs) assay conditions folinic acid, in contrast to ICI D1694, had a relatively small effect on the growth inhibition of CB3717 and the two 7-methylated compounds, and this can be interpreted as these compounds lacking or having a low level of intracellular polyglutamate formation (Table 3). The smallest effect was seen with 7-CH_3 ICI 198583, the proven non-substrate for FPGS in the isolated FPGS system, where even 25μM folinic acid only increased the IC_{50} 3.5-fold. In contrast, folinic acid very effectively antagonised the growth inhibition of 2-NH_2-ICI D1694. Taken together with the L1210:MB3 result above, it would appear that this analogue acts via metabolism to intracellular polyglutamates. However in view of its poorer cytotoxic activity, compared with ICI D1694, the lack of active transport via the RFC probably significantly limits the rate and extent of this metabolism. The reason that this 2-NH_2

Table 3. The effect of folinic acid (leucovorin; LV) on the growth inhibition of ICI D1694, ICI 198583 and related compounds.

	LV concentration, μM	IC_{50}, μM	fold increase in IC_{50}
ICI D1694	0.5	0.43	48
"	25	50	5600
2-NH_2 D1694	0.5	12	19
"	25	>100	>156
7-CH_3 D1694	0.5	5.5	3
"	25	15	9
ICI 198583	0.5	1.5	11
"	25	~6	~43
2-NH_2 " (CB3717)	0.5	33	6
"	25	55	10
7-CH_3 "	0.5	0.37	1.5
"	25	0.87	3.5

L1210 cells were incubated for 48hrs in the presence of the above compounds with or without the addition of 0.5 or 25μM folinic acid

compound apparently can be polyglutamated well while CB3717 cannot, probably relates to improved FPGS substrate activity of this 10-methyl, thiophene compound. Studies in other series have demonstrated that just interchanging 2-CH$_3$ and 2-NH$_2$ has no effect on FPGS substrate activity e.g. CB3717 and ICI 198583 (Table 1). Thus the combination of both the poor transport and "average" FPGS activity of CB3717 results in the slow formation of polyglutamates.

The Importance of the RFC and Polyglutamation to the Activity of ICI D1694 under Short-Exposure Conditions.

The above studies relate to cells exposed to the analogues under continuous exposure conditions. Short-exposure assays can reveal further information as to the importance of rapid transport and rapid polyglutamation to the potent cytotoxic activity of ICI D1694.

Short-exposure Growth Inhibition Assays. If cells are treated for 4hrs with ICI D1694 or related compounds, and then resuspended in drug-free medium for a period of time, those forming sufficient higher chain length polyglutamates within the 4hr period will continue to exert their effects long after drug removal due to the drug-retentive properties of these metabolites. For example, both ICI D1694 and its 2-NH$_2$ are only 13 and 15-fold less active in L1210 cells if they only have a 4hr drug-exposure period followed by resuspension in drug-free medium for 44hrs, consistent with formation of a retained drug-form such as polyglutamates (Table 4). ICI 198583 was 45-fold less active in this system compared with 48hr continuous exposure, but nevertheless still had an IC$_{50}$ of 5.9μM. The two 7-methylated analogues were inactive and can be explained by their lack of or slow polyglutamation proposed above. CB3717 also had no activity after 4hrs exposure to L1210 cells at 100μM, again entirely consistent with very slow metabolism to polyglutamate forms.

Table 4. Short-exposure (4hr) versus continuous exposure assays

	Inhibition of L1210 cell growth, IC$_{50}$ (μM) at 48hrs		$\dfrac{4hr}{continuous}$
	4hr drug exposure	continuous exposure	
ICI D1694	0.13	0.01	13
2-NH$_2$ "	11	0.72	15
7-CH$_3$ "	>100	1.6	>60
ICI 198583	5.9	0.13	45
2-NH$_2$ " (CB3717)	>100	5.5	>18
7-CH$_3$ "	>100	0.19	>530

L1210 cells were incubated in normal serum-containing RPMI medium with the above compounds for 4hrs, washed with medium and then resuspended in drug-free medium for 44hrs. These results are compared with the results for continuous exposure.

In Situ **TS Assays.** Similar short-exposure studies, coupled to the *in situ* TS assay first developed by Yalowich and Kalman et al[11], can also demonstrate the importance of polyglutamation to the activity of ICI D1694. For example, at a 10 x IC$_{50}$

concentration of ICI D1694 (0.1μM), the flux through TS is rapidly inhibited (within 1hr TS activity is <20% of control) (Table 5). If the cells are then resuspended in drug-free medium for 4hrs some activity returns (~40% of control; data not shown) presumably because of efflux of the lower chain length polyglutamates. However if the incubation period is extended to 4hrs, a time when >70% of the polyglutamates are tetraglutamate or longer, TS activity does not return after the cells are resuspended in drug-free medium for a further 4hrs (Table 5). If left for 24hrs in the absence of extracellular drug, some return of activity is seen (~33% of control) (data not shown). However if thymidine is added with the fresh medium for the 24hr period, TS activity returns completely to a control level (data not shown). Presumably the continued cell division in the presence of thymidine allows for dilution out of the intracellular polyglutamates (to~25%) and release of TS inhibition.

Again the analogues of ICI D1694 can underpin interpretation of the above results. The 7-CH$_3$ analogue of ICI D1694, which from all the studies presented so far is concluded not to be polyglutamated to any extent, again rapidly inhibited TS (a 10 x IC$_{50}$ concentration of 16μM resulted in 6% of control activity within 1hr) (Table 5). However if the cells were given a longer incubation period of 4hrs and then resuspended in fresh medium for 4hrs, TS activity returned to a control level. Extending the initial drug-exposure time still further, to 24hrs, and then resuspending in drug-free medium for 4hrs did seem to result in a retained pool of drug, as TS activity was only 40% of control. This may be interpreted as a slow formation of polyglutamates. Moving to the 2-NH$_2$ analogue of ICI D1694 in the *in situ* TS assay, it becomes apparent that again the results support the conclusions above that polyglutamation occurs, but slow transport may limit the extent to which it occurs. In this case TS is not completely inhibited within 1hr at 10 x IC$_{50}$ concentration (35% of control) (Table 5) and if the cells are put in drug-free medium at this time the TS

Table 5. The *in situ* assay for L1210 cells exposed to ICI D1694 and related compounds; to assess recovery of TS activity after the resuspension of cells in drug-free medium.

	drug conc. (10 x IC$_{50}$)	TS activity in intact L1210 cells (rate of ^{3}H release from [5-^{3}H dUrd), % control			
		exposure time			
		1hr	4hrs	4hrs + 4hrs in DFM	24hrs (+dThd) + 4hrs in DFM
ICI D1694	0.1μM	14%	8%	7%	4%
2-NH$_2$ "	7μM	35%	6%	40%	1%
7-CH$_3$ "	16μM	6%	5%	99%	42%
ICI 198583	1.3μM	4%	3%	79%	8%
2-NH$_2$ " (CB3717)	50μM	8%	4%	98%	5%
7-CH$_3$ "	1.9μM	2%	3%	147%	100%

L1210 cells (3-5 x 10^5/ml were incubated for 1 or 4hrs with each compound at a 10 x IC$_{50}$ concentration. After this time 0.3μM [5-^{3}H] dUrd was added and the rate of ^{3}H$_2$O formation was measured over 1hr as previously described[12]. Cells that had been incubated for 4 or 24hrs (the latter in the presence of 20μM dThd to prevent cell death) were washed x1 with medium and then resuspended in fresh drug-free medium for 4hrs before the addition of ^{3}H dUrd.

activity 4hrs later is at control level (data not shown). By extending the initial incubation time to 4hrs, not only is the TS activity only 6% of control, but recovery is only partial after 4hrs in drug-free medium (40% of control) (Table 5). However a 24hr exposure followed by 4hrs in drug-free medium does not result in any recovery of TS activity. Table 5 also includes data for ICI 198583 and its analogues for comparison. ICI 198583, its 2-NH_2 analogue (CB3717) and its 7-CH_3 analogue all inhibit TS to a high extent within 1hr. However ICI 198583, presumably because of its relatively slow rate of polyglutamation compared with ICI D1694, resulted in TS activity returning to 79% of control after a 4hr drug-exposure period followed by 4hrs in drug-free medium. Cells treated with CB3717, however, had normal TS activity under these conditions. Extension of the drug incubation time to 24hrs for either compound was sufficient to prevent TS activity returning after the 4hr drug-free period. This is therefore likely to be due to polyglutamate formation. The 7-CH_3 analogue of ICI 198583 did not continue to inhibit TS under any of the conditions used as might be expected for a compound thought not be subject to any intracellular polyglutamation.

SUMMARY

The uptake of ICI D1694 into L1210 cells is very rapid and evidence strongly suggests that transport is via the reduced-folate/MTX cell membrane carrier (RFC); for example a cell line with a greatly impaired RFC is highly resistant to ICI D1694. Polyglutamates can be found intracellularly within a few minutes, so that experiments initially designed to measure transport were actually measuring transport and polyglutamation. After 30mins, in normal serum-containing tissue culture medium, the concentration of polyglutamates (di, tri and tetra) exceeded that of the parent drug 6-fold. Studies where cells were resuspended in drug-free medium demonstrated that the parent drug and its diglutamate could readily leave the cell. Folinic acid could markedly decrease the polyglutamation of ICI D1694, but had to be given simultaneously with the drug as a 4hr delayed rescue was less effective because substantial polyglutamation had already occurred. This effect was translated into considerable antagonism for cell growth inhibition by simultaneous folinic acid. The importance of the metabolism of ICI D1694 to polyglutamates to its potent cytotoxic activity is demonstrated by compounds related in structure to ICI D1694 but with different properties for the RFC and FPGS. For example, 2-desamino-2-methyl-N^{10}-propargyl-5,8-dideazafolate (ICI 198583) owes its less potent cytotoxic activity to its poorer FPGS substrate activity (Km 40μM compared with 1.3μM for ICI D1694). Replacing the 2-methyl of either compound with amino, which appears to prevent use of the RFC, has a deleterious effect on growth inhibitory activity presumably by limiting the transport of the parent compounds into the cells, thereby slowing the rate of polyglutamate formation. Again a single change to another part of the molecule, that is methylation of the 7-position can have serious consequences on cytotoxic potency, particularly for the ICI D1694 molecule. The 7-methylated compounds are apparently poor or non-substrates for FPGS and therefore retain activity against a cell line unable to polyglutamate antifolates. These same compounds are only slightly affected by co-incubation with folinic acid in L1210 tissue culture, consistent with the failure of these compounds to form intracellular polyglutamates. The results of short-exposure assays and *in situ* TS assays confirms that 7-methylation largely prevents the formation of a retained drug-form (polyglutamates), continuous exposure being necessary to maintain TS inhibition and cause a cytotoxic effect after removal of extracellular drug. We conclude that the rapid accumulation of more active TS inhibitory ICI D1694 polyglutamates that are retained intracellularly is responsible for both the potent cytotoxic activity of the drug under continuous exposure conditions and the persistence of very good activity for a prolonged period after drug removal.

ACKNOWLEDGEMENT

The authors are very grateful to Prof. Hilary Calvert for his helpful comments on this manuscript.

REFERENCES

1. A.L. Jackman, G.A. Taylor, W. Gibson, R. Kimbell, M. Brown, A.H. Calvert, I.R. Judson, and L.R. Hughes, ICI D1694, a quinazoline antifolate thymidylate synthase inhibitor that is a potent inhibitor of L1210 tumour cell growth in vitro and in vivo:a new agent for clinical study, Cancer Res. 51:5579 (1991).
2. E. Sikora, A.L. Jackman, D.R. Newell, and A.H. Calvert, Formation and retention and biological activity of N^{10}-propargyl-5,8-dideazafolic acid (CB3717) polyglutamates in L1210 cells in vitro, Biochem. Pharmacol. 37:4047 (1988).
3. A.L. Jackman, D.R. Newell, W. Gibson, D.I. Jodrell, G.A. Taylor, J.A. Bishop, L.R. Hughes, and A.H. Calvert, The biochemical pharmacology of the thymidylate synthase inhibitor, 2-desamino-2-methyl-N^{10}-propargyl-5,8-dideazafolic acid (ICI 198583), Biochem. Pharmacol. 42:1885 (1991).
4. A.L. Jackman, G.A. Taylor, B.M. O'Connor, J.A. Bishop, R.G. Moran, and A.H. Calvert, Activity of the thymidylate synthase inhibitor 2-desamino-N^{10}-propargyl-5,8-dideazafolic acid and related compounds in murine (L1210) and human (W1L2) systems in vitro and in vivo, Cancer Res. 50:5212 (1990).
5. A.L. Jackman, P.R. Marsham, R.G. Moran, R. Kimbell, B.M. O'Connor, L.R. Hughes, and A.H. Calvert, Thymidylate synthase inhibitors: the in vitro activity of a series of heterocyclic benzoyl ring modified 2-desamino-2-methyl-N^{10}-substituted-5,8-dideazafolates, in:"Adv. Enz. Regul.", G. Weber, ed; Pergamon Press, U.K. (1991).
6. A.L. Jackman, D.I. Jodrell, W. Gibson, and T.C. Stephens, ICI D1694 an inhibitor of thymidylate synthase for clinical study, in:"Purine and Pyrimidine Metabolism in Man V11, Part A", R.A. Harkness et al, eds; Plenum Press, New York, pp19-23 (1991).
7. G.B. Henderson, and E.M. Zevely, Transport of methotrexate in L1210 cells: effect of ions on the rate and extent of uptake, Arch. Biochem. Biophys. 200: 149 (1980).
8. W. Gibson, A.L. Jackman, G.M.F. Bisset, P.R. Marsham, and I.R. Judson, The measurement of ^3H ICI D1694 polyglutamate formation in L1210 cells in vitro by an HPLC ion-pairing method. Brit. J. Cancer, 6, Suppl. 8: 47 (1991).
9. D.W. Fry, J.A. Besserer, and T.J. Boritzki, Transport of the antitumour antibiotic CI-920 into L1210 leukemia cells by the reduced folate carrier system, Cancer Res. 44:3366 (1984).
10. A.L. Jackman, L.R. Kelland, M. Brown, W. Gibson, R. Kimbell, W. Aherne, and I.R. Judson, ICI D1694 resistant cell lines, Proc. Amer. Assoc. Cancer Res. 33: 406 (1992).
11. J.C. Yalowich and T.I. Kalman, Rapid determination of thymidylate synthase activity and its inhibition in intact L1210 leukemia cells in vitro, Biochem. Pharmacol. 34: 2319 (1985).
12. G.A. Taylor, A.L. Jackman, K. Balmanno, L.R. Hughes, and A.H. Calvert, estimation of the in vitro and in vivo inhibitory effects of antifolates upon thymidylate synthase in whole cells, in:"Purine and Pyrimidine Metabolism in Man VI", K, Mikanagi et al, eds; Plenum Press, New York, pp383-388 (1989).

THE HISTORY OF THE DEVELOPMENT AND CLINICAL USE OF CB 3717 AND ICI D1694

Stephen J. Clarke, Ann L. Jackman and Ian R. Judson

Drug Development Section, The Institute of Cancer Research, Sutton, Surrey, UK

DEVELOPMENT OF N^{10}-PROPARGYL-5,8-DIDEAZAFOLIC ACID (CB 3717)

In this chapter we would like to review the historical development and use of two anti-folate thymidylate synthase (TS) inhibitors which have so far reached clinical study, CB 3717 and ICI D1694 (Figure 1). Both agents first entered clinical trial at the Royal Marsden Hospital, the clinical centre attached to the Institute of Cancer Research (ICR), CB 3717 in September 1981 and ICI D1694, a decade later in February 1991.

Thymidylate synthase catalyses the reductive methylation of deoxyuridylate (dUMP) to thymidylate (dTMP) which is the rate limiting step in the *de novo* synthesis of dTTP, the nucleotide specific for DNA synthesis (see Figure 2.). The methyl group is donated by $N^{5,10}$-methylene tetrahydrofolic acid (5, 10-CH_2FH_4). There is also a salvage pathway for the production of dTMP, via thymidine kinase (TK), which can be of significant importance in the presence of a TS inhibitor, especially in rodents where plasma thymidine levels are intrinsically higher than the levels seen in man[1].

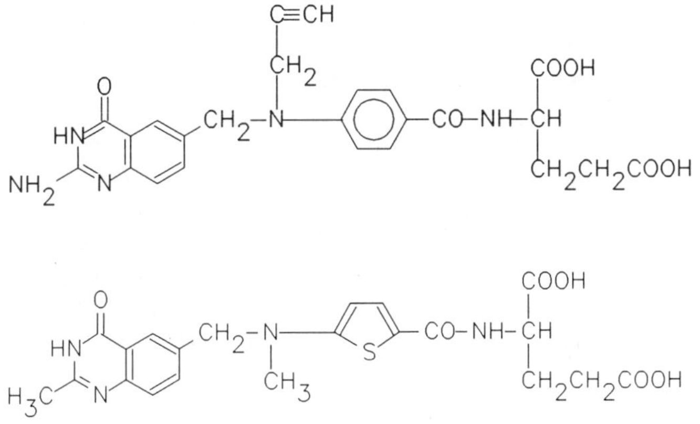

Figure 1. Comparative structures of CB 3717 (above) and ICI D1694 (below)

Novel Approaches to Selective Treatments of Human Solid Tumors: Laboratory and Clinical Correlation Edited by Y. M. Rustum, Plenum Press, New York, 1993

TS is not a new target for an anti-cancer agent as it is one of the loci of the fluoropyrimidine, 5-fluorouracil (5-FU), where the metabolite 5-fluorodeoxyuridylate (FdUMP) forms a ternary complex with TS and $5,10\text{-}CH_2FH_4$. The formation and stability of this ternary complex is enhanced by increased levels of this folate co-factor which allows for more prolonged TS inhibition[2]. This explains the rationale for the addition of folinic acid, a precursor of $5,10\text{-}CH_2FH_4$, in treatment protocols with 5-FU. Other effects of metabolites of 5-FU, including perhaps some toxicities, are due to incorporation into RNA.

Scientists at the ICR sought a folate based inhibitor of TS which it was hoped would avoid those side effects of 5-FU which are due to non-TS related effects. Another advantage of developing a drug based on the folate co-substrate, rather than dUMP, is that the accumulation of dUMP which occurs as a result of successful inhibition of TS cannot compete to overcome the inhibition (as seen with the fluoropyrimidines). Of course antifolate therapy was not new, indeed the predecessor to methotrexate (MTX),

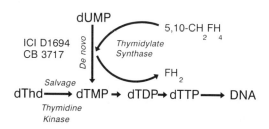

Figure 2. Site of action of thymidylate synthase inhibitors CB 3717 and ICI D1694

aminopterin, was the first antimetabolite to be used in the treatment of cancer. MTX has a multiplicity of effects due to its central role in folate metabolism. As an inhibitor of dihydrofolate reductase (DHFR), MTX inhibits the synthesis of both thymidylate and purines. Purines have importance in general metabolism as well as nucleic acid synthesis and inhibition of their formation can, in a similar way to 5-FU, have effects that may cause unwanted toxicity to tissues other than the tumour.

Quinazoline (5,8 dideaza) analogues of folic acid had already been demonstrated to have TS inhibitory properties by Bird *et al*[3] in 1970 and this area of medicinal chemistry was later taken up by Jones and his colleagues at the ICR. The history of this development is described in more detail elsewhere[4]. A series of N^{10}-substituted 5,8-dideaza analogues of folic acid was synthesised which acted as TS inhibitors intracellularly. One compound, the N^{10}- propargyl analogue, or CB 3717, was chosen for development because of its potent TS inhibition (Ki = 3nM) and its antitumour activity *in vitro* and *in vivo* through TS inhibition[4,5]. Cell lines resistant to methotrexate on the basis of either over production of DHFR or a transport defect were sensitive to CB 3717[5-7].

Over the years a wealth of information has accumulated on the mechanism of action of CB 3717 including evidence of intracellular polyglutamation[8]. Polyglutamation is a natural metabolic process undergone by many of the natural intracellular folates and is essential for intracellular retention of this essential vitamin. Furthermore these polyglutamates can be the preferred substrates for many of the folate-dependent reaction i.e. lower km values. These general properties of polyglutamates are also the properties of some antifolates and it has been shown that their polyanionic nature prevents drug-efflux. Furthermore for CB 3717 they are up to 100-fold better as inhibitors of TS than the parent drug[8].

CLINICAL STUDIES WITH CB 3717

In the initial Phase I trial of CB 3717, performed by Calvert *et al,* 99 patients with a mixture of tumours received treatment which commenced at a dose of 140 mg/m^2 and escalated, stepwise to a maximum dose of 600mg/m$^{2(9)}$. Treatment was initially given as a one hour infusion and repeated 3 weekly (q.3/52). Later, after an assessment of toxicity (nephro and hepatic-see later) a twelve hour infusion q. 3/52 and subsequently a one hour infusion with co-administration of oral prednisolone were utilised in attempts to ameliorate these toxicities.

The dose limiting toxicity was renal which occurred in 70% of patients at doses greater than 450 mg/m^2. The other prominent and more prevalent toxicities were elevations in liver function tests and disabling malaise.

The liver function abnormalities were predominantly a transaminitis with changes occurring more frequently in alanine aminotransferase (ALT)[9]. Lesser abnormalities were seen in alkaline phosphatase and bilirubin. The elevations were more marked after a second course with settling of the changes occurring after a peak value had been reached, in spite of repeated drug administration. The changes were not greater in patients who had abnormal liver function tests prior to commencement of treatment. The changes were seen in 80% of patients treated and did not appear to be dose related. The institution of a twelve hour infusion and co-administration with prednisolone did not affect the incidence of the liver function changes. No patient developed progressive hepatic impairment.

Disabling malaise occurred in 70% of patients and reflected a feeling of anorexia, lethargy and mild nausea which came on after four to five days and resolved after a further three to seven days[9]. These symptoms necessitated the cessation of treatment in 17 patients. The incidence of malaise appeared to correlate with the degree of elevation of ALT, although with both malaise and hepatotoxicity occurring in such a large percentage of patients an association between the two toxicities would be difficult to exclude. Co-administration of prednisolone appeared to ameliorate the malaise.

An irritating maculopapular rash over limbs and trunk was seen in 12 patients[9]. The rash came on soon after commencement of treatment and settled within a week. It did not occur in those patients in whom there was co-administration of steroids. There was evidence of radiation recall in two further patients.

No gut toxicity was reported and myelotoxicity was sporadic and not severe. Five patients had a degree of other mucosal toxicity (sore mouth-2, conjunctivitis-3).

In 76 patients evaluable for anti-tumour response there was some evidence of anti-tumour activity in 21 patients which consisted of 1 complete response (CR), 6 partial responses (PR) and 14 minor responses (MR). The tumour types and numbers of responders were: ovary-9, breast-4, colon-2, non-small cell lung-3, mesothelioma-2 and APUDoma-1. Responses in ovarian cancer included some patients who had platinum resistant tumours. A dose of 400 mg/m^2 was recommended for Phase II trial using this schedule.

In further attempts to overcome the toxicity and perhaps increase anti-tumour affects other Phase I schedules of administration were explored, elsewhere. A Danish group investigated CB 3717 given as a weekly bolus over the dose range of 10-30 mg/m$^{2(10)}$. Again nephrotoxicity was dose limiting with transaminitis and malaise also being seen. There was no bone marrow, gut or skin toxicity seen or any mucositis. No anti-tumour responses were seen. An Italian group assessed CB 3717 as an intravenous bolus given at 1 mg/minute q. 3-4/52 over the dose ranges of 50-400 mg/m^2, but with urinary alkalinization and intravenous hydration being routinely administered at the higher dose levels[11] in an attempt to avoid the nephrotoxicity seen previously. This resulted in some improvement with transient reversible decreases in creatinine clearance being seen in 35% of cycles at 400 mg/m^2. Transaminitis and disabling malaise were again seen. There was a suggestion of anti-tumour response in 3 patients with platinum resistant ovarian cancer.

Table 1. Summary of Phase II trials of CB 3717[12-15]

TUMOUR TYPE	RESULT
Breast	17% PR rate
Hepatoma	43% response rate
Ovary	18% PR rate
Colon	No response
Mesothelioma	6% response rate

Phase II trials of CB 3717 (see Table 1 for summary) were performed in mesothelioma and breast, colon, ovarian and hepatocellular cancers[12-15]. In the phase II trial in breast cancer, at a dose of 400 mg/m^2 (300 mg/m^2 in those with pre-existing renal impairment) q. 3/52 via 1 hour infusion, a 17% partial response rate was seen[13]. These patients predominantly had skin and soft tissue metastases. Most patients had received and progressed on prior chemo or hormonal therapies. In colon carcinoma[14], using the same doses and schedule as the breast cancer trial, 26 patients were treated. Fifty percent of patients had received no prior chemotherapy. No patient exhibited a response. In mesothelioma[12], 18 patients were treated as in the other trials with one patient (6%) exhibiting a partial response. In the hepatocellular carcinoma trial[15], CB 3717 was administered at a dose of 300 mg/m^2 prepared in alkaline solution, preceded and succeeded by alkaline hydration with dosing at 3 weekly intervals. Forty three percent of patients showed evidence of objective response (gauged by a > 50% reduction in serum alpha fetoprotein, maintained for at least 1 month and accompanied by radiological evidence of decrease in tumour size). In the phase II trial in ovarian cancer, which remains unpublished, there was encouraging evidence of anti-tumour response (A. H. Calvert - personal communication). The toxicities seen in the phase II trials mimicked those seen in the phase I trials. Thus in spite of further encouraging activity it was felt that the toxicities of CB 3717, particularly the nephrotoxicity, precluded its further development and further trials were not undertaken. By this time there was evidence that the nephrotoxicity was due to physical properties of the drug and not TS inhibition[16,17]. This suggested and led to a programme of analogue development.

DEVELOPMENT OF TS INHIBITORS THAT LED TO ICI D1694

The cause of the nephrotoxicity with CB 3717 was thought to be due to poor aqueous solubility especially at the acid pH of urine. Increasing the pH of human urine up to 9 led to a 100 fold increase in solubility of CB 3717[16]. Poor aqueous solubility led to crystallisation and accumulation in the kidneys of mice with subsequent tubular damage and cortical scarring[16,18]. This accumulation was seen in murine experiments using [2-^{14}C]-CB 3717[16]. The aetiology of the hepatic changes was less explicable. Abnormalities in liver function seen in animal experiments were not prevented by the co-administration of thymidine, suggesting they were unrelated to TS inhibition. The ^{14}C label experiment had suggested accumulation of CB 3717 in liver as well as kidney and pharmacokinetic studies in the rat had shown biliary precipitation of CB 3717 when plasma levels exceeded 10μg/ml. This plasma level of CB 3717 had been attained in the clinical trial. Thus it was thought possible that the hepatic function abnormalities as well as the nephrotoxicity could be due to poor aqueous solubility. These findings prompted the search for a more water soluble derivative of CB 3717.

The chemical basis for the poor aqueous solubility of CB 3717 was proposed by Jones *et al* to revolve around the 2-amino-3,4-dihydro-4-oxopyrimidine moiety of the drug with inter-molecular hydrogen bonding resulting in insolubility[19]. This prompted the synthesis of 2-desamino CB 3717 to reduce the hydrogen bonding capability, and this indeed proved to be a more water soluble compound than CB3717 at physiological pH[19]. As was predicted desamino-CB 3717 did not produce renal nor hepatic toxicity in rodents[20]. The ability to inhibit TS was 10-fold less for this compound, but suprisingly it had a 10 fold greater potency against L1210 cells than CB 3717 [19,21]. This enhanced potency was found to be due to its use of the reduced-folate carrier/MTX cell membrane carrier (RFC) and indirect evidence suggested that this resulted in better intracellular polyglutamate formation[21]. At this stage ICI Pharmaceuticals, who had had an interest and involvement in the work of the ICR on CB 3717 and some of its analogues, started a joint chemical synthetic programme with the ICR. The initial lead of Jones *et al* on the desamino compound quickly led to the synthesis, at ICI by Hughes *et al,* of 2-substituted analogues, as TS inhibitors. The 2-methyl analogue (2-desamino-2-methyl-N^{10}-propargyl-5,8-dideazafolate; ICI 198583) was found to have improved TS inhibitory activity over the desamino compound (Ki = 10nM) and improved growth inhibitory activity (L1210 IC$_{50}$ = 0.09μM)[22,23]. This compound was now 40-fold more potent than CB 3717 as an inhibitor of cell growth. Use of the ^{3}H compound demonstrated an improved rate of polyglutamate formation of ICI 198583 over CB 3717 which accounts for both its improved cytotoxic activity and antitumour activity in mice[23]. This further improvement in activity over CB 3717 with structural rearrangement prompted an extensive structure activity analysis of ICI 198583 and its derivatives in order to find the most suitable candidate for phase I study in terms of activity and reduced toxicity. The best compound to emerge was ICI D1694 whose structural comparison with CB 3717 is shown in Figure 1[24,25]. ICI D1694 has a Ki for isolated L1210 TS of 62nM and despite this 20-fold poorer potency against isolated TS has a greater cytotoxic potency (500-fold) than CB 3717 due to use of the RFC and its great affinity for folylpolyglutamate synthetase (FPGS)[25]. The rapid and extensive intracellular polyglutamation of ICI D1694 is described by Jackman et al (this volume). ICI D1694 had a broad spectrum of antitumour activity in experimental *in vivo* models, including some human tumour xenografts[25,26]. Of course there were toxicological considerations and ICI D1694 was not found to have the nephrotoxicity associated with CB 3717 while other toxicities were to proliferating tissues[18,27]. High circulating thymidine levels in rodents complicate the assessment of both antitumour activity and toxicity associated with TS inhibitors.[1,27] This assessment is thus different to that of other chemotherapeutic agents and requires a small digression to explain how it was performed with ICI D1694 and its predecessors.

IN VIVO STUDIES WITH ICI D1694

TS Inhibition and Antitumour Activity

The *in vivo* activity of CB 3717[5,21,28], ICI 198583[23] and ICI D1694[25,26] has been published previously and is only reviewed here. As might be expected from the evidence provided in this communication, ICI D1694 is the most active antitumour agent in mice. However first it should be remembered that the unusually high level of plasma thymidine in mice (~ 1-2μM) severely limits the efficacy of TS inhibitors, including ICI D1694, *in vivo* by providing a source of salvagable thymidine for thymidylate synthesis[1,27]. This can be illustrated by the results of the *in situ* TS assay on the ascitic L1210 tumour removed at different times after intravenous bolus injection of the agents (this tumour is refractory to even multiple dose treatment with these agents). The *in situ* assay measures TS inhibition due to non or slowly effluxable drug forms, because this *ex-vivo* assay is performed in medium devoid of drug. Thus two hours exposure to the MTD of CB 3717 (200mg/kg) failed to inhibit the flux through TS more than 40%[21]. ICI 198583 at 50mg/kg inhibited TS >80% two hours after injection although recovery was apparent at 12hrs[23]. Higher doses were more effective, so that with 500mg/kg this inhibition lasted for at least 24hrs. Similarly ICI D1694 inhibited TS to this extent but at a lower dose of 10mg/kg[25]. Considering the rapid plasma clearance of ICI 198583[23] and ICI D1694[29] (15 and 30mins β-half-lives respectively) a significant degree of drug-retention as polyglutamates must be occurring. These results also suggest that CB3717 forms polyglutamates relatively poorly *in vivo*, as was found *in vitro*, but the contribution of the parent drug to TS inhibition with its slower plasma clearance is unknown (90 minute β-half life)[20].

The fact that TS can be inhibited so effectively without significantly inhibiting tumour growth *in vivo* is consistent with thymidine salvage circumventing the TS inhibition. Some tumours grown in the mouse host do respond to treatment with quinazoline TS inhibitors provided a multiple dosing schedule is employed. It has been demonstrated that CB 3717 causes a decrease in plasma thymidine as treatment progresses which seems to be sufficient to reveal antitumour activity[1]. Thus the L1210:ICR tetraploid tumour is sensitive to all three agents with curative doses (to >70% of the mice) of 50, 5 and 0.4mg/kg for CB 3717, ICI 198583 and ICI D1694 respectively[21,23,25]. The activity of these compounds can be prevented by co-administration of thymidine. Another murine tumour, the sub-cutaneous L5178Y lymphoma, also has some sensitivity to ICI D1694 (not to CB 3717) so that 3.3mg/kg twice daily for 5 days gives an 8-9 day growth delay[27]. Again the importance of thymidine salvage is demonstrated with this tumour as a variant of it, the L5178Y TK[-/-] tumour (thymidine salvage incompetent), is highly sensitive to ICI D1694. Stephens *et al* demonstrated that it is curative by a single bolus injection of 10mg/kg. ICI 198583 had to be administered at eight hourly intervals for 5 days (250mg/kg/day) to give a high cure rate[30]. CB 3717 only gave very short growth delays at its MTD in any schedule.

Some human tumour xenografts respond to a repeated dose schedule of these agents, notably the HX62 ovarian tumour which is resistant to platinum complexes. ICI D1694 resulted in 15 days growth delay following 15 daily treatments of 1mg/kg. Similar activity was seen with CB 3717, but only at ~100mg/kg, the MTD for this schedule[31].

Toxicities of ICI D1694

ICI D1694 is therefore not noticably schedule dependent in the absence of thymidine salvage. Of course the use of such TK$^{-/-}$ models makes interpretation of therapeutic index difficult as a single dose of ICI D1694, while curing the tumour, has no toxic side effects. Thus the thymidine salvage competent tumours, L1210:ICR, L5178Y and the HX62 xenograft, have to be used to gauge efficacy and of course a prolonged administration schedule has to be used to overcome the thymidine salvage problem. Under these conditions the mice experience some weight loss, gastro-intestinal toxicity, leucopenia and thrombocytopenia all of which can largely be prevented by co-administration of thymidine suggesting the effects are related to TS inhibition[27]. Folinic acid can also prevent both the toxicities and the antitumour activity of ICI D1694 and *in vitro* data (Jackman *et al*, see this volume) suggests that this is due to interference with transport and/or polyglutamation of the drug.

As the hepatic[32] and kidney toxicities of CB 3717 were not apparently related to TS effects murine models were used to assess these toxicities for ICI D1694. At a dose of 500 mg/kg no toxicities were seen to either organ. However raising the dose to 1g/kg produced some hepatotoxicity (raised plasma ALT with centrilobular necrosis seen on hepatic section) but still no nephrotoxicity.

The thymidine salvage problem in mice means that extrapolation of active or toxic doses to man has to be done with caution. In fact dogs, with a low plasma thymidine level similar to that of man ($\sim 0.1\mu M$), provide a more accurate model for the dose and schedule likely to cause biological effects in man. Indeed ICI D1694 elicited gastro-intestinal and haematological toxicities after single bolus injections (0.1mg/kg or 2mg/m^2 and greater) (T.C. Stephens, ICI Pharmaceuticals; personal communication).

Pharmacology of ICI D1694

The pharmacokinetics in mouse and rat[29] showed that clearance best conformed to 2 compartment open model with a T1/2 β of 30 minutes. At higher doses, in mice, there was probably a third phase of 390 $\pm$ 162 minutes. Excretion in mice and rats was predominantly biliary and there was no evidence for renal or hepatic accumulation as seen with CB 3717.

Thus in summary all the animals studied showed that the toxicities of ICI D1694 were more typical of an anti-metabolite, principally gut and bone marrow toxicities reversible by co-administration of thymidine. There was no evidence of nephrotoxicity or hepatotoxicity.

ICI D1694 CLINICAL STUDY

The phase I trial of ICI D1694 commenced in February 1991 at the Royal Marsden Hospital. Patients have been accrued from that institution and the Rotterdam Cancer Institute, the Netherlands. A subsequent trial has been performed in the US under the auspices of the National Cancer Institute. We shall restrict this discussion to the European trial. The starting dose was 0.1 mg/m^2, which was 20% of the toxic dose low in dogs. Subsequent doses have been given at 0.2, 0.4, 0.6, 1, 1.6, 2.6, 3, and 3.5 mg/m^2. The drug was administered by intravenous infusion over 15 minutes and repeated q. 3/52. Depending on response status the drug was given for a maximum of 6 courses. Sixty one patients, with a broad spectrum of tumour types, have been treated to date. The trial is ongoing with completion expected by the end 1992.

No toxicity was seen below 1.6 mg/m^2. At 1.6 mg/m^2, an elevation in liver enzymes was seen after a second dose. This pattern has also been seen at the higher doses with changes in alanine aminotransferase (ALT) predominating. These changes settle with repeat dosing and return to normal after cessation of treatment. The rapidity of onset and frequency of abnormality of the changes in liver function appear to be dose related. Liver biopsy has not shown any evidence of necrosis nor fibrosis. Unlike with CB 3717 there has been no consistent association of malaise with abnormalities of liver function.

At higher doses the more important toxicities have been gastrointestinal and haematological. Nausea and vomiting which occur 3-5 days after treatment have been seen frequently, but are easily controlled with conventional anti-emetics. Diarrhoea has also been frequent and in 6 patients (5 at 3.0 and 1 at 3.5 mg/m^2) has been severe, leading to dehydration and hypoalbuminaemia and necessitating hospital admission. Myelosuppression, with leucopenia and granulocytopenia predominating, has occurred consistently at 3.0 and 3.5 mg/m^2. Both the gastrointestinal and haematological toxicities appear cumulative, but reversible, in most cases. Neither toxicity has shown any improvement with the use of low dose leucovorin rescue. Other toxicities have included malaise, mucositis, rash, fever and influenza-like symptoms. No nephrotoxicity attributable to ICI D1694 has been seen.

There has been evidence of anti-tumour response in 5 patients, 4 at 3.0 mg/m^2 and 1 at 2.6 mg/m^2. The tumour types have been adenocarcinoma of unknown primary (PR), nasopharyngeal carcinoma (MR), breast (CR) and ovarian cancers (2 x MR).

The pharmacokinetics show a disposition which is best fitted by a 3 compartment model with a protracted gamma phase.

Three and a half mg/m^2 has been the MTD for this schedule of administration and 3.0 mg/m^2 is the dose recommended for phase II trial which will commence in the 3rd quarter of 1992.

SUMMARY

The antifolate thymidylate synthase inhibitors represent an exciting area in new drug development and show that with an understanding of the structural basis for toxicity, new drugs can be synthesised which have a more manageable spectrum of side effects whilst retaining activity. ICI D1694 does not show the nephrotoxicity which affected the development of CB 3717. Myelosuppression and gut toxicity are seen and are more typical of the toxicities one associates with this class of agent. Changes in hepatic enzymes have been seen with both drugs, and are also seen with other anti-folates including MTX, but these changes settle with repeat dosing and with cessation of treatment. We await the results of the planned phase II trials of ICI D1694 with great interest.

ACKNOWLEDGEMENT

The authors would like to acknowledge the assistance of Dr Rupert Smith in preparation of this chapter.

REFERENCES

1. A.L. Jackman, G.A. Taylor, A.H. Calvert and K.R. Harrap, Modulation of Anti-metabolite Effects: Effects of thymidine on the efficacy of the quinazoline-based thymidylate synthetase inhibitor, CB3717. *Biochem Pharmacol*, *33* (1984) 3269-3275.
2. A. Lockshin and P.V. Danenberg, Biochemical factors affecting the tightness of 5-fluorodeoxyuridylate binding to human thymidylate synthetase. *Biochem Pharmacol*, *30* (1981) 247-257.
3. O.D. Bird, J.W. Vaitkus and J. Clarke, 2-Amino-4-hydroxyquinazolines as inhibitors of thymidylate synthetase. *Molec Pharmacol*, *6* (1970) 573-575.
4. A.L. Jackman, T.R. Jones and A.H. Calvert, Thymidylate synthetase inhibitors: experimental and clinical aspects. In F.M. Muggia (ed.), *Experimental and clinical progress in cancer chemotherapy*, Martinus Nijhoff, Boston, 1985, pp. 155-209.
5. T.R. Jones, A.H. Calvert, A.L. Jackman, S.J. Brown, M. Jones and K.R. Harrap, A potent antitumour quinazoline inhibitor of thymidylate synthetase: synthesis, biological properties and therapeutic results in mice. *Europ J Cancer*, *17* (1981) 11-19.
6. H. Diddens, D. Niethammer and R.C. Jackson, Patterns of cross-resistance to the antifolate drugs trimetrexate, metoprine, homofolate, and CB3717 in human lymphoma and osteosarcoma cells resistant to methotrexate. *Cancer Res*, *43* (1983) 5286-5292.
7. Y-C. Cheng, G.E. Dutschman, M.C. Starnes, M.H. Fisher, N.T. Nanavathi and M.G. Nair, Activity of the new antifolate N^{10}-propargyl-5,8-dideazafolate and its polyglutamates against human dihydrofolate reductase, human thymidylate synthetase, and KB cells containing different levels of dihydrofolate reductase. *Cancer Res*, *45* (1985) 598-600.
8. E. Sikora, A.L. Jackman, D.R. Newell and A.H. Calvert, Formation and retention and biological activity of N^{10}-propargyl-5,8-dideazafolic acid (CB3717) polyglutamates in L1210 cells in vitro. *Biochem Pharmacol*, *37* (1988) 4047-4054.
9. A.H. Calvert, D.L. Alison, S.J. Harland, B.A. Robinson, A.L. Jackman, T.R. Jones, D.R. Newell, Z.H. Siddik, E. Wiltshaw, T.J. McElwain, I.E. Smith and K.R. Harrap, A phase I evaluation of the quinazoline antifolate thymidylate synthase inhibitor, N^{10}-propargyl-5,8-dideazafolic acid, CB3717. *J Clin Oncol*, *4* (1986) 1245-1252.
10. S. Vest, E. Bork and H.H. Hansen, A phase I evaluation of N^{10}-propargyl-5,8-dideazafolic acid. *Eur J Cancer Clin Oncol*, *24* (1988) 201-204.
11. C. Sessa, M. Zucchetti, M. Ginier, Y. Willems, M. D'Incalci and F. Cavalli, Phase I study of the antifolate N^{10}-propargyl-5,8-dideazafolic acid, CB3717. *Eur J Cancer Clin Oncol*, *24* (1988) 769-775.
12. B.M.J. Cantwell, M. Earnshaw and A.L. Harris, Phase II study of a novel antifolate, N^{10}-propargyl-5,8-dideazafolic acid (CB3717), in malignant mesothelioma. *Cancer Treat Rep*, *70* (1986) 1335-1336.
13. B.M.J. Cantwell, V. Macaulay, A.L. Harris, S.B. Kaye, I.E. Smith, R.A.V. Milsted and A.H. Calvert, Phase II study of the antifolate N^{10}-propargyl-5,8-dideazafolic acid (CB3717) in advanced breast cancer. *Eur J Cancer Clin Oncol*, *24* (1988) 733-736.
14. M.J. Harding, B.M.J. Cantwell, R.A.V. Milstead, A.L. Harris and S.B. Kaye, Phase II study of the thymidylate synthetase inhibitor CB3717 (N^{10}-propargyl-5,8-dideazafolic acid) in colorectal cancer. *Br J Cancer*, *57* (1988) 628-629.
15. M.F. Bassendine, N.J. Curtin, H. Loose, A.L. Harris and O.F.W. James, Induction

of remission in hepatocellular carcinoma with a new thymidylate synthase inhibitor, CB3717. *J Hepatol, 4* (1987) 349-356.

16. D.R. Newell, D.L. Alison, A.H. Calvert, K.R. Harrap, M. Jarman, T.R. Jones, M. Manteuffel-Cymborowska and P. O'Connor, Pharmacokinetics of the thymidylate synthase inhibitor N^{10}-propargyl-5,8-dideazafolic acid (CB3717) in the mouse. *Cancer Treat Rep, 70* (1986) 971-979.

17. D.L. Alison, D.R. Newell, C. Sessa, S.J. Harland, L.I. Hart, K.R. Harrap and A.H. Calvert, The clinical pharmacokinetics of the novel antifolate N^{10}-propargyl-5,8-dideazafolic acid (CB3717). *Cancer Chemother Pharmacol, 14* (1985) 265-271.

18. D.I. Jodrell, D.R. Newell, S.E. Morgan, S. Clinton, J.P.M. Bensted, L.R. Hughes and A.H. Calvert, The renal effects of N^{10}-propargyl-5,8-dideazafolic acid (CB3717) and a non-nephrotoxic analogue ICI D1694, in mice. *Br J Cancer, 64* (1991) 833-838.

19. T.R. Jones, T.J. Thornton, A. Flinn, A.L. Jackman, D.R. Newell and A.H. Calvert, Quinazoline antifolates inhibiting thymidylate synthase: 2-desamino derivatives with enhanced solubility and potency. *J Med Chem, 32* (1989) 847-852.

20. K.R. Harrap, A.L. Jackman, D.R. Newell, G.A. Taylor, L.R. Hughes and A.H. Calvert, Thymidylate synthase: a target for anticancer drug design. In G. Weber (ed.), *Advances in Enzyme Regulation*, Pergamon, Oxford, 1989, pp. 161-179.

21. A.L. Jackman, G.A. Taylor, B.M. O'Connor, J.A. Bishop, R.G. Moran and A.H. Calvert, Activity of the thymidylate synthase inhibitor 2-desamino-N^{10}-propargyl-5,8-dideazafolic acid and related compounds in murine (L1210) and human (W1L2) systems in vitro and in L1210 in vivo. *Cancer Res, 50* (1990) 5212-5218.

22. L.R. Hughes, A.L. Jackman, J. Oldfield, R.C. Smith, K.D. Burrows, P.R. Marsham, J.A. Bishop, T.R. Jones, B.M. O'Connor and A.H. Calvert, Quinazoline antifolate thymidylate synthase inhibitors: alkyl, substituted alkyl, and aryl substituents in the C2 position. *J Med Chem, 33* (1990) 3060-3067.

23. A.L. Jackman, D.R. Newell, W. Gibson, D.I. Jodrell, G.A. Taylor, J.A. Bishop, L.R. Hughes and A.H. Calvert, The biochemical pharmacology of the thymidylate synthase inhibitor, 2-desamino-2-methyl-N^{10}-propargyl-5,8-dideazafolic acid (ICI 198583). *Biochem Pharmacol, 42* (1991) 1885-1895.

24. P.R. Marsham, L.R. Hughes, A.L. Jackman, A.J. Hayter, J. Oldfield, J.M. Wardleworth, J.A. Bishop, B.M. O'Connor and A.H. Calvert, Quinazoline antifolate thymidylate synthase inhibitors: heterocyclic benzoyl ring modifications. *J Med Chem, 34* (1991) 1594-1605.

25. A.L. Jackman, G.A. Taylor, W. Gibson, R. Kimbell, M. Brown, A.H. Calvert, I.R. Judson and L.R. Hughes, ICI D1694, a quinazoline antifolate thymidylate synthase inhibitor that is a potent inhibitor of L1210 tumor cell growth in vitro and in vivo: a new agent for clinical study. *Cancer Res, 51* (1991) 5579-5586.

26. T.C. Stephens, B.E. Valcaccia, M.L. Sheader, L.R. Hughes and A.L. Jackman, The thymidylate synthase (TS) inhibitor ICI D1694 is superior to CB3717, 5-fluorouracil(5-FU) and methotrexate (MTX) against a panel of human tumor xenografts. *Proc Amer Assoc Cancer Res, 32* (1991) 328.

27. A.L. Jackman, D.I. Jodrell, W. Gibson and T.C. Stephens, ICI D1694, an inhibitor of thymidylate synthase for clinical study. In R.A. Harkness, G. Elion and N. Zollner (eds.), *Purine and pyrimidine metabolism in man VII*, Plenum Press, New York, 1991, pp. 19-23.

28. N.J. Curtin, A.L. Harris, O.F.W. James and M.F. Bassendine, Inhibition of the growth of human hepatocellular carcinoma in vitro and in athymic mice by a quinazoline inhibitor of thymidylate synthase, CB3717. *Br J Cancer, 53* (1986) 361-368.

29. D.I. Jodrell, D.R. Newell, W. Gibson, L.R. Hughes and A.H. Calvert, The pharmacokinetics of the quinazoline antifolate ICI D1694 in mice and rats. *Cancer Chemother Pharmacol, 28* (1991) 331-338.
30. T.C. Stephens, J.A. Calvete, D. Janes, L.R. Hughes, A.L. Jackman and A.H. Calvert, Assessment of quinazoline thymidylate synthase (TS) inhibitors using a thymidine kinase deficient cell line (L5178Y TK-/-). *Proc Amer Assoc Cancer Res, 30* (1989) 477.
31. T.C. Stephens, J.A. Calvete, D. Janes, S.E. Waterman, B.E. Valcaccia, L.R. Hughes and A.H. Calvert, Antitumour activity of a new thymidylate synthase (TS) inhibitor, D1694. *Proc Amer Assoc Cancer Res, 31* (1990) 342.
32. D.R. Newell, D.L. Alison, A.L. Jackman, C. Sessa, A.H. Calvert and K.R.Harrap, Clinical and preclinical pharmacokinetic studies with the thymidylate synthetase (TS) inhibitor N10 propargyl-5,8-dideazafolic acid (CB3717). *Proc Amer Assoc Cancer Res, 26* (1985) 350.

DISCUSSION OF DR. JACKMAN'S/DR. SORENSEN'S PRESENTATION

Dr. Mihich: I was wondering whether Dr. Jackman knew first hand or second hand what happened to the comparison of D-1694 and if FU/leucovorin, in the case of FU/leucovorin there is a piling up of dUMP pools but there is also TS inhibition and there is a debate how much of the effect is due to thymineless condition and how much is due to DNA damage due to perhaps to the piling up of the dUMP pools. And the question that I have, has anybody compared the thymineless type of death that you seem to see in your compound with the type of death that occurs after FU/leucovorin?

Dr. Jackman: D-1694 direct inhibition of thymidylate synthase is by complex formation with dUMP. The dUMP rises after inhibition of TS could be hundreds of fold so the proposed mechanism of cell death that we're looking at and is misincorporation perhaps of dUTP into DNA which is proposed mechanism of CB3717. Dr. Aherne at our Institute is looking at that. 3717 cause DNA strand breaks and also causes apoptosis. Dr. Rustum do you want to talk about your studies?

Dr. Rustum: We have a paper that was just accepted in Cancer Research on the DNA damage induced by D-1694. The effect of D-1694 on induction of DNA damage is a delayed effect. In other words, if you expose cells for 2 hours, short-term exposure to drug, wash the cells free of drug, put them in drug-free media and measure the induction of single- and double-strand breaks at various times thereafter you find that maximum level of DNA damage occurs approximately around 20 hours. Under these conditions, thymidylate synthase was rapidly inhibited by greater than 90%. So, maximum DNA damage did not correspond in time with TS inhibition. Which one of these effects is the most critical event responsible for cell death is not known at this time.

Dr. Sorenson: I just want to respond to 1 or 2 things that Dr. Young said earlier about phase II dose and prior leucovorin. What we're doing at NCI at the moment is that we're entering patients previously untreated who have not received leucovorin for the previous year and we're also looking at red blood cell folate levels to try and correlate, if we can, correlate red blood cell folate level with tolerance to the therapy. We've done this in about 6 patients so far and I can say that we haven't been able to correlate them in the sense that some people with high red blood cell folates have actually had grade 3 neutropenia and people with normal or low red blood cell folates have tolerated the therapy. So, red blood folate may not be sensitive enough to attest to as to what's going on.

Dr. Calvert: I've got one comment and one question. I think, the comment is aimed to clinical Phase I presentations I'm not sure that they're really showing as much differences as I thought they did before. You've both got some toxicities. There may be some differences in the severity or the incidence of diarrhea but my guess is that on the whole you're going to come out within 10% or so of the same dose on the two studies. I don't like it if most of the patients are not dropping their blood count because it gives me the feeling that it may be due to individual variations of handling of the drug. Patients are simply not getting the antimetabolite effect.

Dr. Sorenson: First of all, a comment on Dr. Moran's first point about anemia. The one patient who got 11 cycles has had some anemia that we are evaluating. This is when she went home she got, as well getting neutropenic, she was also anemic to about a hemaglobin of 6.9. So we're getting studies on her and we should have some of this data. But in general we haven't seen anemia developing in our patients. Remember I think it's really dangerous to make conclusions about response particularly, but also about overall toxicity patterns when you've got so few patients at the highest doses. But in any case regarding the neutropenia, that actually is an interesting thing that I have noticed. The patients who get Grade III neutropenia it goes down to Grade III some patients don't have any change in their white count. We haven't really seen an increase in proportion of patients with grade 1, grade 2 and grade 3 neutropenia. So, that may be a problem in a predictive point of view.

Audience: Since about 90% of your patients have had prior therapy with both 5-fluorouracil and leucovorin, is it possible that you are pre-selecting patients who would not not respond either because of overproduction of TS or the inability to sustain polyglutamate? You might also be skewing the toxicity evaluation by taking that patient population too.

Dr. Sorenson: I agree with you completely that lack of responses does not concern me in this exact patient population right now because they could well have become TS resistant to that form of attack.

Dr. Houghton: Comment please on the choice of schedule of D1694 administration. The animal data clearly show that you have to have daily administration for at least 5 days before you start seeing responses. So, were you not surprised you've actually seen responses with your schedule.

Dr. Sorenson: Well, actually I prefer Dr. Jackman's comment on that and since I've been involved with this I've been interested in other schedules but you obviously have to start somewhere.

Dr. Jackman: I think it's very important. In man you've already got at least a 10-fold lower thymidine level and we believe it is so low that bolus administration should be enough in the same way that bolus administration was enough in the TK⁻ tumor. So, it's a thymidine masking effect and that was why we were so cautious and would not recommend daily treatment in man.

Dr. Jackman: I think that 0.6 μM is a high estimate. It's about .1 or even lower.

P53: A DETERMINANT OF THE CELL CYCLE
RESPONSE TO DNA DAMAGE

Michael B. Kastan

The Johns Hopkins Oncology Center
Baltimore, Md. 21287

Historically, most efficacious chemotherapuetic regimens have been developed empirically (i.e. by trial and error) rather than by a rational understanding of the differences between normal cells and tumor cells in the molecular and cellular responses to chemotherapeutic agents. Dosing and scheduling of agents optimally should be based on a detailed understanding of such differences between the responses of normal cells and tumor cells in order to maximize therapeutic index with antineoplastic agents. Molecular characterization of cell cycle checkpoints following DNA damage should provide insights into both: 1) mechanisms of cellular transformation, since these checkpoints appear to limit heritable genetic changes following DNA damage; and 2) mechanisms of tumor cell kill following chemotherapy, since these checkpoints appear to enhance cell survival following DNA damage (Hartwell and Weinert, 1989). Recent characterization in our laboratory of the p53 tumor suppressor gene as a determinant of the cell cycle response to certain types of DNA damage (Kastan et al, 1991; Kuerbitz et al, 1992) should have therapeutic implications, especially since p53 is the most commonly mutated gene in human cancers identified thus far (Vogelstein, 1990; Hollstein et al., 1991).

Experiments from numerous laboratories had identified the p53 gene product as an inhibitor of cellular proliferation (e.g. Baker et al., 1990), however the physiologic role of this growth suppressor gene was unclear. Recently, we noted that levels of p53 protein transiently increase by a post-transcriptional mechanism following γ-irradiation in temporal association with a transient arrest of cells in the G_1 phase of the cell cycle (Kastan et al, 1991). A dependence of this arrest on wild-type p53 function was suggested by the observation that cells with wild-type p53 genes exhibited the arrest, while cells with mutant or absent p53 genes lacked the G_1 arrest. The G_2 arrest was not affected by the status of the p53 gene. Inhibition of the rise in p53 protein and the G_1 arrest by caffeine and cycloheximide demonstrated that these cell cycle checkpoints are active cellular processes responding to DNA damage and are not simply due to the presence of damaged DNA which cannot be replicated.

A definitive role for p53 in this process has been clarified by the demonstrations that: 1) constitutive expression of a transfected mutant p53 gene in cells with wild-type endogenous p53 genes abrogated the G_1 arrest following γ-irradiation, while insertion of a wild-type p53 gene into tumor cells with no intact p53 genes

Novel Approaches to Selective Treatments of Human Solid Tumors: Laboratory and Clinical Correlation Edited by Y. M. Rustum, Plenum Press, New York, 1993

partially restored this arrest (Kuerbitz et al, 1992); and 2) that normal fibroblasts from mice in which both normal p53 alleles have been deleted by homologous recombination lose the G_1 arrest following γ-irradiation (Kastan et al, submitted, 1992). We are currently focusing our efforts on characterizing the biochemical steps in this pathway, including the post-transcriptional mechanism the cell uses to increase p53 protein levels following DNA damage, and the mechanism(s) by which the altered p53 protein leads to a G_1 arrest. These investigations have already led to the identification of two other gene products involved in this signal transduction pathway which controls the G_1 arrest following γ-irradiation.

Since normal cells will virtually always have wild-type p53 genes, and therefore exhibit a G_1 arrest following certain types of DNA damage, while a significant percentage of tumor cells (particularly solid tumors of the breast, colon, lung, ovaries, brain, etc. [see Hollstein et al, 1991 for review]) will have mutant p53 genes and will

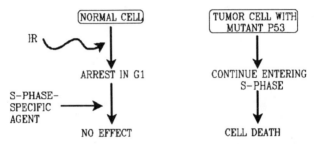

Figure 1. A potential schema for scheduling anti-neoplastic agents to maximize therapeutic index based on p53 status. The tumor will be treated locally or systemically with an agent, such as ionizing radiation (IR), that induces a p53-dependent G_1 arrest. Normal cells should arrest in G_1, while tumor cells with mutant p53 genes will continue to progress into S-phase. Appropriate timing of addition of a second agent which selectively kills cells which continue to progress through S-phase should lead to more selective killing of tumor cells with relative sparing of the arrested normal cells.

lack the G_1 arrest, it should be feasible to schedule DNA damaging antineoplastic agents such that toxicity to normal cells is minimized while tumor cell kill is simultaneously maximized. For example (see Figure 1), this could potentially be accomplished by first using an agent which induces this pathway and causes cells with wild-type p53 function to arrest in G_1; cells with abnormal p53 genes would continue to progress through S-phase following this treatment. Subsequent use of an agent which would selectively kill the cells which continued through S-phase (in this case, the tumor cells with mutant p53 genes), could have additive or synergistic killing of the tumor cells, while relatively sparing the arrested normal cells. Thus, taking advantage of this "natural" difference between normal cells and tumor cells and of the knowledge that p53 functions as a cell cycle checkpoint determinant should provide a rational basis for optimal scheduling of anti-neoplastic agents in some settings.

REFERENCES

Baker, S.J., Markowitz, S., Fearon, E. R., Willson, J.K.V., and Vogelstein, B., 1990, Suppression of human colorectal carcinoma cell growth by wild-type p53, *Science* 249: 912.

Hartwell, L.H. and Weinert, T.A., 1989, Checkpoints: controls that ensure the order of cell cycle events, *Science* 246: 629.

Hollstein, M., Sidransky, D., Vogelstein, B., and Harris, C.C., 1991, p53 mutations in human cancers, *Science* 253: 49.

Kastan, M.B., Onyekwere, O., Sidransky, D., Vogelstein, B., and Craig, R.W., 1991, Participation of p53 protein in the cellular response to DNA damage, *Cancer Research*, 51: 6304.

Kuerbitz, S.J., Plunkett, B.S., Walsh, W.V., and Kastan, M.B., 1992, Wild-type p53 is a cell cycle checkpoint determinant following irradiation, *Proc. Natl. Acad. Sci. USA*, 89: 7491.

Vogelstein, B., 1990, A deadly inheritance, *Nature* 348: 681.

DISCUSSION OF DR. KASTAN'S PRESENTATION

Dr. Moran: Did I understand you to say you have done the embryotic stem experiment to knock out both copies of P53?

Dr. Kastan: Right.

Dr. Moran: Does that give you live embryo out of that?

Dr. Kastan: Yes. It was published by a group at M.D. Anderson this past year in Nature and Fineberg and Jack's group has found the same thing. It has absolutely no effect on development whatsoever that's discernible at this point. The embryo is perfect. The mice are perfectly normal. The only abnormality is that they develop tumors at an incredibly high rate at very young ages and that would all be consistent with this model that the only time the P-53 dependent cell cycle check point occurs is when there is a lesion in the DNA that initiates this pathway. The reason that all the work in the past using constitutively expressed P-53 in tumor cells stops every tumor cell from growing is because it's overexpressed and that's what it does. But normally in cells it's not playing a role in regulating that process. So, that would all be consistent with this being the function of P-53.

Dr. DeCabrio: Was there any indication that the G_1 arrest exists in the yeast at all?

Dr. Kastan: The answer to the first question is no there was no G_1 arrest measureable in yeast depending on whose lab you're talking to. Some labs think they're beginning to be able to measure it but it's not a well described phenomena it's a matter of great debate. The mutation is clearly only effects the G_2 arrest and if there is G_1 arrest occurring in yeast it's very difficult to pick up. But I also want to point out there's no P-53 analog that's been identified in yeast either so this may be a cell cycle check-point that's occurred later in evolution.

Dr. Mihich: I know that trying to use a simple model as possible which is correct but have you any evidence of this particular pathway in relation to repair or lack of repair that occurs after damage with other agents not x-irradiation? The reason why I'm asking this is because for instance, Dr. Beerman and I'm sure there are others, have shown that whereas x-irradiation has the same sensitivity of DNA in nucleus and in its normal structures is the same to radiation can be very different to several drugs. So, that the question is would this model be applicable to all types of DNA damage or do you have information that would show differential effects?

Dr. Kastan: That's a very good question. I'll try to address that by saying we had looked at a lot of different DNA damage in the agents and its only a selective few that actually induce this process. I think it's premature for me to tell you which ones do and which ones don't because the time courses could be different and the dose responses could be different until we test a whole slew of doses and time course I don't want to say for sure. But it looks very clear that most types of DNA damage, such as bulky adducts, probably do not induce this pathway. Certainly small base damage does not.

Dr. Rustum: Dr. Kastan, last night we were talking about the aspect of DNA damage and kinetics of DNA damage and my question for today is you have demonstrated a cause/effect relationship between the alteration or increase of P-53 and blocking the cells in G_1 phase. Which one of these is the causative for cell death? Would radiation effect the onset of DNA damage?

Dr. DeCabrio: It's not clear at all yet whether this pathway dictates cell death. In fact, preliminary data suggests that it may be cell type specific. Some cell types may use this for programmed cell death but most cell types won't. But, as a general rule of thumb with very preliminary data, it looks like there's G_1 arrest or lack thereof does not dictate cell survival by itself following these types of DNA damage.

Audience: In the heterozygous alleles is there any way of regulating the different alleles the different rates within the cell?

Dr. DeCabrio: You mean in the knock-out mice? That's a very difficult thing to do. People are obviously working very hard in understanding what regulates transcription and expression of P-53. It would be a very important question for patients with Li Fraumeny syndrome that are identical to the knock-out mice where they have one abnormal P-53 allele and one normal one in their germ line.

Dr. Kufe: Dr. Kastan have you seen any phosphorylation of P-53 in these studies?

Dr. Kastan: We're in the process of doing those right now. It's a difficult experiment to do because since the levels are going up P-32 levels into the protein are likely to go up. So if we see a 3-5 fold increase in the levels of P-32 then the level per amount of protein is probably going to be about the same so we were waiting to really characterize everything we could about the process before we started doing those biochemical studies.

Dr. Kufe: When you put the mutant P-53 in and you don't see any change in protein levels following radiation, is that acting as the dominant negative then in sopping up whatever events stabilizes the P-53 protein?

Dr. Kastan: Clearly, mutant P-53 blocks the function of wild type P-53 by binding to the P-53 protein acts as an oligomer probably a tetramer and binds to DNA and activates transcription and so presumes mechanism by which mutant P-53 is dominant/negative by the protein binding to the wild type form of the protein and high stocheometric amounts. Mutant P-53 protein has to be overexpressed in order for it to be dominant/negative and it's thought to be because it blocks adequate oligimerization of the complex and it doesn't allow it to function.

THERAPEUTIC IMPLICATIONS OF MOLECULAR GENETICS

Stanley R. Hamilton

Department of Pathology
The Johns Hopkins University School of Medicine and Hospital
Baltimore, MD 21205-2196

INTRODUCTION

Molecular genetics and molecular biology have produced fantastic gains in the understanding of cellular mechanisms involved in neoplasia. Clinical application of these gains, however, remains in its infancy at present. One area of intense interest is gene therapy, the treatment of patients to correct germline or acquired abnormalities in genes, including those involved in neoplasia (reviewed in reference 1). The variety of altered genes in neoplasia provides numerous potential targets for this therapeutic approach.

Recombinant DNA technology has already been applied or can be applied in many aspects of cancer therapy (Table 1). Among the most promising approaches is immunomodulation to enhance the immunogeneity of tumor cells to the patient's immune response. This chapter will concentrate on potential therapeutic approaches directed at specific molecular genetic alterations. Colorectal neoplasia will be addressed since this tumor is the second most common cause of cancer deaths in the United States and is one of the most extensively studied at the molecular genetic level.

Table 1. Recombinant DNA Technology for Therapy.

Recombinant drugs
Cytokines, growth factors and antagonists,
  monoclonal antibodies, toxin immunoconjugates,
  toxin-ligand conjugates, antigen binding proteins
Informational drugs
  Oligodeoxynucleotides, ribozymes, specific proteases
Genetic immunomodulation
  Cytokines into immune cells or tumor cells
  Tumor virus vaccines
Normal tissue protection
  Stem cell cytotoxic drug resistance
  Colony-stimulating factors
Drug targeting
  Virally directed enzyme prodrug therapy
Gene replacement therapy

Novel Approaches to Selective Treatments of Human Solid Tumors: Laboratory and Clinical Correlation Edited by Y. M. Rustum, Plenum Press, New York, 1993

The molecular genetic alterations in human colorectal neoplasia involve both stimulatory oncogenes and tumor suppressor genes that undergo inactivation (reviewed in references 2-7). Multiple clonal genetic abnormalities accumulate during the development of colorectal carcinomas in their precursor adenomas.[8] Among the oncogene abnormalities, ras gene mutations which activate the K-ras or N-ras protocogene are frequent and typically occur relatively early in the adenoma-carcinoma sequence. Other oncogenes are also abnormal, including c-src,c-myc, and c-myb.

GENE THERAPY AND ONCOGENES

The potential for gene therapy of colorectal neoplasia through oncogene targets has been shown in vitro with antisense oligodeoxy-nucleotide technology directed at c-myb in cell lines.[9] Antisense oligodeoxynucleotides are small synthetic nucleotide sequences designed to be complementary to specific DNA or RNA sequences. Introduction of antisense oligodeoxynucleotides into cells allows binding to genes to inhibit transcription or to mRNA to inhibit translation. Inhibition of c-myb via antisense oligodeoxynucleotides in three colorectal cancer cell lines with detectable c-myb mRNA expression resulted in reduced tumor cell proliferation and reduced tritiated thymidine incorporation into DNA along with reduced c-myb mRNA expression. By contrast, a colorectal cancer cell line without c-myb mRNA expression was not inhibited.

The potential problems of the antisense oligodeoxynucleotide therapeutic approach include permeability of cells to the synthetic sequences, stability, targeting, and therapeutic index (differential effects in tumor cells as compared with non-neoplastic cells).[1] Whether or not downregulation of oncogenes in human cancers in vivo can be accomplished to treat patients effectively is an important and unanswered question. In addition, intertumoral and even intratumoral heterogeneity for the target oncogene can be expected to impact on the potential clinical utility.

GENE THERAPY AND SUPPRESSOR GENES

In human colorectal neoplasia, several tumor suppressor genes are often abnormal.[2-7] These include the APC (Adenomatous Polyposis Coli) gene[10] and MCC (Mutated in Colorectal Carcinoma) gene[11] on the long arm of chromosome 5, the DCC (Deleted in Colorectal Carcinoma) gene[12] on the long arm of chromosome 18, and the p53 (named for the molecular weight of its protein product) gene[13-19] on the short arm of chromosome 17. Germline mutation of the APC gene is responsible for adenomatous polyposis syndrome and the phenotypic variant Gardner syndrome which has extraintestinal manifestations.[20-23] Abnormality of the APC gene can be identified in the majority of patients with adenomatous polyposis syndrome. Most of the genetic abnormalities lead to truncation of the gene product due to occurrence of deletion, insertion leading to downstream nonsense codons, or nonsense mutation. The predicted amino acid sequence of the gene product indicates a large protein with 2843 amino acids which has probable G protein binding sites and coiled-coil motif favoring a cytoplasmic localization as a structural protein.

The APC gene appears to be involved in ordinary colorectal neoplasia as well as in adenomatous polyposis syndrome because the gene is commonly abnormal in sporadic adenomas and carcinomas.[10] Because the majority of colorectal carcinomas and their precursor adenomas have genetic alterations of APC which would be expected to inactivate the gene, the alterations appear to occur early in the adenoma-carcinoma sequence.

The MCC gene has been much less extensively studied. It has a probable G protein-binding region and predicted coiled-coil motif as does the gene product of the nearby APC gene, but MCC is much less frequently mutated in sporadic colorectal tumors.

The potential utility of the APC and MCC genes as targets for gene therapy has been addressed in a microcell-mediated whole chromosome transfer study.[24] A whole chromosome 5 was inserted into a colorectal cancer cell line with multiple genetic abnormalities including the presence of only one mutated copy of APC and only one normal copy of MCC. The modified cell line had dramatically different morphology than the parental line. In addition, the clones showed dramatically reduced tumorigenicity in nude mice as compared to the parental line and to a control with chromosome transfer of an irrelevant (chromosome 15). Similar results were obtained by another group of investigators using a different colorectal cancer cell line.[25]

The DCC gene encodes a large protein with amino acid sequence homology to neural cell adhesion molecule (NCAM). The gene product appears to be a cell surface glycoprotein on goblet cells and may be involved in cell-cell and cell-matrix interations in adhesion and differentiation. Deletion of DCC is frequent in colorectal carcinomas and adenomas which have developed carcinoma. Thus, alteration appears to be a relatively late event in colorectal neoplasia. A whole chromosome 18 transfer study into the cell line with multiple genetic abnormalities including only one copy of DCC demonstrated no alteration in morphology but reduced tumorigenicity in the clones.[24] The effects were not nearly as dramatic as for transfer of whole chromosome 5. In another colorectal cancer cell line whole chromosome 18 altered morphology and suppressed tumorigenicity.[25] Transfection of wild-type DCC gene into a cell line with DCC deletion resulted in decreased colony formation and smaller colonies as compared to the parental line.

The p53 gene has been extensively studied in a variety of human cancers.[16-19] In colorectal carcinoma, mutation of one copy of p53 and deletion of the other copy is a frequent finding in colorectal carcinomas, but far less frequent in adenomas.[14] In addition, immunohistochemical studies demonstrate diffuse overexpression of p53 gene product, which is usually associated with p53 gene mutation, in carcinomas but often not in the adenomas in which they arose. These findings suggest that p53 plays a key role in the conversion of the benign precursor lesion to the malignant tumor. (See chapter by Dr. Kastan for additional information on p53). In vitro therapeutic approaches to colorectal neoplasia directed at p53 have included whole chromosome 17 transfer and transfection of the p53 gene itself. In a whole chromosome 17 transfer study, no clones could be obtained, indicating dramatic tumor suppression.[24] With transfection of wild-type p53 gene into two cell lines with deletion and mutation of p53 and into a third cell line with no structural abnormality of p53 but very low level of expression of the wild-type protein, colony formation in soft agar was dramatically inhibited.[26] In addition, colorectal cancer cells expressing wild-type p53 after transfection showed dramatic suppression of tritiated thymidine into DNA indicating inhibition of proliferation. As a consequence, p53 represents an important target for gene therapy in human colorectal cancer, but also in a wide variety of other human cancers due to its high frequency of abnormality.

In addition to abnormalities of APC, MCC, DCC, and p53, allelotyping demonstrates allelic deletions suggesting possible tumor suppressor genes on many other chromosome sites in human colorectal cancers,[27] including the short arms of chromosome 1 and 8 and the long arm of chromosome 22. As a consequence, additional target genes may be identified in the future.

FUTURE PROSPECTS

Correction of suppressor gene abnormalities <u>in vivo</u> poses substantial technical hurdles. The processing steps involved in gene therapy include escape of degradation by extracellular nucleases, absorption onto and uptake into target cells, transport from the cytoplasm to the nucleus, integration into host chromosomes, avoidance of mutation of the inserted gene, expression of the transgene, and finally its transcriptional control.[1] The complexity of the process is self-evident. Gene replacement therapy requires effective delivery systems. Whereas physical methods of gene transfer can be used <u>in vitro</u>, <u>in vivo</u> gene therapy is far more difficult. At present, viral-mediated systems employing retroviruses or modified adenovirus or Herpes simplex virus are under intense investigation. Low efficiency of expression of transfected genes occurs in mammalian cells. The length of DNA which can be inserted and expressed is relatively short, and the expression is often short-lived. Heterogeneity of the response of cell types occurs. Insertion of a wild-type gene to replace a defective germline gene such as APC in adenomatous polyposis syndrome or into virtually all cells of a tumor to correct a somatic defect remains to be accomplished in experimental models. Thus, development of pharmacologic agents which mimic wild-type suppressor gene function or eliminate oncogene function at some point along the pathways important in the neoplastic process may be a more feasible strategy.

REFERENCES

1. A.A. Gutierrez, N.R. Lemoine, K. Sikora, Gene therapy for cancer. Lancet 339:715 (1992).
2. E.R. Fearon, Genetic alterations underlying colorectal tumorigenesis. Cancer Surveys 12:119 (1992).
3. E.C. Fearon, and P.A. Jones, Progressing toward a molecular description of colorectal cancer development. FASEB 6:2783 (1992).
4. S.R. Hamilton, Molecular genetics of colorectal carcinoma. Cancer Supplement 70:1216 (1992).
5. A.K. Rustgi, D.K. Podolsky, The molecular baiss of colon cancer. Ann. Rev. Med. 43:61 (1992).
6. D.J. Ahnen, Genetics of colon cancer (review). West J. Med. 154:700 (1991).
7. E.R. Fearon, and B. Vogelstein, A genetic model for colorectal tumorigenesis. Cell 61:759 (1990).
8. B. Vogelstein, E.R. Fearon, S.R. Hamilton, S.E. Kern, A.C. Preisinger, M. Leppert, Y. Nakamura, R. White, A.M.M. Smiths, J. Bos, Genetic alterations during colorectal-tumor development. New Engl. J. Med. 319:525 (1988).
9. C. Melani, L. Rivoltini, G. Parmiani, B. Calabretta, M.P. Colombo, Inhibition of proliferation by c-myb antisense oligodeoxynucleotides in colon adenocarcinoma cell lines that express c-myb. Cancer Res 51:2897 (1991).
10. S.M. Powell, N. Zilz, Y. Beazer-Barclay, T. M. Bryan, S.R. Hamilton, S. N. Thibodeau, B. Vogelstein, K.W. Kinzler. APC mutations occur early during colorectal tumorigenesis. Nature 359:235 (1992).
11. K.W. Kinzler, M.C. Nilbert, B. Vogelstein, T.M. Bryan, D.B. Levy, K.J. Smith, A.C. Preisinger, S.R. Hamilton, P. Hedge, A. Markham, M. Carlson, G. Joslyn, J. Groden, R. White, Y. Miki, Y. Miyoshi, I. Nishisho, Y. Nakamura. Identification of a gene located at chromosome 5q21 that is mutated in colorectal cancers. Science 251:1366 (1991).
12. E.R. Fearon, K.R. Cho, J.M. Nigro, S.E. Kern, J.W. Simons, J.M. Ruppert, S.R. Hamilton, A.P. Preisinger, G. Thomas, K.W. Kinzler, B. Vogelstein, Identification of a chromosome 18q gene which is altered in colorectal cancers. Science 247:49 (1990).
13. S. J. Baker, E.R. Fearon, J. M. Nigro, S.R. Hamilton, A.C. Preisinger, J.M. Jessup, P. vanTuinen, D.H. Ledbetter, D.F. Barker, Y. Nakamura, R. White, B. Vogelstein. Chromosome 17 deletions and p53 gene mutations in colorectal carcinomas. Science 244:217-221 (1989).

14. S. J. Baker, A.C. Preisinger, J.M. Jessup, C. Paraskeva, S. Markowitz, J.K.V. Willson, S.R. Hamilton, B. Vogelstein, p53 gene mutations occur in combination with 17p allelic deletions as late events in colorectal tumorigenesis. Cancer Res 50:7717 (1990).

15. J. Cunningham, J.A. Lust, D.J. Schaid, G.D. Bren, H.A. Carpenter, E. Rizza, J.S. Kovach, S.N. Thibodeau, Expression of p53 and 17p allelic loss in colorectal carcinoma. Cancer Res. 52:1974 (1992).

16. A.J. Levine, The p53 tumor suppressor gene and product. Cancer Surveys 12:59 (1992).

17. D.P. Lane, p53, guardian of the genome. Nature 358:15 (1992).

18. S.J. Ullrich, C.W. Anderson, W.E. Mercer, E. Appella, The p53 tumor suppressor protein, a modulator of cell proliferation. J. Biol. Chem. 267:15259 (1992).

19. J.W. Shay, H. Werbin, W.D. Funk, W.E. Wright, Cellular and molecular advances in elucidating p53 function. Mutation Res. 277:163 (1992).

20. K.W. Kinzler, M.C. Nilbert, L-K. Su, B. Vogelstein, T.M. Bryan, D.B. Levy, K.J. Smith, A.C. Preisinger, P. Hedge, D. McKechnie, R. Finniear, A. Markham, J. Groffen, M.S. Bogusi, C.F. Altohul, A. Horii, H. Ando, Y. Miyoshi, Y. Miki, I. Nishisho, Y. Nakamura, Identification of FAP locus genes from chromosome 5q21. Science 253:661 (1991).

21. I. Nishisho, Y. Nakamura, Y. Miyoshi, Y. Miki, H. Ando, A. Horii, K. Koyama, J. Utsunomiya, S. Baba, P. Hedge, A. Markham, A.J. Krush, G. Petersen, S.R. Hamilton, M.C. Nilbert, D.B. Levy, T.M. Bryan, A.C. Preisinger, K.J. Smith, L-K. Su, K.W. Kinzler, B. Vogelstein, Mutations of chromosome 5q21 genes in FAP and colorectal cancer patients. Science 253:665 (1991).

22. G. Joslyn, M. Carlson, A. Thliveris, H. Albertsen, L. Gelbert, W. Wamowitz, J. Groden, J. Stevens, L. Spirio, M. Robertson, L. Sargeant, K. Krapcho, E. Wolff, R. Burt, J.P. Hughes, J. Warrington, J. McPherson, J. Wasmuth, D. LePasliet, H. Abderrahim, D. Cohen, M. Leppert, R. White, Identification of deletion mutations and three new genes at the familial polyposis locus. Cell 66:601 (1991).

23. J. Groden, A. Thliveris, W. Samowitz, M. Carlson, L. Gelbert, H. Albertsen, G. Joslyn, J. Stevens, L. Spirio, M. Robertson, L. Sargeant, K. Krapcho, E. Wolff, R. Burt, J. P. Hughes, J. Warrington, J. McPherson, J. Wasmuth, D. LePaslier, H. Abderahim, D. Cohen, M. Leppert, R. White, Identification and characterization of the familial adenomatous polyposis coli gene. Cell 66:589 (1991).

24. M.C. Goyette, K. Cho, C.L. Fasching, D.B. Levy, K.W. Kinzler, C. Paraskeva, B. Vogelstein, E.J. Stanbridge, Progression of colorectal cancer is associated with multiple tumor suppressor gene defects but inhibition of tumorigenicity is accomplished by correction of any single defect via chromosome transfer. Mol. Cell Biol. 12:1387 (1992).

25. K. Tanaka, M. Oshimura, R. Kikuchi, M. Seki, T. Hayashi, M. Miyaki, Suppression of tumorigenicity in human colon cancer cells by introduction of normal chromosome 5 or chromosome 18. Nature 349:340 (1991).

26. S.J. Baker, S. Markowitz, E.R. Fearon, J.K. Willson, B. Vogelstein, Suppression of human colorectal carcinoma cell growth by wild-type p53. Science 249:912 (1990).

27. B. Vogelstein, E.R. Fearon, S.E. Kern, S.R. Hamilton, A.C. Preisinger, Y. Nakamura, R. White, Allelotype of colorectal caricnomas. Science 244:207 (1989).

DISCUSSION OF DR. HAMILTON'S PRESENTATION

Dr. Kufe : I was curious about your c-myb anti-sense studies and the concentrations you need to inhibit growth and whether that's something realistic therapeutically.

Dr. Hamilton: Those studies were done in vitro by an Italian group and were published in Cancer Research last year and it appears that these are at the least pharmacologic doses. Obviously the problem with this technology is getting the active compound into the cells and functioning in the site where they need to be occurring. At this point, I think that it's fairly obvious the major stumbling block to this very elegant form of therapy is going to be the technology to be able to get genes into cells and make them function once they're in there, particularly in mammalian cells because of the limitations on length of DNA that can be put in and the frequent short-lived expression that occurs such as happened in the P-53 studies that Dr. Suzy Baker and others have done.

Dr. Rustum: Dr. Hamilton since your group has been involved with this for quite some time now is there any correlation between any of the genetic alterations and response to chemotherapy in colorectal cancer? I have seen some of your preliminary data presented about 6 months ago. They were quite interesting. Would you like to comment about that?

Dr. Hamilton: At this point in time, the allelic deletions on 17 P/ involving P-53 and on 18Q and DCC are being studied by several different groups as prognostic markers. The response to therapy aspect of it is really just beginning. We published an initial preliminary study showing that cases with allelic deletion had a poor 5 year survival rate irrespective of therapy and we currently are involved in collaborative studies with the Eastern Cooperative Oncology Group trying to further define the nature of the various chemotherapeutic regimens that are commonly being used in relationship to the molecular genetic alterations. That's the long answer. The short answer is no.

Dr. Mihich: In some of the methodologies, there is a problem of selectivity. You listed several of those for instance the Tommy Cheng type of approach of having the insertion of TK with the virus. How do you assure that it will only go to the target cell and not to the normal cell and how will it achieve an increase in selectivity in this regard? The same pertains to some of the other examples that you brought up.

Dr. Hamilton: Yes, that's exactly right. I think that the problems and the concerns about the retroviral delivery systems are evident in the deliberations that have gone on in terms of the initial in-born area metabolism studies at the NIH that obviously this is a point of great concern and it's probably unrealistic to think that there's going to be a perfect system. What one would hope is that you can eventually arrive at a system which has some degree of redundancy to it by the incorporation of appropriate relatively tissue-specific promotors and vectors that are hopefully relatively tropic for specific cell types. One might be able to achieve a reasonable outcome but as I say what's obvious in looking at this problem is the technology that has to be overcome in being able to use this in any sort of meaningful clinical fashion in vivo.

SUMMARY

Dr. Mihich:

A summary by definition is brief but to summarize 3 days of discussions is not simple. I think that the meeting could be defined as being divided in two portions; one portion had to do with the concept of application of our chemical pharmacology information to the rationale design of new treatments. This is a goal we have driven towards, some of us, for many many years. In fact, decades and I think that this conference showed that this is possible that it is a reality in drug design and treatment design. The other portion is what we heard this morning which has to do with the future, the new leads and the possibilities that we may have in the future to explore what is really an explosion of knowledge in the area of the molecular biology of the cancer cell and of the normal cell. Now let's deal with the first part first. I think that one of the rewarding things for some of us here has been that this concept of metabolic modulation which was born in our Department through the work of Alex Bloch, Maire Hakala, and Joe Rustum and was brought to the clinic through the aggressiveness and courage of Dr. George Mathe and Dr. David Machover this concept clearly has proven to be a viable concept in determining increased effectiveness of certain agents particularly antimetabolites. Now this concept is also abused sometimes but was not abused at this meeting to my satisfaction because we are not dealing with combination chemotherapy in the simple term we are dealing here with the modification of a target cell biochemistry such that the activity over an effective agent is increased. That is rather different from two active agents that are synergizing with each other. Now what did we talk about? We talked about the modulation of 5-fluorouracil as a major example and modulation by leucovorin, PALA, interferons and platinum. Platinum we used as a modulator and not necessarily as an antiproliferative cytotoxic agent. This question that has really irked us for a number of years about the mode of action of 5-FU is continuing to be present with us without an overt solution. What is the most important proximal effect in the cytotoxic activity of 5-FU whether modulated or not modulated, is it inhibition of thymidylate synthase and its consequences or is it incorporation into RNA and its consequences? This is not resolved yet and even though there are many indications here that we heard about in these two days that perhaps both phenomenon are usefully interacting in determining death at least of certain cell type. The particularly interesting aspects in the area of RNA was what Dr. Bruce Dolnick was telling us about the specificity of the messenger RNA that can be effective which provides an example of the possibility in the future to utilize drugs for specific intervention on certain gene expression may at the post-transcriptional level perhaps later on as we heard this morning even at the transcriptional level. Now another point that was raised during the meeting was the comparison between the 5-FU leucovorin treatment with the antifols as far as inhibition of cells but with particular emphasis on thymidylate synthetase. If one looks at the data in tissue culture it seems that there are many similarities almost identities. The effects on thymidylate synthetase are similar the duration of effect is different the augmentation of the pools of dUMP is equally enormous at least in tissue culture and with such a magnitude that the fact that the 5-FU/leucovorin has a relatively shorter inhibition of TS as compared to the antifols direct expressed specific inhibitors it may not be very important and if the effect is through a dUMP related damage of DNA because if it is true that these pools are so enormously increase such that the ratio between pools and enzyme is irrelevant given the fact that the enzyme is increased and increased perhaps differently in the two cases may not be so critical. This should be looked at because I think it is important to decide once and forever whether this secondary damage of DNA is really critical for the action of 5-FU and of the inhibitor of thymidylate synthase in general. Indications are strong but the final answer I don't think it is in yet. Also the issue about these antifols which Dr. Rick Moran was particularly prospecting a good future for depends essentially on what will happen in vivo. In vitro all the argument that Rick it brought up in terms of elevation of dUMP favoring the activity of these enzymes these low reduced folate pools that are characteristic of certain tumors solid tumors is favoring the binding of these inhibitors and all of these are things that indeed occur in vitro the question will be how much of these changes will occur in vivo in different tissues and what is the basis for selectivity and what will be the differences in selectivities between these different approaches in terms of TS inhibition. Now we talked then later about well I should say that both the antifols and the 5-FU/leucovorin should benefit from combination with at least some interferons we can do interferons in a minute because there is some discrepancy there between some of the formation that Dr. Janet Houghton gave us and some information that Dr. Chu gave us but they may be more apparent than real. But anyway to the extent that interferon is limiting in some systems the rise of TS after TS inhibition both of these treatments both the FU/LV and the antifol should benefit from and this of course needs to be studied. In fact, one of the good aspects of this kind of meeting is that we come with some questions we get some answers and we leave with more questions and this is a sign of success of the meeting. I think that in relation to PALA, Danny had to leave he told me he had to catch a plane a few minutes ago, in terms of PALA there is clearly an effect there and as I brought up the day before yesterday to me at least, it is intriguing to compare in experimental systems at least PALA combination with high dose thymidine combination with FU. The two agents are very different biochemically. Thymidine spares the catabolism of FU incidentally someone said interferon does it too which was an interesting observation and high dose thymidine is competing for the kinase with FU therefore there is less FU being formed there is feedback inhibition by thymidylate for the reductase or another pathway of preformation is inhibited and as a result a lot of FU goes into RNA and very little goes into FUDP and TS inhibition. Thymidine was a failure clinically. Now was it a failure because we didn't know how to use it cause we didn't know 6 years ago as much as we know now about the system or was it a failure because of this biochemical feature that it has as compared to PALA which indeed is pushing 5-FU into RNA but is also allowing the formation of FUMP in TS inhibition. So, this will be experimentally I think a nice comparison also to understand the relative role of TS inhibition and F-RNA phenomenon because the two would be different with the two agents, that is experimental work. And also there is a possibility that the patterns of modulation by these agents may be different cell types. This is one thing that I felt maybe would have been postponed to the next meeting some years from now. That is we did not talk too much about heterogeneity of cells and within the same cell population or among tumor cells and this is a rather important feature, important consideration when it comes to alternative pathways and it was brought up in relation to Dr. Houghton and Dr. Chu's studies was whether differences seen by those two authors due to differences in interferon types used, interferon-#, interferon-γ or was it a difference in cell types that were studied and both possibilities are open. Both data earlier we have to decide which if generality for each of them and if it a matter of different interferon it will be extremely interesting. As you remember, those of you who are here, Dr. Houghton found that interferon induced an increase in DNA damage by the FU/LV situation and Dr. Chu found that interferon exerted a translational level a control on the synthesis of TS whereby reducing the level of TS. Now if as you said before, if what is important is DNA damage more than TS levels then that issue is not terribly important, but that's an open question. Now we did not hear too much about the rate of TS turnover we discussed augmentation of TS, translation of control by interferon but what is a natural rate of TS turnover in different tumor cells or normal cells? Is that the basis for possible differences or possible selectivities? I do not know. That is why it is so important to check the issue of DNA damage as being, which is a consequence of TS inhibition, as being the proximal phenomenon. It is very important because that could overwhelm all other kind of consideration at the level of the enzyme inhibition. We talked about platinum and the platinum I mean as you know platinum as a modulator by decreasing methionine increasing the pools uptake increasing the pools of reduced folates and therefore possible increasing the effectiveness of FU and leucovorin. In that regard, moving to the clinical level for a moment there were differences in concepts and possibly results between different groups in terms of scheduling of these two agents. There was the Frei group and Boston group is saying that there is 65% response in head and neck cancer is related to the co-existance of the two agents at the same time. That is the cell has to see both FU and platinum at the same time to be able to achieve the clinical result. The other groups who are giving it in sequence the issue is not yet resolved which was the optimal sequence between the two. So that is where more work needs to be done. Now it was very interesting to me what Dr. Rustum was saying about FUdR and FUdR metabolic pathways being modified by kinetics essentially. The area under the curve of FUdR determines which will determine different schedule etc. favoring one direction towards FUdMP or the other direction towards RNA. I think that is interesting and it gives an intriguing example of how such a relatively multifactorial but simple pharmacolgical modification can effect a target cell pathway regulation in effect. That again is a first example but should be pursued, clarified and consolidated. We did touch on oral vs i.v. leucovorin, i.v. push vs infusion incidentally I can't resist telling the few clinicians who are left that they should really not use unless they are proposing a revolution of the English language they should not use i.v. bottles because bottles if you look at your dictionary is a bulk material per oral good that is the Latin definition of bottles. Even my French colleagues, who should know better, are using i.v. bottles. So that was a just a side comment. But we need to compare i.v. push with i.v. infusion and it seems that in some cases there was both clinical and pre-clinical report of a favoring therapeutic results after i.v. infusion and in other cases particularly in relation to reduced folate pools as Dr. Priest was talking there may be a difference with i.v. push. So that seems to be a necessity. Also the oral vs i.v. infusion there was some concept that the tubes were equivalent in terms of levels of 5-FU/LV achievable and that should be clarified in very, very tight studies in the clinic. Now there was not, well I think that it was almost resolved but again a side-by-side clinical was not carried out that the d is an innert form of leucovorin and that dL and L are similar given the appropriate to those comparisons. That however was not compared side-by-side. There was not much discussed in terms of lack of responsiveness except for the elegant studies of Dr. Berger who was looking at isoenzyme of TS as determined by print mutation but we could have discussed more it seems to me on the question of resistance which is in part related to heterogeneity of cells. This is something for the next meeting. Now I think I mentioned enough given the late hour about the antifols but I am very curious to see what will happen with these agents because they have also limitations. Limitation in uptake since they are picked up by the folate pathways, limitation in polyglutamylation they are very good substrates but still they require polyglutamylation and there is this question about the mechanism. I should have mentioned that because when I was mentioning interferon that from a theoretical point of view at least, it would be very interesting to understand what is the molecular basis for interferon interferring with translational phenonmen and I think that is a good Ph.D. thesis for the future. Now, in terms of advanced colorectal carcinoma the modulation of 5-FU although it confirmed the concept of metabolic modulation rather disapointing in terms of survival from many groups here and abroad it became apparent that survival under those conditions is not greatly increased, not greatly prolonged. However, great promise is coming up in the adjuvant setting and we heard a lot about current and ongoing studies as adjuvant with 5-FU and leucovorin and this seems to be very promising at this moment. Now, the PALA story at the clinical level was also interesting and it was just starting there was good news in breast carcinoma, particularly in combination also with leucovorin which makes an interesting combination with or without MMPR and Dr. Graham was saying that there is great variation and they're talking about heterogeneity again a great variation of Atcase among different tumors of a different patient and that was very relevant to the rationale determination of the dose of PALA that should be given. So these are all points open for further consolidation and others to understand their relevance. There were some interesting results on chronobiology I must tell you that I have been a little bit skeptical about the relevance of that in practice but I was impressed by those data there were differences that we saw that could be irrelavant at least in model systems it may not be relevant in human life but it is certainly relevant in model systems, and what a beautiful day when it was presented to us. There is more work that needs to be done in terms of the mechanism of platinum as a modulator the data Dr. Saijo gave us are very interesting but we have to find out how much the effect of platinum in relation to pyrimidine uptake and thymidine levels etc. is relevant to the biological effects and chemotherapeutic effects of 5-FU. UFt which is a built-in metabolic modulation combination is being started in this country now as you heard and has some promising or interesting results in Japan.I think that probably I've spent a quarter of an hour to discuss the first part of the meeting but I would like to touch a little bit on this morning also because this morning we had a glimpse of things that many of us have thought in recent years more and more about. It was interesting, it is of course very interesting that one can use tumor markers as a potential prognostic and not to speak about diagnostic, prognostic factors and this system of checking some markers of patients is interesting. But in terms of intervention and at least as a therapist I always try to think about intervention and given consideration to the fact that we only project the future because the future in many areas are not here yet because of the difficulty that we discussed later in the morning. But there is a future, there's a future in terms of intervention on tumor suppressor gene now if and when we understand what are the products of tumor suppressor genes that interact with transcription factors then and if we assume there's the lack of those interactions are responsible for the lack of tumor suppression then there is an avenue to see how we could interfere with transcription factor. Either with products of tumor suppressor gene or with drugs and there are ways now to, for instance, to interact with certain transcription factor in terms of attachment to DNA through DNA interacting agents and this is a new revisiting of some of the agents we have taken for granted for being simply cytotoxic. The idea of having monoclonals and antisense against mutated oncogenes for selected treatment of target tumors is excellent and has problems; has problems that we heard this morning about in terms of antisense, this is true for genes too, susceptibility to nucleases, kinetics, entrance in the cell, selectivity of which cell to enter in and one can try several devices with viral with attachment to other molecules and this has been touched on this morning. This is for the next 10 years to worry about. The contol of cell cycle the interaction between certain genes and cyclines in controlling the transcription of gene function which are essential for progression along the third cycle. It is an exciting area especially when you think about kinases and the practicality of having a biochemical and medicinal chemistry thinking inserted onto the molecular biology thinking. Because after all, everything ends up being biochemistry. I'm not a biochemist so I'm not pushing water through my own mill. The idea of apoptosis I mean I'm impressed by the work published by Evans and by Moshe Oren on these oncogenes being involved in modifying cell control such that program cell death can be initiated. I think that is an interesting route to pursue and we hope to hear more about it and the complexity and therefore the opportunities for specific intervention are increased by this Boston and other people findings of interaction of say P53 or RB with various protein that are from various viruses which seems to be required for the suppressive action or for the controlling action of these genes and therefore provide additional point of interference. But mind you this is day dreaming in this moment in a practical sense but we have to start in that direction somewhere. It is day dreaming but sometimes our clinicians who are courageous and not inhibited by the desire to know more and more and more about mechanisms this is sometimes our standing block, did already try cis-retionic acid plus interferon in head and neck tumor and that my provide the tool because that is an interferon with progression in head and neck and it did seem to have an effect and therefore it could provide a tool, a probe, to study this system in humans. I mention the kinases already and the regulation of cell cycle. The antisense the issue is complicated we mentioned already the MDR transfection some specific gene transfection to cells I think is rather difficult as we discussed in terms of solid tumor targets. When it comes to stem cells and stem cell disease either for protection of the bone marrow by transfecting stem cells with the MDR or by reconstitution of suppressive function say in conjunction with bone marrow transplantation of possibly residual cells in the bone marrow, I think that has more possibilities. But for the solid tumor we are still a little bit in difficulty and Fornay someone referred to Fornay's data from Turin about the IL2 gene introduction. An increasing heterogeneicity of that might also be a possibility but it is again facing the problem of selectivity, how to do it in that tumor or not. So, I've rambling around a little all I can say is that I learned a lot and I was also very happy to see how much of our efforts of the past twenty years and thinking have reaped fruits have been borne by this but also how much needs to be done and certainly this meeting in its first part has given us a sense of the promise for the future of biochemical pharmacological approaches in the rationale design of clinical cancer chemotherapy and therapeutics not only chemotherapy but therapeutics including some biological factors. What we heard this morning really makes us happy to be alive as scientists because it is an exciting time for all of us. Thank you.

ABBREVIATIONS

ACTase	aspartate carbamoyltransferase
ALT	alanine aminotransferase
6-AN	6-aminonicotinamide
Anth	anthracycline
APC Gene	adenomatous polyposis coli gene
ATP	adenosine triphosphate
AUC	area under the concentration time curve
GISCAD	Italian Group for the Study of Digestive Tract Cancer
MLM	bleomycin
CDDP	cisplatin
CF*	citrovorum factor
C.I.	continuous infusion
CNS	central nervous system
CR	complete tumor regression
$CH_2H_4PteGlu$	5,10-methylenetetrahydrofolate
5,10-CH_2THF (CH_2FH_4)	5,10-methylenetetrahydrofolate
5-CH_3THF (5-CH_3FH_4)	5-methyltetrahydrofolate
5-CHO-THF* (5-CHOFH)	5-formyltetrahydrofolate
DCC Gene	deleted in colorectal carcinoma gene
DHF	dihydrofolate
DHFR	dihydrofolate reductase
D.I.	dose intensity
DNA DSB	DNA double strand breaks
DOX	doxorubicin
DP	dypiridamole
DPD	dehydropyrimidine dehydrogenase
dThd-Pase	thymidine phosphorylase
dTMP	deoxythymidine monophosphate
dTTP	deoxythymidine triphosphate
dUMP	deoxyuridine monophosphate
EPI	epirubicin
FA*	folinic acid
F-DNA	fluorouridine incorporation into DNA
FdUDP	fluorodeoxyuridine diphosphate
FdUrd (FUdR)	5-fluoro-2′deoxyuridine
FdUMP	FdUrd monophosphate
FdUTP	fluoroxyuridine triphosphate
FHX (Regimen)	5-fluorouracil+hydroxyurea+radiotherapy
FHX-L (Regimen)	5-fluorouracil+hydroxyurea+ radiotherapy+leucovorin
FPGS	folylpolyglutamate synthetase
F-RNA	fluorouridine incorporation into RNA
FT	ftorafur (tegafur)
FUH_2	fluorodihydrouracil
FUra (5-FU)	5-fluorouracil
FUTP	FUra triphosphate
Fx	fractionation
HPLC	high performance liquid chromatography
HU	hydroxyurea
IC_{50}	concentration of drug to inhibit growth by 50%
ICR	Institute of Cancer Research
IFN	interferon

IL	interleukin
IR	ionizing radiation
IV	intravenous
l-OHP	oxaliplatin
LV*	leucovorin
MCC Gene	mutated in colorectal carcinoma gene
MER	methanol extracted residue
MMC	mitomycin C
MMPR	6-methylmercaptopurine
MR	minor response
MTD	maximum tolerated dose
MTX	methotrexate
MX	mitoxantrone
N^5-HCO-H_4PteGlu	5-formyltetrahydrofolate
NC	no change
N-CAM	neural cell adhesion molecule
NCCTG	North Central Cancer Treatment Group
OTT	overall treatment time
PALA	N-(phosphonacetyl)-l-aspartate
PBM (Regimen)	cisplatin+bleomycin+methotrexate
PD	progressive disease
PFL (Regimen)	cisplatin+5-fluorouracil+leucovorin
PR	partial tumor regression
PRPP	phosphoribosyl-pyrophosphate
PS	performance status
Pts	patients
RFC	reduced-folate carrier
RT	radiotherapy
SACCCS	Surgical Adjuvant Colorectal Cancer Chemotherapy
SWOG	Southwest Oncology Group
THF (FH_4)	tetrahydrofolate
TK	thymidine kinase
TMP	thymidylate
TS	thymidylate synthase
UFT	ftorafur/uracil (1:4)
UTP	uridine triphosphate
VDS	vindesine
WBC	white blood cell

* citrovorum factor, folinic acid, and leucovorin are all used to describe racemic (6R,S) 5-formyltetrahydrofolate (5-HCO-H_4PteGlu). LV is the preferred abbreviation for this volume.

AUTHOR INDEX

SUBJECT INDEX

Since this symposium dealt with the topic of chemotherapy using the combination of 5-fluorouracil and leucovorin (called by one or another of its synonyms), the index dose not include citations to every contribution under each of these headings. Citations were included only in the cases where the editor decided that they were warranted. Similarly, since leucovorin is called by many different names (5-formyltetrahydrofolate, citrovorum factor, folinic acid) each reference dose not appear under all the titles. Abbreviations used are those defined on p. 311.